Ear, Nose, and Throat Disorders
SOURCEBOOK

Second Edition

Health Reference Series

Second Edition [handwritten: last CKO: Nov 2017 46 CKOS]

[handwritten: new edition:]

Ear, Nose, and Throat Disorders

SOURCEBOOK

Basic Consumer Health Information about Disorders of the Ears, Hearing Loss, Vestibular Disorders, Nasal and Sinus Problems, Throat and Vocal Cord Disorders, and Otolaryngologic Cancers, Including Facts about Ear Infections and Injuries, Genetic and Congenital Deafness, Sensorineural Hearing Disorders, Tinnitus, Vertigo, Ménière Disease, Rhinitis, Sinusitis, Snoring, Sore Throats, Hoarseness, and More

Along with Reports on Current Research Initiatives, a Glossary of Related Medical Terms, and a Directory of Sources for Further Help and Information

Edited by
Sandra J. Judd

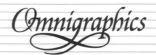

Omnigraphics

615 Griswold Street • Detroit, MI 48226

Bibliographic Note
Because this page cannot legibly accommodate all the copyright notices, the Bibliographic Note
portion of the Preface constitutes an extension of the copyright notice.

Edited by Sandra J. Judd

Health Reference Series

Karen Bellenir, *Managing Editor*
David A. Cooke, M.D., *Medical Consultant*
Elizabeth Barbour, *Research and Permissions Coordinator*
Cherry Stockdale, *Permissions Assistant*
Laura Pleva Nielsen, *Index Editor*
EdIndex, Services for Publishers, *Indexers*

* * *

Omnigraphics, Inc.

Matthew P. Barbour, *Senior Vice President*
Kay Gill, *Vice President—Directories*
Kevin Hayes, *Operations Manager*
David P. Bianco, *Marketing Director*

* * *

Peter E. Ruffner, *Publisher*

Frederick G. Ruffner, Jr., *Chairman*

Copyright © 2007 Omnigraphics, Inc.

0-7808-0872-X

Library of Congress Cataloging-in-Publication Data

Ear, nose, and throat disorders sourcebook : basic consumer health information about
disorders of the ears, hearing loss, vestibular disorders, nasal and sinus problems, throat
and vocal cord disorders, and otolaryngologic cancers, including facts about ear
infections and injuries, genetic and congenital deafness, sensorineural hearing disorders,
tinnitus, vertigo, minihre disease, rhinitis, sinusitis, snoring, sore throats, hoarseness,
and more; along with reports on current research initiatives, a glossary of related
medical terms, and a directory of sources for further help and information / edited by
Sandra J. Judd. -- 2nd ed.
    p. cm. -- (Health references series)
    Summary: "Provides basic consumer health information about various disorders of the
ear, nose, and throat. Includes index, glossary of related terms, and other resources"--
Provided by publisher.
    Includes bibliographical references and index.
    ISBN 0-7808-0872-X (hardcover : alk. paper)   1. Otolaryngology--Popular works.
I. Judd, Sandra J.
    RF59.E18 2006
    617.5'1--dc22
                                                                            2006019114

Table of Contents

Visit www.healthreferenceseries.com to view *A Contents Guide to the Health Reference Series*, a listing of more than 12,000 topics and the volumes in which they are covered.

Part II: Hearing Disorders

Part VI: Cancers of the Ears, Nose, and Throat

Preface

About This Book

Ailments of the ears, nose, and throat are some of the most common illnesses troubling Americans today. Consider the following statistics:

- Three out of four children will have experienced an ear infection by the age of three.

- At least twelve million Americans have tinnitus, or ringing in the ears, with one million experiencing it so severely that it impacts their daily lives.

- Twenty-eight million Americans suffer some form of hearing loss, and the hearing of thirty million more is at risk because of exposure to dangerous noise levels.

- Thirty-seven million Americans suffer from sinusitis each year.

- More than seven million Americans experience vocal disorders.

- Cancers of the head and neck account for 3–5% of all cancers and result in thousands of deaths annually.

Ear, Nose, and Throat Disorders Sourcebook, Second Edition provides readers with updated health information about the causes, symptoms, diagnosis, and treatment of diseases and disorders that affect the ears, nose, sinuses, throat, and voice, including ear infections, otosclerosis, cholesteatoma, hearing loss, tinnitus, vestibular disorders, vertigo, Ménière disease, rhinitis, sinusitis, deviated septum, sleep apnea, sore throat, laryngitis, tonsillitis, swallowing disorders, and otolaryngologic cancers. Current research initiatives are also described, along with a glossary of related terms and directory of resources for further help and information.

How to Use This Book

This book is divided into parts and chapters. Parts focus on broad areas of interest. Chapters are devoted to single topics within a part.

Part I: Disorders of the Ears begins with an introduction to the anatomy and function of the ear. It describes disorders that commonly affect the ear, including ear infections and injuries, and discusses the most frequently used diagnostic tests.

Part II: Hearing Disorders provides a detailed look at the most common types of hearing loss. It explains how hearing is tested in newborns, children, and adults, and looks at ways to protect hearing. The part concludes with facts about electronic hearing devices, including hearing aids and cochlear implants, and methods of communicating with people who are deaf or hard of hearing.

Part III: Vestibular Disorders looks at disorders affecting the sense of balance and the diagnostic tests commonly used to detect them. The ways in which aging, allergies, and other environmental factors impact the vestibular system are explained, and methods of vestibular rehabilitation are described.

Part IV: Disorders of the Nose and Sinuses describes nasal and sinus anatomy, and it details the disorders that most commonly affect the nose and sinuses. Frequently used diagnostic tests and surgical procedures are also explained.

Part V: Disorders of the Throat and Vocal Cords offers information about sore throats, disorders of the tonsils and adenoids, laryngitis and other laryngeal problems, swallowing disorders, and disorders of the voice and vocal cords.

Part VI: Cancers of the Ears, Nose, and Throat provides a detailed look at nasopharyngeal, esophageal, laryngeal, and other cancers that affect the ears, nose, and throat. Each cancer-related chapter includes a discussion of risk factors, symptoms, diagnosis, staging, and treatment. This part concludes with a summary of recent research findings regarding cancers of the ear, nose, and throat.

Part VII: Additional Help and Information provides a glossary of terms related to the ears, nose, and throat and a directory of organizations that can provide further information.

Bibliographic Note

This volume contains documents and excerpts from publications issued by the following U.S. government agencies: Centers for Disease Control and Prevention; National Cancer Institute (NCI); National Institute of Allergy and Infectious Diseases (NIAID); National Institute of Dental and Craniofacial Research (NIDCR); National Institute on Deafness and Other Communication Disorders (NIDCD); National Institutes of Health; National Library of Medicine; Osteoporosis and Related Bone Diseases National Resource Center; and the U.S. Food and Drug Administration.

In addition, this volume contains copyrighted documents from the following organizations and individuals: A.D.A.M., Inc.; American Academy of Audiology; American Academy of Facial Plastic and Reconstructive Surgery; American Academy of Family Physicians; American Academy of Otolaryngology–Head and Neck Surgery; American Association for Clinical Chemistry; American Hearing Research Foundation; American Rhinologic Society; Australian Hearing; Better Health Channel (Victoria Australia); Donna M. D'Alessandro, M.D.; Milton J. Dance Jr. Head and Neck Rehabilitation Center, Greater Baltimore Medical Center; Gale Group; Timothy C. Hain, M.D.; Hearing Loss Association of America; League for the Hard of Hearing; National Jewish Medical and Research Center; National Sleep Foundation; National Spasmodic Dysphonia Association; Nemours Foundation; New York Eye and Ear Infirmary; Northwestern Nasal and Sinus; Northwestern University Center for Voice; Pediatric Otolaryngology Head and Neck Surgery Associates, P.A.; Primary Children's Medical Center; Royal National Institute for Deaf People; Setliff Sinus Institute; Tampa Bay Hearing and Balance Center; Three Rivers Endoscopy Center; University of Maryland Medicine; University of Pennsylvania Hospital Balance Center; University of Rochester Health Promotion Office; University of Washington Virginia Merrill Bloedel Hearing Research Center; and Vestibular Disorders Association.

Full citation information is provided on the first page of each chapter. Every effort has been made to secure all necessary rights to reprint the copyrighted material. If any omissions have been made, please contact Omnigraphics to make corrections for future editions.

Acknowledgements

Thanks go to the many organizations, agencies, and individuals who have contributed materials for this *Sourcebook* and to medical consultant Dr. David Cooke and document engineer Bruce Bellenir. Special thanks go to managing editor Karen Bellenir and research and permissions coordinator Liz Barbour for their help and support.

About the Health Reference Series

The *Health Reference Series* is designed to provide basic medical information for patients, families, caregivers, and the general public. Each volume takes a particular topic and provides comprehensive coverage. This is especially important for people who may be dealing with a newly diagnosed disease or a chronic disorder in themselves or in a family member. People looking for preventive guidance, information about disease warning signs, medical statistics, and risk factors for health problems will also find answers to their questions in the *Health Reference Series*. The *Series*, however, is not intended to serve as a tool for diagnosing illness, in prescribing treatments, or as a substitute for the physician/patient relationship. All people concerned about medical symptoms or the possibility of disease are encouraged to seek professional care from an appropriate health care provider.

Locating Information within the Health Reference Series

The *Health Reference Series* contains a wealth of information about a wide variety of medical topics. Ensuring easy access to all the fact sheets, research reports, in-depth discussions, and other material contained within the individual books of the series remains one of our highest priorities. As the *Series* continues to grow in size and scope, however, locating the precise information needed by a reader may become more challenging.

A Contents Guide to the Health Reference Series was developed to direct readers to the specific volumes that address their concerns. It presents an extensive list of diseases, treatments, and other topics of general interest compiled from the Tables of Contents and major index headings. To access *A Contents Guide to the Health Reference Series*, visit www.healthreferenceseries.com.

Medical Consultant

Medical consultation services are provided to the *Health Reference Series* editors by David A. Cooke, M.D. Dr. Cooke is a graduate of Brandeis University, and he received his M.D. degree from the University of Michigan. He completed residency training at the University of Wisconsin Hospital and Clinics. He is board-certified in Internal Medicine. Dr. Cooke currently works as part of the University of Michigan Health System and practices in Ann Arbor, MI. In his free time, he enjoys writing, science fiction, and spending time with his family.

Our Advisory Board

We would like to thank the following board members for providing guidance to the development of this series:

Dr. Lynda Baker,
Associate Professor of Library and Information Science,
Wayne State University, Detroit, MI

Nancy Bulgarelli,
William Beaumont Hospital Library, Royal Oak, MI

Karen Imarisio,
Bloomfield Township Public Library, Bloomfield Township, MI

Karen Morgan,
Mardigian Library, University of Michigan-Dearborn,
Dearborn, MI

Rosemary Orlando,
St. Clair Shores Public Library, St. Clair Shores, MI

Health Reference Series *Update Policy*

The inaugural book in the *Health Reference Series* was the first edition of *Cancer Sourcebook* published in 1989. Since then, the *Series* has been enthusiastically received by librarians and in the medical community. In order to maintain the standard of providing high-quality health information for the layperson the editorial staff at Omnigraphics felt it was necessary to implement a policy of updating volumes when warranted.

Medical researchers have been making tremendous strides, and it is the purpose of the *Health Reference Series* to stay current with the most recent advances. Each decision to update a volume is made on an individual basis. Some of the considerations include how much new information is available and the feedback we receive from people who use the books. If there is a topic you would like to see added to the update list, or an area of medical concern you feel has not been adequately addressed, please write to:

Editor
Health Reference Series
Omnigraphics, Inc.
615 Griswold Street
Detroit, MI 48226
E-mail: editorial@omnigraphics.com

Part One

Disorders of the Ears

Chapter 1

Looking at the Ears

Chapter Contents

Section 1.1

How Do We Hear?

Your ears pick up sound, which travels in invisible waves through the air. Sound occurs when a moving or vibrating object causes the air around it to move.

Sound waves travel down the ear canal and hit the eardrum in the middle ear. This causes the eardrum to vibrate. Three tiny bones in your middle ear link the vibrating eardrum to the cochlea in the inner ear.

The cochlea is filled with liquid that carries the vibrations to thousands of tiny hair cells sitting on a membrane that stretches the length of the cochlea. The hair cells on the membrane fire off tiny electrical signals. These electrical signals travel up the cochlea nerves of the auditory pathway to the brain. All this happens in a fraction of a second.

The Parts of Your Ear

Your ear is made up of a conductive pathway that includes the outer and middle ear and the neural nerve pathway that includes the inner ear and auditory nerve.

The Outer Ear

The outer ear consists of the:

- external flap of skin (pinna) and cartilage;
- ear canal that leads down to the eardrum.

The pinna is the external flap of skin that helps you know the direction of sound. It serves to collect or funnel sounds into your ear canal yet it is not very important for good hearing.

The ear canal varies in size and shape from person to person. It runs nearly horizontally toward the center of the head for about one inch (in adults) and ends at the eardrum.

The skin along the outer part of the canal has tiny hairs and produces a waxy substance called cerumen. This earwax discourages foreign objects from entering the ear and keeps the skin of the canal from drying out.

The Middle Ear

The middle ear consists of the:

- eardrum;
- air-filled cavity that includes three middle ear bones;
- oval and round window membranes;
- eustachian tube.

The Eardrum and Middle Ear Bones

The cone-shaped eardrum is stretched across the ear canal and is quite stiff, yet flexible. Behind the eardrum three bones are connected to form the ossicular chain. They are the:

- hammer (malleus); • anvil (incus); • stirrup (stapes).

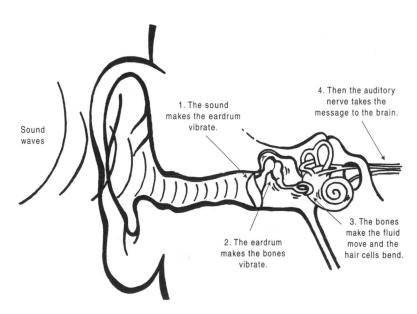

Figure 1.1. *How we hear (figure re-drawn for Omnigraphics by Alison DeKleine, with permission from Australian Hearing).*

The hammer is connected to the eardrum on one end and through the anvil to the stirrup at the other end. The stirrup is the smallest bone in the body, smaller than a grain of rice. It rests against the oval window membrane leading into the inner ear.

The stirrup moves in and out of the oval window membrane like a piston as the drum moves in response to sound.

The round window membrane is located just below the oval window and is flexible. When the stirrup moves in and out it pushes the fluid in the cochlea and the round window allows the fluid to be displaced.

The middle-ear cavity, filled with air, is connected to the back of the nose and throat by the eustachian tube. This tube adjusts the air pressure in the middle-ear space to match the air pressure on the outside of the eardrum and is normally closed. In a plane, when you take off or land, it helps to yawn or swallow because these actions usually open the eustachian tube to adjust the air pressure in the middle ear space.

The Inner Ear

The inner ear is made up of the:

* cochlea;
* semicircular canals.

The cochlea is a tiny spiral-shaped structure, about the size of a pea. It is nestled in the bone of the skull and filled with fluid. A thin membrane with around fifteen thousand microscopic hair cells sits in this fluid. Each cell is tuned to a particular sound or frequency.

The tiny hair cells connect to the cochlea nerve that sends messages to the brain.

The semicircular canals are mainly responsible for the sense of balance.

About Australian Hearing

Australian Hearing was established by the Australian government in 1947 to assist World War II veterans with ear damage and to care for Australian children who experienced hearing loss following the rubella epidemic of the late 1940s. It is one of the largest and most comprehensive providers of hearing services in the world. Australian Hearing is also home to the internationally renowned National Acoustic Laboratories, a leading research facility into hearing loss and treatment innovations. Find Australian Hearing on the Internet at www .hearingcom.au.

Section 1.2

Ear Examination

From *Gale Encyclopedia of Medicine 2nd Edition*, by Altha Roberts Edgren, 2, Thomson Gale, © 2002, Thomson/Gale. Reprinted by permission of The Gale Group.

Definition

An otoscope is a hand-held instrument with a tiny light and a cone-shaped attachment called an ear speculum, which is used to examine the ear canal. An ear examination is a normal part of most physical examinations by a doctor or nurse. It is also done when an ear infection or other type of ear problem is suspected.

Purpose

An otoscope is used to look into the ear canal to see the ear drum. Redness or fluid in the eardrum can indicate an ear infection. Some otoscopes can deliver a small puff of air to the eardrum to see if the eardrum will vibrate (which is normal). This type of ear examination with an otoscope can also detect a buildup of wax in the ear canal, or a rupture or puncture of the eardrum.

Precautions

No special precautions are required. However, if an ear infection is present, an ear examination may cause some discomfort or pain.

Description

An ear examination with an otoscope is usually done by a doctor or a nurse as part of a complete physical examination. The ears may also be examined if an ear infection is suspected due to fever, ear pain, or hearing loss. The patient will often be asked to tip the head slightly toward the shoulder so the ear to be examined is pointing up. The doctor or nurse may hold the ear lobe as the speculum is inserted into the ear, and may adjust the position of the otoscope to get a better view of the ear canal and eardrum. Both ears are usually examined, even if there seems to be a problem with just one ear.

Preparation

No special preparation is required prior to an ear examination with an otoscope. The ear speculum, which is inserted into the ear, is cleaned and sanitized before it is used. The speculums come in various sizes, and the doctor or nurse will select the size that will be most comfortable for the patient's ear.

Aftercare

If an ear infection is diagnosed, the patient may require treatment with antibiotics. If there is a buildup of wax in the ear canal, it might be rinsed or scraped out.

Risks

This type of ear examination is simple and generally harmless. Caution should always be used any time an object is inserted into the ear. This process could irritate an infected external ear canal and could rupture an eardrum if performed improperly or if the patient moves.

Normal Results

The ear canal is normally skin-colored and is covered with tiny hairs. It is normal for the ear canal to have some yellowish-brown earwax. The eardrum is typically thin, shiny, and pearly-white to light gray in color. The tiny bones in the middle ear can be seen pushing on the eardrum membrane like tent poles. The light from the otoscope will reflect off of the surface of the eardrum.

Abnormal Results

An ear infection will cause the eardrum to look red and swollen. In cases where the eardrum has ruptured, there may be fluid draining from the middle ear. A doctor may also see scarring, retraction of the eardrum, or bulging of the eardrum.

Chapter 2

The Pinna (External Ear)

Chapter Contents

Section 2.1

Small Ear (Microtia)

Information provided by Thomas Romo, III, M.D. and Anthony Sclafani, M.D., FACS. Reprinted with permission from the New York Eye and Ear Infirmary, © 2006. All rights reserved.

What is microtia?

Microtia by definition means small ear and is a congenital birth defect that occurs in one out of every eight thousand to ten thousand natural births. Certain populations such as American Indians have a one in twenty-five hundred occurrence rate. This congenital birth defect of the ear can be quite disturbing to the new family, who are hoping to have one of the most joyous times of their life.

What causes microtia?

It is important to inform the family members that this birth defect is usually a noninducible type of congenital malformation and that patient counseling is critical to prevent the guilt that is usually associated with this type of birth defect. Therefore, this ear deformity is not routinely caused by actions of the mother in the prenatal period, including ingestion of caffeine, alcohol, or routine medications. Two very strong medications, Thalidomide and Accutane, can produce microtia auricular deformity but are also associated with other major deformities such as heart abnormalities and intestinal and neurological deficits. There is a rare familial genetic pattern for microtia but no specific genetic dominance or expression has been identified and therefore genetic counseling is not routinely needed for these patients.

It is critical that the first physicians who are in contact with the parents of the neonate who has a microtia deformity inform the parents of the correct treatment options. This helps to allay their fears and dispel some of the unrealistic expectations regarding treatment options that are purported in the lay press. Microtia is usually broken down into four categories:

- **Grade I** is a slightly small ear with identifiable structures and a small but present external ear canal.

- **Grade II** is a partial or hemi-ear with a closed off or stenotic external ear canal producing a conductive hearing loss.

- **Grade III** is absence of the external ear with a small peanut vestige structure and an absence of the external ear canal and eardrum.

- **Grade IV** is absence of the total ear or anotia.

The deficit associated with microtia is that the child cannot hear well on the side of the head that presents with the microtia. The child routinely has an absence of the external ear or pinna as well as an absent external canal and eardrum. The patient routinely has a small middle ear cavity with fusion of the small middle ear bones or ossicles, an open or patten eustachian tube, and normal inner ear. Therefore, these children have a maximum conductive hearing loss. Because it is critical for children to have normal hearing in order to have normal speech, and bilateral hearing for the ability to detect directionality, the surgical treatment of microtia is to provide reconstitution of the external ear, ear canal, and middle ear structures.

How is microtia treated?

Each patient undergoes a thorough evaluation to detect the level of external ear, external ear canal, middle ear, and facial and bite deformities. The workup for these patients consists of a hearing test, CT scan of the temporal bone to detect the exact course of facial nerve and delineation of the amount of middle ear and external canal deformity, and x-rays of the face and mandible to detect hemi-facial deformities and bite irregularities. Following this evaluation, which usually commences at the five- to six-year-old age level, a treatment option is recommended to the parents of the child with the ear deformity. Patients who have the most common auricular deformity, Grade III, require a four- to five-stage reconstruction procedure performed over a one- to two-year period.

The primary procedure consists of harvesting cartilage from the opposite side of the chest from the ear deformity. This cartilage is then carved into the shape and framework of a normal ear structure copied after the normal contralateral ear. The ear framework is then inset into a pocket behind the peanut vestige and the overlying skin is shrink wrapped around the framework utilizing suction drains. This procedure requires the patient to remain in the hospital two to three days before being discharged home with drains in place that are removed one week postoperatively. Following the primary procedure, three months later, the second stage consists of removing the upper portion of the peanut vestige and then flipping the lower earlobe portion posterior and hooking this up to the reconstructed ear framework. This is an outpatient procedure where the patient goes home on the same day. This now provides the patient with a realistic looking ear, but one that is still tethered to the side of the head.

The third stage consists of lateralizing or moving the framework from the side of the head. This is accomplished by elevating the framework and then placing a skin graft and additional cartilage behind the framework to allow for permanent lateralization. At this point, the patient has a relatively natural looking ear.

The fourth-stage operation consists of elevation of a drill-out procedure where the external ear canal is actually created by the neuro-otologist. This canal is carried down until the location of the bony tympanic plate is detected. The bony plate is removed and a new tympanic membrane or eardrum is made from muscle lining, and this is connected to the middle ear ossicles. The newly formed canal is lined with a skin graft and attached to the external framework. This procedure requires the patient to be in the hospital for two to three days and is performed two to three months following the second stage. At this point the patient now has almost normal hearing and a natural ear framework on the side of the head.

Alternatively, a bone-anchored hearing aid (BAHA) can be placed to allow for hearing amplification surgery.

The fifth stage is a customizing procedure including construction of a preauricular canal tragus and any other finesse procedures needed to be done. If a patient has an underlying maxillofacial or hemi-facial deformity, these procedures are performed by the oromaxilla facial surgeon during the first, second and third stages of the auricular reconstruction.

Section 2.2

Cauliflower Ear

This information was provided by KidsHealth, one of the largest resources online for medically reviewed health information written for parents, kids, and teens. For more articles like this one, visit www.KidsHealth.org, or www.TeensHealth.org. © 2004 The Nemours Center for Children's Health Media, a division of The Nemours Foundation.

Have you ever seen someone whose ear looks bumpy and lumpy? The person might have cauliflower ear. That sure is a funny name. Let's find out more about it.

Cauliflower ear occurs after someone gets a hit or repeated hits to the ear. Wrestlers and boxers are more likely to have cauliflower ear because their ears may be hit while they're in a match. These blows can damage the shape and structure of the outside of the ear.

For cauliflower ear to form, the ear has to be struck hard enough for a large blood clot (lump of blood) to develop under the skin. Another way cauliflower ear can happen is when the ear's skin is stripped away from the cartilage, the flexible material that gives a normal ear its shape.

This cartilage needs oxygen and nutrients carried by the flow of blood. A tear, severe bruise, or blood clot can block the blood flow. If that happens, the cartilage can die. Without cartilage to keep its firm, rounded shape, the ear shrivels a bit and the cauliflower look begins to appear. Once this happens, the person's ear may look like this permanently.

You may be wondering if there's any way to prevent cauliflower ear. Wearing the right headgear when playing sports—especially contact sports—is a must. Helmets can not only save you from developing cauliflower ear but protect you from serious head injury as well. Always wear a helmet if you are biking, blading, riding your scooter, or playing any sport where helmets or other forms of headgear are recommended or required (like football, baseball, hockey, boxing, or wrestling).

If someone receives a sharp blow to the ear, there are ways to prevent cauliflower ear. A doctor can drain the blood from the ear through a cut and then reconnect skin to the cartilage by applying a tight bandage. Sometimes stitches are needed to sew the ear if the skin is badly ripped. The doctor may sometimes give the patient antibiotics to prevent an infection. If it's caught and treated early enough, a person usually will not get cauliflower ear.

And then they can stick to just eating the kind of cauliflower that's on their dinner plates!

Section 2.3

Otoplasty (Ear Plastic Surgery)

Reprinted with permission from the American Academy
of Facial Plastic and Reconstructive Surgery, www.aafprs.org.

Probably no other physical characteristic cries out for facial plastic surgery more than protruding ears. Children, long the victims of cruel nicknames like "Dumbo" or "Mickey Mouse," are the most likely candidates for otoplasty, but this surgery can be performed at any age after the ears have reached full size, usually around five to six years of age. Even if the ears are only mildly distorted, the condition can lead to self-consciousness and poor adaptation to school. When it comes to otoplasty, conventional wisdom is the earlier the better.

Adults may also benefit from this procedure, which improves self-esteem with relative ease. Often, adults choose this surgery in conjunction with other facial plastic surgical procedures. Not only is it possible to "pin back" ears, but ears can also be reshaped, reduced in size, or made more symmetrical.

If you are wondering how otoplasty can improve the way you look, you need to know how otoplasty is performed and what you can expect from this procedure. This section can address many of your concerns.

Successful facial plastic surgery is a result of good rapport between patient and surgeon. Trust, based on realistic expectations and exacting medical expertise, develops in the consulting stages before surgery. Your surgeon can answer specific questions about your specific needs.

Is Otoplasty for You?

General good health and realistic expectations are prerequisites. It is also important to understand the surgery. Otoplasty will not alter hearing ability. What is important for successful otoplasty is that the ears be in proportion to the size and shape of the face and head.

When considering otoplasty, parents must be confident that they have their child's best interests at heart. A positive attitude toward the surgery is an important factor in all facial plastic surgery, but it is especially critical when the patient is a child or adolescent.

Adult candidates for otoplasty should understand that the firmer cartilage of fully developed ears does not provide the same molding capacity as in children. A consultation with a facial plastic surgeon can help parents decide what is best for their child, not only aesthetically, but also psychologically and physically. Timing is always an important consideration. Having the procedure at a young age is highly desirable in two respects: the cartilage is extremely pliable, thereby permitting greater ease of shaping; and secondly, the child will experience psychological benefits from the cosmetic improvement.

Making the Decision for Otoplasty

Your choice of a qualified facial plastic surgeon is of paramount importance. During the consultation, the surgeon will examine the structure of the ears and discuss possibilities for correcting the problems. Even if only one ear needs "pinning back," surgery will probably be recommended on both ears to achieve the most natural, symmetrical appearance.

After the surgeon and patient decide that otoplasty is indicated, your surgeon will discuss the procedure. Following a thorough medical history, your surgeon will explain the kind of anesthesia required, surgical facility, and costs. Typically, your surgeon will suggest a general anesthesia for young patients and a local anesthetic combined with a mild sedative for older children and adults. Under normal conditions, otoplasty requires approximately two hours.

Understanding the Surgery

Surgery begins with an incision just behind the ear, in the natural fold where the ear is joined to the head. The surgeon will then remove the necessary amounts of cartilage and skin required to achieve the right effect. In some cases, the surgeon will trim the cartilage, shaping it into a more desirable form, and then pin the cartilage back with permanent sutures to secure the cartilage.

In other instances, the surgeon will not remove any cartilage at all, using stitches to hold the cartilage permanently in place. After sculpting the cartilage to the desired shape, the surgeon will apply sutures to anchor the ear until healing occurs to hold the ear in the desired position.

What to Expect after the Surgery

Soft dressings applied to the ears will remain for a few days. Most patients experience some mild discomfort. If you are accustomed to sleeping on your side, your sleep patterns may be disrupted for a week or so because you cannot put any pressure on the ear areas. Head-bands are sometimes recommended to hold the ears in the desired position for two weeks after the surgery.

The risks are minimal. There will be a thin white scar behind the ear after healing. Because this scar is in a natural crease behind the ear, the problem of visibility is inconsequential. Anything unusual should be reported to the surgeon immediately.

Facial plastic surgery makes it possible to correct many facial flaws that can often undermine one's self-confidence. By changing how you look, cosmetic surgery can help change how you feel about yourself.

Insurance does not generally cover surgery that is purely for cosmetic reasons. Surgery to correct or improve birth defects or traumatic injuries may be reimbursable in whole or in part. It is the patient's responsibility to check with the insurance carrier for information on the degree of coverage.

Chapter 3

Ear Infections

Chapter Contents

Section 3.1

Swimmer's Ear

From "Pediatric Common Questions, Quick Answers," by Donna M. D'Alessandro, M.D., Lindsay Huth, B.A., and Susan Kinzer, M.P.H., revised October 2004. © Donna M. D'Alessandro, M.D. All rights reserved. For additional information, visit http://www.virtualpediatric hospital.org.

What is otitis externa?

- Otitis externa is also called "swimmer's ear" or an "outer ear infection."

- It is an infection of the outer ear canal.

What causes it?

- The infection is caused by bacteria or fungi.

- Water often has bacteria in it.

- After swimming, water sometimes stays pooled in the ear.

- Bacteria may start to grow and cause an infection.

- Bacteria are most likely to be found in rivers, lakes, and ponds.

- Swimming pools can also cause infection. The chlorine can dry out the skin and the ears can get more easily infected.

- It is most common in the summer months (when children swim the most).

Who can get it?

- It is most common in children and young adults who swim or dive a lot.

- Children who have stuck something in the ear, possibly cutting or scratching it, are more likely to get an ear infection.

- Children who have ears with dry skin or lots of wax in their ears are more likely to get an infection.

What are the signs and symptoms?

- The first symptom is often an itching in the ear.
- The ear may feel plugged.
- The most common symptom is ear pain.
- The pain often gets worse when the outer part of the ear or ear-lobe is touched.
- Pus, a greenish-yellow fluid, may drain from the ear.
- There may be some hearing loss.
- Children may have a fever.
- Neck glands may become swollen.

Is it contagious?

No. It is not contagious.

How is it treated?

- If your child has symptoms of an ear infection, take her to the doctor.
- The doctor may prescribe eardrops.
- Have your child tilt her head to the side so her infected ear is facing up. Put in the drops.
- If the doctor prescribes oral antibiotics (by mouth), have your child take them as long as advised, even if her symptoms start to get better before the medicine is gone.
- The doctor might recommend acetaminophen for pain.
- Putting a warm cloth or heating pad against her ear may help ease pain.
- While your child has the infection, keep water, soap, shampoo, and other irritating items out of her ear.
- She may need to use a shower cap or earplugs.

- Avoid swimming for two weeks after the infection is gone. If your child swims sooner than that, use tightly fitting earplugs.

How long does it last?

- Pain may last or even increase for the first twelve to twenty-four hours after treatment begins.

- With treatment, the pain usually goes away in three to four days.

- The infection is usually gone after two weeks.

Can it be prevented?

- Do not stick objects in the ear (such as cotton swabs, bobby pins, or pencils), even to try to clean it.

- The objects may scratch the skin and open it up for infection.

- Keep the ears clean and dry.

- Put petroleum jelly on pieces of cotton to use as earplugs for swimming or showering.

- To dry out the ears, put rubbing alcohol on a piece of cotton and place it in the ear.

- You can also dry the ears out with eardrops from the store, like Swim-Ear or Aqua Ear.

- Children who have ears with dry skin or lots of wax in their ears may need to get their ears cleaned out by a doctor. Do this every year before swimming season.

When should I call the doctor?

- Call the doctor if your child has symptoms of an ear infection.

- Call the doctor if she still has symptoms of an ear infection after two weeks of treatment.

- Call the doctor if your child has any hearing loss.

- Call the doctor if fluid drains from the ear, especially if it is thick, a strange color, bloody, or if it smells bad.

- Call the doctor if you have questions or concerns about your child's treatment or condition.

Quick Answers

- Otitis externa is also sometimes called "swimmer's ear" or an "outer ear infection."

- After swimming, water sometimes stays pooled in the ear. If there is bacteria in the water, it could cause infection.

- It is most common in children and young adults who swim or dive a lot.

- The infection may cause itching, a feeling of plugged ears, some hearing loss, or pain.

- It is not contagious.

- If your child has symptoms of an ear infection, take her to the doctor. The doctor may prescribe eardrops or antibiotics.

- With treatment, pain usually goes away in three to four days. The infection is usually gone after two weeks.

- To prevent ear infections, avoid sticking objects in the ear, even cotton swabs. Keep the ears clean and dry.

- Call the doctor if you have questions or concerns about your child's treatment or condition.

References

American Academy of Otolaryngology. Swimmers Ear: Itchy Ears and Ear Fungus. Sinus Care Center. 1993 (cited 2002 March 18).

Pediatrics. External Otitis: Treatment and Prevention. (cited 2002 March 18).

Rutherford, K. External Otitis (Swimmer's Ear). KidsHealth. 2001 May (cited 2002 March 18).

Section 3.2

Otitis Media

Reprinted from "Otitis Media (Ear Infection)," National Institute on Deafness and Other Communication Disorders, National Institutes of Health, NIH Publication No. 97-4216, July 2002.

What is otitis media?

Otitis media is an infection or inflammation of the middle ear. This inflammation often begins when infections that cause sore throats, colds, or other respiratory or breathing problems spread to the middle ear. These can be viral or bacterial infections. Seventy-five percent of children experience at least one episode of otitis media by their third birthday. Almost half of these children will have three or more ear infections during their first three years. It is estimated that medical costs and lost wages because of otitis media amount to $5 billion a year in the United States. Although otitis media is primarily a disease of infants and young children, it can also affect adults.

How do we hear?

The ear consists of three major parts: the outer ear, the middle ear, and the inner ear. The outer ear includes the pinna—the visible part of the ear—and the ear canal. The outer ear extends to the tympanic membrane or eardrum, which separates the outer ear from the middle ear. The middle ear is an air-filled space that is located behind the eardrum. The middle ear contains three tiny bones, the malleus, incus, and stapes, which transmit sound from the eardrum to the inner ear. The inner ear contains the hearing and balance organs. The cochlea contains the hearing organ, which converts sound into electrical signals, which are associated with the origin of impulses carried by nerves to the brain where their meanings are appreciated.

Why are more children affected by otitis media than adults?

There are many reasons why children are more likely to suffer from otitis media than adults. First, children have more trouble fighting infections. This is because their immune systems are still developing. Another reason has to do with the child's eustachian tube. The eustachian tube is a small passageway that connects the upper part of the throat to the middle ear. It is shorter and straighter in the child than in the adult. It can contribute to otitis media in several ways.

The eustachian tube is usually closed but opens regularly to ventilate or replenish the air in the middle ear. This tube also equalizes middle ear air pressure in response to air pressure changes in the environment. However, a eustachian tube that is blocked by swelling of its lining or plugged with mucus from a cold or for some other reason cannot open to ventilate the middle ear. The lack of ventilation may allow fluid from the tissue that lines the middle ear to accumulate. If the eustachian tube remains plugged, the fluid cannot drain and begins to collect in the normally air-filled middle ear.

One more factor that makes children more susceptible to otitis media is that adenoids in children are larger than they are in adults. Adenoids are composed largely of cells (lymphocytes) that help fight infections. They are positioned in the back of the upper part of the throat near the eustachian tubes. Enlarged adenoids can, because of their size, interfere with the eustachian tube opening. In addition, adenoids may themselves become infected, and the infection may spread into the eustachian tubes.

Bacteria reach the middle ear through the lining or the passageway of the eustachian tube and can then produce infection, which causes swelling of the lining of the middle ear, blocking of the eustachian tube, and migration of white cells from the bloodstream to help fight the infection. In this process the white cells accumulate, often killing bacteria and dying themselves, leading to the formation of pus, a thick yellowish-white fluid in the middle ear. As the fluid increases, the child may have trouble hearing because the eardrum and middle ear bones are unable to move as freely as they should. As the infection worsens, many children also experience severe ear pain. Too much fluid in the ear can put pressure on the eardrum and eventually tear it.

What are the effects of otitis media?

Otitis media not only causes severe pain but may result in serious complications if it is not treated. An untreated infection can travel from the middle ear to the nearby parts of the head, including the brain. Although the hearing loss caused by otitis media is usually temporary, untreated otitis media may lead to permanent hearing impairment. Persistent fluid in the middle ear and chronic otitis media can

reduce a child's hearing at a time that is critical for speech and language development. Children who have early hearing impairment
from frequent ear infections are likely to have speech and language
disabilities.

How can someone tell if a child has otitis media?

Otitis media is often difficult to detect because most children affected by this disorder do not yet have sufficient speech and language
skills to tell someone what is bothering them. Common signs to look
for are:

- unusual irritability;
- difficulty sleeping;
- tugging or pulling at one or both ears;
- fever;
- fluid draining from the ear;
- loss of balance;
- unresponsiveness to quiet sounds or other signs of hearing difficulty such as sitting too close to the television or being inatten-
  tive.

Can anything be done to prevent otitis media?

Specific prevention strategies applicable to all infants and children
such as immunization against viral respiratory infections or specifically against the bacteria that cause otitis media are not currently
available. Nevertheless, it is known that children who are cared for
in group settings, as well as children who live with adults who smoke
cigarettes, have more ear infections. Therefore, a child who is prone
to otitis media should avoid contact with sick playmates and environmental tobacco smoke. Infants who nurse from a bottle while lying
down also appear to develop otitis media more frequently. Children
who have been breast-fed often have fewer episodes of otitis media.
Research has shown that cold and allergy medications such as antihistamines and decongestants are not helpful in preventing ear infections. The best hope for avoiding ear infections is the development
of vaccines against the bacteria that most often cause otitis media.
Scientists are currently developing vaccines that show promise in
preventing otitis media. Additional clinical research must be completed to ensure their effectiveness and safety.

How does a child's physician diagnose otitis media?

The simplest way to detect an active infection in the middle ear is to look in the child's ear with an otoscope, a light instrument that allows the physician to examine the outer ear and the eardrum. Inflammation of the eardrum indicates an infection. There are several ways that a physician checks for middle ear fluid. The use of a special type of otoscope called a pneumatic otoscope allows the physician to blow a puff of air onto the eardrum to test eardrum movement. (An eardrum with fluid behind it does not move as well as an eardrum with air behind it.)

A useful test of middle ear function is called tympanometry. This test requires insertion of a small, soft plug into the opening of the child's ear canal. The plug contains a speaker, a microphone, and a device that is able to change the air pressure in the ear canal, allowing for several measures of the middle ear. The child feels air pressure changes in the ear or hears a few brief tones. While this test provides information on the condition of the middle ear, it does not determine how well the child hears. A physician may suggest a hearing test for a child who has frequent ear infections to determine the extent of hearing loss. The hearing test is usually performed by an audiologist, a person who is specially trained to measure hearing.

How is otitis media treated?

Many physicians recommend the use of an antibiotic (a drug that kills bacteria) when there is an active middle ear infection. If a child is experiencing pain, the physician may also recommend a pain reliever. Following the physician's instructions is very important. Once started, the antibiotic should be taken until it is finished. Most physicians will have the child return for a follow-up examination to see if the infection has cleared.

Unfortunately, there are many bacteria that can cause otitis media, and some have become resistant to some antibiotics. This happens when antibiotics are given for coughs, colds, flu, or viral infections where antibiotic treatment is not useful. When bacteria become resistant to antibiotics, those treatments are then less effective against infections. This means that several different antibiotics may have to be tried before an ear infection clears. Antibiotics may also produce unwanted side effects such as nausea, diarrhea, and rashes. See the final question below for more on this subject.

Once the infection clears, fluid may remain in the middle ear for several months. Middle ear fluid that is not infected often disappears after three to six weeks. Neither antihistamines nor decongestants are recommended as helpful in the treatment of otitis media at any stage in the disease process. Sometimes physicians will treat the child with an antibiotic to hasten the elimination of the fluid. If the fluid persists for more than three months and is associated with a loss of hearing, many physicians suggest the insertion of "tubes" in the affected ears. This operation, called a myringotomy, can usually be done on an outpatient basis by a surgeon, who is usually an otolaryngologist (a physician who specializes in the ears, nose, and throat). While the child is asleep under general anesthesia, the surgeon makes a small opening in the child's eardrum. A small metal or plastic tube is placed into the opening in the eardrum. The tube ventilates the middle ear and helps keep the air pressure in the middle ear equal to the air pressure in the environment. The tube normally stays in the eardrum for six to twelve months, after which time it usually comes out spontaneously. If a child has enlarged or infected adenoids, the surgeon may recommend removal of the adenoids at the same time the ear tubes are inserted. Removal of the adenoids has been shown to reduce episodes of otitis media in some children, but not those who are under four years of age. Research, however, has shown that removal of a child's tonsils does not reduce occurrences of otitis media. Tonsillotomy and adenoidectomy may be appropriate for reasons other than middle ear fluid.

Hearing should be fully restored once the fluid is removed. Some children may need to have the operation again if the otitis media returns after the tubes come out. While the tubes are in place, water should be kept out of the ears. Many physicians recommend that a child with tubes wear special earplugs while swimming or bathing so that water does not enter the middle ear.

What research is being done on otitis media?

Several avenues of research are being explored to further improve the prevention, diagnosis, and treatment of otitis media. For example, research is better defining those children who are at high risk for developing otitis media and conditions that predispose certain individuals to middle ear infections. Emphasis is being placed on discovering the reasons why some children have more ear infections than other children. The effects of otitis media on children's speech and language development are important areas of study, as is research to develop more accurate methods to help physicians detect middle ear infections. How the defense molecules and cells involved with immunity respond to bacteria and viruses that often lead to otitis media is also under investigation. Scientists are evaluating the success of certain drugs currently being used for the treatment of otitis media and are examining new drugs that may be more effective, easier to administer, and better at preventing new infections. Most important, research is leading to the availability of vaccines that will prevent otitis media.

What is the current thinking on the use of antibiotic therapy for otitis media?

There is ongoing scientific discussion about the use and potential overuse of antibiotic therapy for otitis media. For further information, please note the following publications.

Berman S, Byrns PJ, Bondy J, Smith PJ, Lezotte D. Otitis media-related antibiotic prescribing patterns, outcomes, and expenditures in a pediatric Medicaid population. *Pediatrics*. 4 Oct 1997. 100(4): 585–92.

Culpepper L, Froom J. Routine antimicrobial treatment of acute otitis media: is it necessary? *JAMA*. 26 Nov 1997. 278(20): 1643–45.

Dagan R, Leibovitz E, Leiberman A, Yagupsky P. Clinical significance of antibiotic resistance in acute otitis media and implication of antibiotic treatment on carriage and spread of resistant organisms. *Pediatr Infect Dis J*. 19 May 2000. 19(5 Suppl): S57–S65.

Dowell SF, Butler JC, Giebink GS, Jacobs MR, Jernigan D, Musher DM, Rakowsky A, Schwartz B. Acute otitis media: management and surveillance in an era of pneumococcal resistance—a report from the Drug-Resistant Streptococcus pneumoniae Therapeutic Working Group. *Pediatr Infect Dis J*. Jan 1999. 18(1): 1–9.

Ehrlich GD, Veeh R, Wang X, Costerton JW, Hayes JD, Hu FZ, Daigle BJ, Ehrich MD, Post JC. Mucosal biofilm formation on middle-ear mucosa in the chinchilla model of otitis media. *JAMA*. April 2002. 287(13): 1710–15.

Glasziou PP, Hayem M, Del Mar CB. Antibiotics for acute otitis media in children. *Cochrane Database Syst Rev*. 2000. 2: CD000219.

Kozyrskyj AL, Hildes-Ripstein GE, Longstaffe SE, Wincott JL, Sitar DS, Klassen TP, Moffatt ME. Treatment of acute otitis media with a shortened course of antibiotics: a meta-analysis. *JAMA*. 3 Jun 1998. 279(21): 1736–42.

Little P, Gould C, Moore M, Warner G, Dunleavey J, Williamson I. Predictors of poor outcome and benefits from antibiotics in children

27

with acute otitis media: pragmatic randomised trial. *BMJ*. 6 July 2002. 325(7354): 22–24.

Maw R, Wilks J, Harvey I, Peters TJ, Golding J. Early surgery compared with watchful waiting for glue ear and effect on language development in preschool children: a randomised trial. *Lancet*. 20 Mar 1999. 353 (9157): 960–63.

McCaig LF, Besser RE, Hughes JM. Trends in antimicrobial prescribing rates for children and adolescents. *JAMA*. 19 June 2002. 287(23): 3096–102.

Otitis Media with Effusion in Young Children, Clinical Practice Guideline No. 12, AHCPR Publication No. 94-0622. Agency for Healthcare Research and Quality, Rockville, MD. July 1994.

Perz JF, Craig AS, Coffey CS, Jorgensen DM, Mitchel E, Hall S, Schaffner W, Griffin MR. Changes in antibiotic prescribing for children after a community-wide campaign. *JAMA*. 19 June 2002. 287(23): 3103–9.

Pichichero ME. Acute otitis media: part II. Treatment in an era of increasing antibiotic resistance. *Am Fam Physician*. 15 April 2000. 61(8): 2410–16.

Rosenfeld RM, Vertrees JE, Carr J, Cipolle RJ, Uden DL, Giebink GS, Canafax DM. Clinical efficacy of antimicrobial drugs for acute otitis media: metaanalysis of 5400 children from thirty-three randomized trials. *J Pediatrics*. Mar 1994. 124(3): 355–67.

Stine AR. Is amoxicillin more effective than placebo in treating acute otitis media in children younger than 2 years? *J Fam Pract*. May 2000. 49(5): 465–66.

Section 3.3

Chronic Middle Ear Infection

From "Pediatric Common Questions, Quick Answers," by Donna M. D'Alessandro, M.D., Lindsay Huth, B.A., and Susan Kinzer, M.P.H., revised October 2004. © Donna M. D'Alessandro, M.D. All rights reserved. For additional information, visit http://www.virtualpediatrichospital.org.

What is a chronic middle ear infection?

- A chronic middle ear infection lasts a long time. Symptoms are usually harder to notice than those seen with an acute ear infection. Acute ear infections last a shorter time but symptoms are usually worse.

- In a chronic ear infection, fluid (effusion) is usually trapped in the middle ear.

- Chronic middle ear infections are more serious than middle ear infections. Symptoms could cause permanent damage.

What causes a chronic middle ear infection?

- A chronic middle ear infection is caused when bacteria or viruses that get in the nose or throat reach the middle ear through the Eustachian tube (a small tube in the ear).

- Allergies, colds, or swelling and scarring from other ear infections can block the tube.

- If the tube is blocked, fluid can't drain from the ear.

- When fluid is in the ear, it's easier for the ear to get infected again.

Who can get chronic middle ear infections?

- Children who have had other ear infections or a cold are more likely to get a chronic infection.

- Children are more likely than adults to get ear infections.

- Ear infections are most common in the winter and early spring.
- Children are more likely to get ear infections if they go to day-care, use a pacifier, have allergies, take a bottle to bed, or are around people who smoke.
- Boys are more likely than girls to get an ear infection.

What are the symptoms of a chronic middle ear infection?

Symptoms are less severe than an acute ear infection. They may last a long time but be hard to notice. They can affect one or both ears.

- Fluid in the middle ear makes it hard to hear.
- The ear may ache or feel plugged.
- Children who are too young to tell you how they feel may pull or rub their ear.
- Pus may drain from the ear.

Are chronic middle ear infections contagious?

- No. Chronic middle ear infections are not contagious.

How are chronic middle ear infections treated?

Fluid may drain without treatment in a few months. If not, your child needs to see a doctor. The following things usually take place:

- The doctor will look in your child's ears to check for redness and fluid.
- The doctor may take tests to help decide if there is an ear infection.
- The doctor may prescribe an antibiotic to kill the infection and medicine to help with your child's cold, allergies, pain, or fever.
- Acetaminophen (such as Tylenol, Panadol, or Tempra) can be used to help pain and fever.
- Do not use aspirin.
- Make a follow-up appointment with the doctor to make sure the ear infection is gone.
- Treatment may last months. The doctor might recommend an operation to help prevent future infections.

- In the operation, a small opening would be made in the eardrum to help drain fluid.

How long does a chronic middle ear infection last?

- Fluid may stay in the middle ear for weeks or months.
- Hearing will get better as the fluid drains.
- Children can play outside while they have the infection.

Can chronic middle ear infections be prevented?

- Treat an acute ear infection as soon as possible so it is less likely to become a chronic infection.
- Go back to the doctor after treatment to make sure the infection is gone.
- Young children should not lie down with bottles or have bottles propped up. Holding children up as they are fed helps prevent infection.

When should I call the doctor?

- Call the doctor if you think your child has an ear infection.
- Call the doctor if your child gets new symptoms or symptoms get worse.
- Call the doctor if your child has a rash or diarrhea with the ear infection.
- Earaches could also be due to tooth problems, an ear canal injury (from a cotton swab), earwax, or something stuck in the ear. Call the doctor if your child has one of these problems.
- Call the doctor if you have questions or concerns about your child's illness.

Quick Answers

- A chronic middle ear infection is a long-lasting infection in the middle ear.
- It is caused by bacteria, viruses, or fluid in the middle ear.
- Children who have had other ear infections or a cold are more likely get a chronic infection.

- The infection may make it hard to hear or make the ears feel plugged.

- Chronic middle ear infections are not contagious.

- Fluid may drain without treatment. If not, your child needs to see a doctor.

- Treatment may last months.

- To help prevent chronic middle ear infections, treat middle ear infections as soon as possible, take all of the medicine, and follow up to make sure the infection is gone.

- Call the doctor if you have questions or concerns about your child's illness.

References

American Academy of Family Physicians. Ear Infections. 2001 July (cited 2001 September 17). Available from: URL: http://www.family doctor.org/handouts/684.html.

American Academy of Family Physicians. Ear Infection: What is Otitis Media with Effusion? 2000 (cited 2001 September 17). Available from: URL: http://www.familydoctor.org/handouts/330.html.

Casano, PJ M.D. Earache & Otitis Media. American Academy of Otolaryngology: Head and Neck Surgery Public Service Brochure. 1995 (cited 2001 July 27). Available from: URL: http://www.sinuscarecenter .com/om aao.html.

Children's Hospital, Boston. Middle Ear Infection (Otitis Media). 1989 August (cited 2001 July 27). Available from: URL: http://www.vh.org/ Patients/IHB/Peds/Infectious?otitis/OtitisMedia1.html.

MedlinePlus. Otitis Media—Chronic. 2001 May 16 (cited 2001 September 17). Available from: URL: http://www.nlm.nih.gov/medlineplus/ ency/article/000619.htm.

Rutherford Kim M.D. Acute Otitis Media. KidsHealth. 2001 June (cited 2001 July 27); Available from: URL: http://www.kidshealth.org/ pageManager.jsp?dn=KidsHealth&lic=1&ps=107&cat_id+article _set=22743.

Section 3.4

Mastoiditis

The mastoid bone is a part of the skull behind the ear which has small air cells or sinuses that connect to the middle ear. Mastoiditis is an infection that affects the mastoid bone. The infection typically starts first in the middle ear and spreads into the mastoid. Infection in the mastoid may destroy the thin bone of the air cells. Progressive infection trapped in the mastoid, mastoiditis, may cause serious complications.

Early symptoms of mastoiditis include ear pain and pressure, drainage of pus from the ear, and hearing loss. As acute mastoiditis worsens, the pus becomes creamy, pain waxes and wanes through the day, and swelling behind the ear may appear. Fever is variable, commonly worse as the pain and pressure increase. Meningitis, brain spinal-fluid infection, or brain abscess may complicate unmanaged mastoiditis. Since the facial nerve runs through the mastoid, facial paralysis sometimes occurs on the affected side. Permanently impaired hearing, eardrum membrane perforation, and cholesteatoma may also develop as a result of chronic mastoiditis. After an ear examination by the physician, a CAT scan reveals whether the mastoid infection is likely to respond to antibiotics alone or antibiotics plus surgery.

When possible, an audiogram documents the degree of associated hearing loss. The evaluation may happen in the emergency room or the physician's office, depending on how acutely ill the person is. Less severe acute mastoiditis typically resolves with oral antibiotics. More severe acute mastoiditis, especially if associated with complications, may require intravenous antibiotics. When the air cell bony walls have been destroyed by progressive infection, when swelling behind the ear develops, or other serious complications arise, surgery is usually necessary. Persisting infection that fails to respond to antibiotics may require surgery, as well. Surgery to clean out mastoid infection is called a mastoidectomy. When an eardrum (tympanic membrane) hole is also present, it may be repaired simultaneously with a tympanoplasty.

In the developed world, other serious complications of mastoiditis are rare. Life-threatening problems include obstruction of a major vein from the brain, the sigmoid sinus. Sigmoid sinus occlusion causes severe fevers and headache, commonly in association with meningitis. Mastoid infection may spread into the neck, causing marked swelling on the side of the neck along with fever and exquisite tenderness. Infection in the neck left untreated can impair breathing and spread into the chest. In areas of the world where tuberculosis is common, tuberculous mastoiditis may occur as well. Rarely, tumors and disorders of the blood cell system or immune system may also look like mastoiditis.

Section 3.5

Ear Tubes

Painful ear infections are a rite of passage for children—by the age of five, nearly every child has experienced at least one episode. Most ear infections either resolve on their own (viral) or are effectively treated by antibiotics (bacterial). But sometimes, ear infections or fluid in the middle ear may become a chronic problem leading to other issues such as hearing loss, behavior, and speech problems. In these cases, insertion of an ear tube by an otolaryngologist (ear, nose, and throat surgeon) may be considered.

What are ear tubes?

Ear tubes are tiny cylinders placed through the eardrum (tympanic membrane) to allow air into the middle ear. They also may be called tympanostomy tubes, myringotomy tubes, ventilation tubes, or PE (pressure equalization) tubes. These tubes can be made out of plastic, metal, or Teflon and may have a coating intended to reduce the possibility of infection. There are two basic types of ear tubes: short-term and long-term. Short-term tubes are smaller and typically stay in place for six months to a year before falling out on their own. Long-term tubes are larger and have flanges that secure them in place for a longer period of time. Long-term tubes may fall out on their own, but removal by an otolaryngologist is often necessary.

Who needs ear tubes?

Ear tubes are often recommended when a person experiences repeated middle ear infection (acute otitis media) or has hearing loss caused by the persistent presence of middle ear fluid (otitis media with effusion). These conditions most commonly occur in children, but can also be present in teens and adults and can lead to speech and balance problems, hearing loss, or changes in the structure of the eardrum. Other less common conditions that may warrant the placement of ear tubes are malformation of the eardrum or eustachian tube, Down syndrome, cleft palate, and barotrauma (injury to the middle ear caused by a reduction of air pressure), usually seen with altitude changes such as flying and scuba diving.

Each year, more than half a million ear tube surgeries are performed on children, making it the most common childhood surgery performed with anesthesia. The average age of ear tube insertion is one to three years old. Inserting ear tubes may:

- reduce the risk of future ear infection,
- restore hearing loss caused by middle ear fluid,
- improve speech problems and balance problems, and
- improve behavior and sleep problems caused by chronic ear infections.

How are ear tubes inserted?

Ear tubes are inserted through an outpatient surgical procedure called a myringotomy. A myringotomy refers to an incision (a hole) in the eardrum or tympanic membrane. This is most often done under a surgical microscope with a small scalpel (tiny knife), but it can also be accomplished with a laser. If an ear tube is not inserted, the hole would heal and close within a few days. To prevent this, an ear tube is placed in the hole to keep it open and allow air to reach the middle ear space (ventilation).

What is the procedure for ear tube surgery?

A light general anesthetic (laughing gas) is administered for young children. Some older children and adults may be able to tolerate the procedure without anesthetic. A myringotomy is performed and the fluid behind the ear drum (in the middle ear space) is suctioned out. The ear tube is then placed in the hole. Ear drops may be administered after the ear tube is placed and may be necessary for a few days. The procedure usually lasts less than fifteen minutes and patients awaken quickly. Sometimes the otolaryngologist will recommend removal of the adenoid tissue (lymph tissue located in the upper airway behind the nose) when ear tubes are placed. This is often considered when a repeat tube insertion is necessary. Current research indicates that removing adenoid tissue concurrent with placement of ear tubes can reduce the risk of recurrent ear infection and the need for repeat surgery.

What should be expected after surgery?

After surgery, the patient is monitored in the recovery room and will usually go home within an hour if no complications are present. Patients usually experience little or no postoperative pain, but grogginess, irritability, and/or nausea from the anesthesia can occur temporarily. Hearing loss caused by the presence of middle ear fluid is immediately resolved by surgery. Sometimes children can hear so much better that they complain that normal sounds seem too loud. The otolaryngologist will provide specific postoperative instructions for each patient, including when to seek immediate attention and follow-up appointments. He or she may also prescribe antibiotic ear drops for a few days.

To avoid the possibility of bacteria entering the middle ear through the ventilation tube, physicians may recommend keeping ears dry by using earplugs or other water-tight devices during bathing, swimming, and water activities. However, recent research suggests that protecting the ear may not be necessary, except when diving or engaging in water activities in unclean water such as lakes and rivers. Parents should consult with the treating physician about ear protection after surgery.

What are the possible complications?

Myringotomy with insertion of ear tubes is an extremely common and safe procedure with minimal complications. When complications do occur, they may include:

- **Perforation:** This can happen when a tube comes out or a long-term tube is removed and the hole in the tympanic membrane (eardrum) does not close. The hole can be patched through a minor surgical procedure called a tympanoplasty or myringoplasty.

- **Scarring:** Any irritation of the eardrum (recurrent ear infections), including repeated insertion of ear tubes, can cause scarring called tympanosclerosis or myringosclerosis. In most cases, this causes no problems with hearing.

- **Infection:** Ear infections can still occur in the middle ear or around the ear tube. However, these infections are usually less frequent, result in less hearing loss, and are easier to treat—often only with ear drops. Sometimes an oral antibiotic is still needed.

- **Ear tubes come out too early or stay in too long:** If an ear tube expels from the eardrum too soon (which is unpredictable), fluid may return and repeat surgery may be needed. Ear tubes that remain too long may result in perforation or may require removal by the otolaryngologist.

Consultation with an otolaryngologist (ear, nose, and throat surgeon) may be warranted if you or your child has experienced repeated or severe ear infections, ear infections that are not resolved with antibiotics, hearing loss due to fluid in the middle ear, or barotrauma, or have an anatomic abnormality that inhibits drainage of the middle ear.

Section 3.6

Alternative Treatments for Ear Infections

Excerpted from "Otitis Media," © 2006 A.D.A.M., Inc.
Reprinted with permission.

The goals for treating ear infections include curing the infection, relieving pain and other symptoms, and preventing recurrent ear infections. If a bacterial infection is present, antibiotics are necessary (see section "Medications").

With that said, antibiotics tend to be overused for the treatment of ear infections. Many studies suggest that uncomplicated ear infections in children over two years old can resolve within one week without antibiotics. In general, antibiotics are overused in the Western culture, leading to the growth and development of organisms that are resistant to these drugs. Finally, many ear infections are caused by a virus, not a bacterium; antibiotics are intended to treat bacterial infections.

Antibiotics should generally be used in children under two years old. Those older than two should be assessed individually and antibiotics given selectively.

Luckily, there are many alternative ways to treat the symptoms of ear infections and to prevent persistent and recurrent ear infections. For example, herbal ear drops and homeopathic remedies can be helpful for treating or preventing ear infections.

Lifestyle

Applying warm compresses (for example, using a warm cloth or hot water bottle filled with warm water) may help relieve pain.

Medications

- Antibiotics are prescribed to treat a bacterial infection. It is essential that the instructions for taking the drug (that is, how much, how often, and for how long) be followed carefully. The entire course of the antibiotic must be completed in order to avoid a relapse. The antibiotic most often prescribed for acute otitis media is amoxicillin, unless your child is allergic to penicillin, in which case there are several others from which your doctor will choose. If your doctor suspects a resistant organism (see earlier explanation), a different antibiotic will be selected. For chronic otitis media (that is, recurrent and persistent ear infections) or if your child has a perforated eardrum or develops infection after tympanostomy tubes have been placed (see Surgery and Other Procedures), antibiotic ear drops may be prescribed instead of oral antibiotics and continued for a long period of time (like a few months).

- Nasal sprays, nose drops, oral decongestants, or, occasionally, oral antihistamines may be used to promote drainage of fluid through the eustachian tubes.

- Ear drops may be prescribed to relieve pain.

- Over-the-counter oral medications for pain and/or fever may be used, like ibuprofen or acetaminophen. Aspirin should not be used in children.

- Rarely, oral corticosteroids may be prescribed to reduce inflammation.

Surgery and Other Procedures

If there is fluid in the middle ear and the condition persists, even with antibiotic treatment, a healthcare provider may recommend myringotomy (surgical opening of the eardrum) to relieve pressure and allow drainage of the fluid. This may or may not involve the insertion of tympanostomy tubes (often referred to as ear tubes). In this procedure, a tiny tube is inserted into the eardrum, keeping open a small hole through which fluids can drain to the outside. Tympanostomy tube insertion is done under general anesthesia. Usually the tubes fall out by themselves or are removed in your provider's office.

If your adenoids and tonsils are enlarged, surgical removal may be considered, especially if you have chronic, recurrent ear infections. Similarly, surgical repair of a ruptured eardrum may be necessary to prevent recurrent ear infections.

Nutrition and Dietary Supplements

Foods rich in antioxidants and other important chemicals that help boost immune function are important to include in your child's daily diet. Such foods include fresh, darkly colored fruits and vegetables. Eating plenty of omega-3 fatty acids (a group of essential fatty acids that tend to reduce inflammation) may be important as well. Sources of omega-3 include fish, walnuts, and flaxseeds. Children should not have these foods prior to ages two to three years old.

Because supplements (like those described below) may have side effects or interact with medications, they should be taken only under the supervision of a knowledgeable healthcare provider.

Lactobacillus: A probiotic or "friendly"/healthy bacteria, may reduce the incidence of respiratory infections, like colds and sinusitis, and their associated complications such as ear infections. More research in this area would be helpful.

Xylitol: A sugar alcohol produced naturally in birch, strawberries, and raspberries has properties that fight pneumococcus, a bacteria that commonly causes ear and upper respiratory infections. Some studies are reporting that children who chew gum (if they are old enough) or take a syrup containing xylitol experience fewer ear infections than children who do not take xylitol. More research is needed on this subject.

Herbs

The use of herbs is a time-honored approach to strengthen the body and treat disease. Herbs, however, contain active substances that can trigger side effects and interact with other herbs, supplements, or medications. For these reasons, herbs should be taken with care and only under the supervision of a practitioner knowledgeable in the field of herbal medicine.

Calendula, St. John's Wort, Mullein Flower, Garlic: Herbal specialists will often prescribe herbal ear drops containing one or all of these ingredients for ear pain or infection. In a study conducted in Israel, 103 children with ear infections were given herbal ear drops or drops containing pain-relieving medications. The herbal ear drops contained a variety of herbal extracts including calendula, St. John's wort, mullein flower, and garlic. The researchers found that the combination of herbs in the ear drops was as effective as the medication ear drops in reducing the children's ear pain.

Echinacea: The Native American medicinal plant known as coneflower (*Echinacea angustifolia / Echinacea pallida / Echinacea purpurea*) is one of the most popular herbs in America today. Used primarily to reduce the symptoms and duration of the common cold and flu and to alleviate the symptoms associated with them, such as sore throat (pharyngitis), cough, and fever, many herbalists also recommend echinacea to help boost the activity of the immune system and to help the body fight infections. For this reason, professional herbalists may recommend echinacea to treat ear infections.

Eucalyptus: Parts of the eucalyptus plant have the ability to fight infection, reduce inflammation, and lower fever. For this reason, eucalyptus is often found in remedies used to treat the common cold. Similarly, some herbalists prescribe a tincture made from eucalyptus leaves for chronic ear infections. It is important to note that children under six years old should not take eucalyptus leaves or oil by mouth and children under two should not apply the oil to the face or nose. Therefore, use of eucalyptus ear drops should be reserved for children older than two years and oral eucalyptus for children older than six years.

Other: Some preliminary animal studies suggest that capsaicin, an active ingredient found in cayenne, may help prevent the development of ear infections for those at risk. Much more research is needed before knowing if this same benefit applies to people. Also, capsaicin has been used in homeopathic doses to treat ear infections.

In test tube laboratory studies, tea tree oil demonstrates ability to fight many of the organisms that cause ear infections. Whether this will translate into helpful treatment for otitis media in people is unknown at this time, however. Like capsaicin, much more research is needed, particularly since one early animal study raises the possibility that tea tree oil may cause hearing damage in guinea pigs.

Chiropractic

Chiropractors report and preliminary evidence suggests that spinal manipulation treatments may benefit some children with otitis media. In one study involving 315 children with otitis media, a total of five spinal manipulations significantly improved symptoms after eleven days.

Homeopathy

Although not many studies have examined the effectiveness of specific homeopathic therapies in general, there have been several studies evaluating the use of homeopathy for ear infections. Some of the homeopathic remedies included in such studies or that a professional homeopath might consider for the treatment of ear infections are listed below. Before prescribing a remedy, homeopaths take into account a person's constitutional type. A constitutional type is defined as a person's physical, emotional, and psychological makeup. An experienced homeopath assesses all of these factors when determining the most appropriate treatment for each individual.

- **Aconitum:** For throbbing ear pain that comes on suddenly after exposure to cold or wind; and in children with high fever and whose ears have a bright red coloring.

- **Belladonna:** For sudden onset of infection with piercing pain that often spreads to the neck, flushed face including reddened ears, agitation (even impaired consciousness and nightmares), wide-eyed stare, high fever, and swollen glands; this remedy is most appropriate for children who feel relief when sitting upright and from warm compresses to the ear; this remedy should not be used in children whose symptoms have persisted for more than three days.

- **Chamomilla:** For intense ear pain and extreme irritability and anger (including screaming); this remedy is most appropriate for children who are difficult to comfort unless being rocked or carried by a person who is walking back and forth.

- **Hepar Sulfuricum:** for sharp pains and a smelly, yellowish-green discharge that occur in the middle and late stages of an ear infection, particularly when the child is extremely moody and clearly angry; this remedy is most appropriate for individuals whose symptoms are worsened by cold air and improved by warmth.

- **Lycopodium:** For right-sided ear pain that is worse in the late afternoon and early evening; the child will generally say that his ears feel stuffed up and he may hear a ringing or buzzing sound; the appropriate individual tends to be insecure and need others around, although the personality type may act like a bully as a defense mechanism.

- **Mercurius:** Good for chronic ear infections; for acute or chronic pain that is worse at night and may extend down into the throat; relief comes from nose blowing; and the appropriate child may sweat or drool a lot and have bad breath.

- **Pulsatilla:** For infection following exposure to cold or damp weather; the ear is often red and may have a yellowish/greenish discharge; ear pain worsens when sleeping in a warm bed and is relieved somewhat by cool compresses; this remedy is most appropriate for children who tend to be gentle, weepy, and mildly whiny and are easily soothed by affection.

- **Silica:** For chronic or late-stage infection when the child feels chilly, weak, and tired; sweating may also be present.

Warnings and Precautions

For a child under two, let the doctor know right away if he or she is experiencing a fever, even if no other symptoms are present. Also, if high fever or severe pain is present in a child, of any age, the doctor should be seen right away as well.

Let your health care provider know if your child's symptoms (namely, pain, fever, or irritability) do not improve within twenty-four to forty-eight hours.

If severe pain suddenly stops hurting, this may indicate a ruptured eardrum.

It is possible that swimming will exacerbate an ear infection, particularly the pain from changes in pressure if swimming under water. If a ruptured eardrum is present, swimming is out of the question and even without a rupture, diving and swimming underwater should be avoided with an ear infection. If your child has ear tubes, use earplugs or cotton balls coated with petroleum jelly when swimming to prevent infection.

Prognosis and Complications

Generally, an ear infection is a simple, nonserious condition without complications. Most children will have minor, temporary hearing loss during and right after an ear infection. This is due to fluid lingering in the ear. Permanent hearing loss is extremely rare, but the risk increases if the child has a lot of ear infections. Other potential complications from otitis media include:

- Ruptured or perforated eardrum;

- Chronic, recurrent ear infections;

- Enlarged adenoids or tonsils;

- Mastoiditis (an infection of the bones around the skull);

- Meningitis (an infection of the brain);
- Formation of an abscess or a cyst (called cholesteatoma) from chronic, recurrent ear infections;
- Speech or language delay in a child who suffers lasting hearing loss from multiple, recurrent ear infections; again, this is very unusual.

Supporting Research

Barnett ED, Levatin JL, Chapman EH, et al. Challenges of evaluating homeopathic treatment of acute otitis media. *Pediatr Infect Dis J*. 2000;19(4):273–75.

Basak S, Turkutanit S, Sarierler M, Metin KK. Effects of capsaicin pre-treatment in experimentally-induced secretory otitis media. *J Laryngol Otol*. 1999;113(2):114–17.

Bitnun A, Allen UD. Medical therapy of otitis media: use, abuse, efficacy and morbidity. *J Otolaryngol*. 1998;27(suppl 2):26–36.

Bizakis JG, Velegrakis GA, Papadakis CE, Karampekios SK, Helidonis ES. The silent epidural abscess as a complication of acute otitis media in children. *Int J Pediatr Otorhinolaryngol*. 1998;45:163–66.

Blumenthal M, Goldberg A, Brinckmann J. *Herbal Medicine: Expanded Commission E Monographs*. Newton, MA: Integrative Medicine Communications; 2000:118–23.

Brown CE, Magnuson B. On the physics of the infant feeding bottle and middle ear sequela: ear disease in infants can be associated with bottle feeding. *Int J Pediatr Otorhinolaryngol*. 2000;54(1):13–20.

Cohen R, Levy C, Boucherat M, Langue J, de la Rocque F. A multicenter, randomized, double-blind trial of 5 versus 10 days of antibiotic therapy for acute otitis media in young children. *J Pediatr*. 1998; 133:634–39.

Cummings S, Ullman D. *Everybody's Guide to Homeopathic Medicines*. 3rd ed. New York, NY: Penguin Putnam; 1997: 127–29.

Eskola J, Kilpi T, Palmu A, et al. Pneumococcal conjugate vaccine against acute otitis media. *NEJM*. 2001;344(6):403–9.

Fallon JM. The role of the chiropractic adjustment in the care and treatment of 332 children with otitis media. *J Clin Chiropractic Pediatr*. 1997;2(2):167–83.

Frei H, Thurneysen A. Homeopathy in acute otitis media in children: treatment effect or spontaneous resolution? *Br Homeopath J*. 2001; 90(4):178–79.

Friese KH. Acute otitis media in children: a comparison of conventional and homeopathic treatment. *Biomedical Therapy*. 1997;15(4): 462–66.

Gehanno P, Nguyen L, Barry B, et al. Eradication by ceftriaxone of streptococcus pneumoniae isolates with increased resistance to penicillin in cases of acute otitis media. *Antimicrob Agents Chemother*. 1999;43:16–20.

Hatakka K, Savilahti E, Ponka A, et al. Effect of long term consumption of probiotic milk on infections in children attending day care centres: double blind, randomised trial. *BMJ*. 2001;322(7298):1327.

Ilicali OC, Keles N, Deger K, Savas I. Relationship of passive cigarette smoking to otitis media. *Arch Otolaryngol Head Neck Surg*. 1999;125(7): 758–62.

Jacobs J, Springer DA, Crothers D. Homeopathic treatment of acute otitis media in children: a preliminary randomized placebo-controlled trial. *Pediatr Infect Dis J*. 2001;20(2):177–83.

Jonas WB, Jacobs J. *Healing with Homeopathy: The Doctors' Guide*. New York, NY: Warner Books; 1996: 171–72.

Kruzel T. *The Homeopathic Emergency Guide*. Berkeley, Calif: North Atlantic Books; 1992:243–45.

Kemper AR, Krysan DJ. Reevaluating the efficacy of naturopathic ear drops. *Arch Pediatr Adolesc Med*. 2002;156(1):88–89.

Klein JO. Changes in management of otitis media: 2003 and beyond. *Pediatr Ann*. 2002;31(12):824–26, 829.

Klein JO. Pneumococcal vaccines for infants and children—past, present, and future. *Curr Clin Top Infect Dis*. 2002;22:252–65.

Manis D, Greiver M. New conjugated pneumococcal vaccine. Does it decrease the incidence of acute otitis media? *Can Fam Physician*. 2002;48:1777–79.

Newall CA, Anderson LA, Phillipson JD. *Herbal Medicines: A Guide for Health Care Professionals*. London, England: The Pharmaceutical Press; 1996:108.

Sarrell EM, Mandelberg A, Cohen HA. Efficacy of naturopathic extracts in the management of ear pain associated with acute otitis media. *Arch Pediatr Adolesc Med*. 2001;155(7):796–99.

Stathis SL, O'Callaghan DM, Williams GM, Najman JM, Andersen MJ, Bor W. Maternal cigarette smoking during pregnancy is an independent predictor for symptoms of middle ear disease at five years' post-delivery. *Pediatrics*. 1999;104(2):e16.

Uhari M, Kontiokari T, Koskela M, Niemela M. Xylitol chewing gum in prevention of acute otitis media: double-blind randomised trials. *Br Med J*. 1996;313:1180–84.

Ullman D. *Homeopathic Medicine for Children and Infants*. New York, NY: Penguin Putnam; 1992: 78–81.

Ullman D. *The Consumer's Guide to Homeopathy*. New York, NY: Penguin Putnam; 1995: 178–79.

Wright ED, Pearl AJ, Manoukian JJ. Laterally hypertrophic adenoids as a contributing factor in otitis media. *Int J Pediatr Otorhinolaryngol*. 1998;45:207–14.

Zhang SY, Robertson D. A study of tea tree oil ototoxicity. *Audiol Neurootol*. 2000;5(2):64–68.

Chapter 4

Ear Injuries

Chapter Contents

Section 4.1

Perforated Eardrum

A perforated eardrum is a hole or rupture in the eardrum, a thin membrane that separates the ear canal and the middle ear. The medical term for eardrum is tympanic membrane. The middle ear is connected to the nose by the eustachian tube, which equalizes pressure in the middle ear.

A perforated eardrum is often accompanied by decreased hearing and occasional discharge. Pain is usually not persistent.

Causes of Eardrum Perforation

The causes of perforated eardrum are usually from trauma or infection. A perforated eardrum can occur:

- if the ear is struck squarely with an open hand;
- with a skull fracture;
- after a sudden explosion;
- if an object (such as a bobby pin, Q-tip, or stick) is pushed too far into the ear canal;
- as a result of hot slag (from welding) or acid entering the ear canal.

Middle ear infections may cause pain, hearing loss, and spontaneous rupture (tear) of the eardrum, resulting in a perforation. In this circumstance, there may be infected or bloody drainage from the ear. In medical terms, this is called otitis media with perforation.

On rare occasions a small hole may remain in the eardrum after a previously placed PE (pressure equalizing) tube either falls out or is removed by the physician.

Most eardrum perforations heal spontaneously within weeks after rupture, although some may take up to several months. During the healing process the ear must be protected from water and trauma. Those eardrum perforations that do not heal on their own may require surgery.

Effects on Hearing from Perforated Eardrum

Usually, the larger the perforation, the greater the loss of hearing. The location of the hole (perforation) in the eardrum also affects the degree of hearing loss. If severe trauma (e.g., skull fracture) disrupts the bones in the middle ear that transmit sound or causes injury to the inner ear structures, the loss of hearing maybe quite severe.

If the perforated eardrum is due to a sudden traumatic or explosive event, the loss of hearing can be great and ringing in the ear (tinnitus) may be severe. In this case the hearing usually returns partially, and the ringing diminishes in a few days. Chronic infection as a result of the perforation can cause major hearing loss.

Treatment of the Perforated Eardrum

Before attempting any correction of the perforation, a hearing test should be performed. The benefits of closing a perforation include prevention of water entering the ear while showering, bathing, or swimming (which could cause ear infection); improved hearing; and diminished tinnitus. It also may prevent the development of cholesteatoma (skin cyst in the middle ear), which can cause chronic infection and destruction of ear structures.

If the perforation is very small, otolaryngologists may choose to observe the perforation over time to see if it will close spontaneously. They also might try to patch a cooperative patient's eardrum in the office. Working with a microscope, your doctor may touch the edges of the eardrum with a chemical to stimulate growth and then place a thin paper patch on the eardrum. Usually with closure of the tympanic membrane improvement in hearing is noted. Several applications of a patch (up to three or four) may be required before the perforation closes completely. If your physician feels that a paper patch will not provide prompt or adequate closure of the hole in the eardrum, or attempts with paper patching do not promote healing, surgery is considered.

There are a variety of surgical techniques, but all basically place tissue across the perforation, allowing healing. This procedure is called tympanoplasty. Surgery is typically quite successful in closing the perforation permanently and improving hearing. It is usually done on an outpatient basis.

Your doctor will advise you regarding the proper management of a perforated eardrum.

Section 4.2

Tympanoplasty: Surgical Repair of the Perforated Eardrum

What is a tympanoplasty?

A tympanoplasty is a surgical procedure that repairs or reconstructs the eardrum (tympanic membrane) to help restore normal hearing. This procedure may also involve repair or reconstruction of the small bones behind the tympanic membrane (ossiculoplasty) if needed. Both the eardrum and middle ear bones (ossicles) need to function well together for normal hearing to occur.

What are the indications for a tympanoplasty?

This procedure is usually not performed (or needed) in children under four years of age. A tympanoplasty is recommended when the eardrum is torn (perforated), sunken in (atelectatic), or otherwise abnormal and associated with hearing loss. Abnormalities of the eardrum and middle ear bones can occur through injury, otitis media, congenital (at birth) deformities, or chronic ear conditions such as a cholesteatoma.

How successful is tympanoplasty in restoring normal hearing?

Return to a normal range of hearing after tympanoplasty is dependent upon the extent of the abnormality. Surgeries that involve repair of the eardrum only usually have a success rate of 85 to 90 percent.

A second operation may be necessary in some cases if the hearing is not restored to an acceptable level.

Are there any other options aside from tympanoplasty?

Tympanoplasty in most cases is an elective procedure, meaning that it can be scheduled whenever the patient is ready to have it done. Another option instead of this procedure includes the use of a hearing aid. When the tympanic membrane has a hole (perforation) in it, earplugs are usually recommended to protect the middle ear from infection. In a few cases, such as a significant infection or a cholesteatoma, this procedure may prevent more significant damage to the ear and the surgery may need to be performed more urgently.

What is done in preparation for a tympanoplasty?

Usually other ear, nose, and throat conditions are treated before a tympanoplasty is considered. For example, if an adenoidectomy is indicated, this surgery is usually completed before tympanoplasty.

Otitis media of any type should not be present at the time of surgery, as infection in the ear makes the operation much more difficult and may ruin the reconstruction. If your surgeon has suggested certain medications prior to surgery, these should be taken without exception to ensure a successful outcome.

A hearing test is performed to document any hearing deficiency. The more significant the hearing loss, the sooner the procedure should be performed. The eardrum will also be examined before surgery using a special operating microscope.

What is involved with a tympanoplasty?

A tympanoplasty is performed with the patient fully asleep (under general anesthesia). A surgical cut (incision) is usually made behind the ear, the ear is moved forward, and the eardrum is then carefully exposed. The eardrum is then lifted up (tympanotomy) so that the inside of the ear (middle ear) can be examined. If there is a hole in the eardrum, it is cleaned (debrided) and the abnormal area can be cut away. A piece of fascia (tissue under the skin) from the temporalis muscle (behind the ear) is then cut and placed under the hole in the eardrum to create a new intact eardrum. This tissue is called a graft. The graft allows your child's normal eardrum skin to grow across the hole.

If needed, reconstruction of the middle ear bones (ossiculoplasty) or cholesteatoma removal may also be performed at this time.

This surgery usually requires an overnight hospital stay. The child has a dressing (large bandage) over the surgical site. This is removed the next morning and the patient is discharged home. Occasionally, in older children, or those undergoing a less involved procedure, same-day surgery is possible.

Eardrops may be prescribed after discharge.

The most important part of this surgery for the parent is your part in restricting activity as outlined by your surgeon. By following these instructions very closely, you can make sure your child's result is the best it can be.

What are the risks and complications of a tympanoplasty?

Because this surgery takes place in and around the ear, there are special risks for this surgery in addition to the usual risks of infection and bleeding. Because each child's situation is different, your surgeon will relate to you just how likely these complications are to occur.

- **Hearing Loss:** A tympanoplasty is performed to help restore normal hearing. However, some hearing loss (more common with ossiculoplasty) may still be present after the procedure. An operation is termed successful if the hearing is restored within ten to fifteen decibels of normal.

- **Facial Nerve Injury and Paralysis:** Because the facial nerve runs close to the surgical site, injury, although uncommon, can occur. This may result in temporary facial muscle weakness or loss of taste on one side of the tongue.

- **Dizziness:** This complication after surgery is rare and is more likely to occur when mastoidectomy is performed for cholesteatoma when the cholesteatoma has eroded the balance system.

- **Loss of Graft:** Because this operation involves grafting using your child's own tissue, very rarely this tissue will not survive long enough for the hole in the eardrum to heal completely. In this case, another operation may be necessary. Because the success rate of this surgery is so high, re-operation also has a very high success rate.

Your surgeon will schedule follow-up visits after surgery to look at the eardrum, to check hearing, and to ensure normal healing. It is important to keep these appointments, as they will help to maximize the success of the procedure.

Section 4.3

Barotrauma

Reprinted from "Barotrauma," by Brandon G. Bentz, M.D., and C. Anthony Hughes, M.D., last revised April 2002. © 2002 American Hearing Research Foundation. Reprinted with permission.

What is barotrauma?

Barotrauma refers to injury sustained from failure to equalize the pressure of an air-containing space with that of the surrounding environment. The most common examples of barotrauma occur in air travel and scuba diving. Although the degree of pressure changes are much more dramatic during scuba diving, barotraumatic injury is possible during air travel.

Barotrauma can affect several different areas of the body, including the ear, face, and lungs. Here we will focus on barotrauma as it relates to the ear.

What are the symptoms of barotrauma?

Symptoms of barotrauma include "clogging" of the ear, ear pain, hearing loss, dizziness, ringing of the ear (tinnitus), and hemorrhage from the ear.

Dizziness (or vertigo) may also occur during diving from a phenomenon known as alternobaric vertigo. It is caused by a difference in pressure between the two middle ear spaces, which stimulates the vestibular (balance) end organs asymmetrically, thus resulting in vertigo. The alternobaric response can also be elicited by forcefully equalizing the middle ear pressure with the Politzer maneuver, which can cause an unequal inflation of the middle ear space.

What is inner ear decompression sickness?

Inner ear decompression sickness (IEDCS) is an injury that closely resembles inner ear barotrauma; however, the treatment is different. This injury is more common among commercial and military divers who breathe a compressed mixture of helium and oxygen. Symptoms include hearing loss, ringing of the ears, and/or dizziness during ascent or shortly thereafter.

IEDCS most often occurs during decompression (ascent), or shortly after surfacing from a dive. In contrast, barotrauma most often occurs during compression (descent) or after a short, shallow dive. Patients with IEDCS should be rapidly transported to a hyperbaric chamber for recompression. A significant correlation exists between early recompression and recovery.

What causes barotrauma?

Barotrauma is caused by a difference in pressure between the external environment and the internal parts of the ear. Since fluids do not compress under pressures experienced during diving or flying, the fluid-containing spaces of the ear do not alter their volume under these pressure changes. However, the air-containing spaces of the ear do compress, resulting in damage to the ear if the alterations in ambient pressure cannot be equalized.

Barotrauma can affect the outer, middle, or inner ear.

Outer Ear: The outer ear is an air-containing space that can be affected by changes in ambient pressure. During diving, water normally replaces the air in the external ear canal. An obstruction such as wax, a bony growth, or earplugs can create an air-containing space that can change in volume in response to changes in ambient pressure. During descent, the volume of this space decreases causing the tympanic membrane to bulge outward (toward the outer ear canal). This can cause pain, small hemorrhages in the eardrum, or blebs (small blisters).

Middle Ear: The most common problem that occurs in diving and flying is the failure to equalize pressure between the middle ear and the ambient environment. Equalization of pressure occurs through the eustachian tube, which is the soft tissue tube that extends from the back of the nose to the middle ear space. The extent of injury depends upon the degree and speed of the ambient pressure changes. The greatest relative pressure changes in diving occur near the surface. Therefore, the largest proportional volume changes, and thus the most injuries, occur at shallow depths.

As a diver descends to only 2.6 feet with difficulty equalizing the pressure of his middle ear space, the tympanic membrane and ossicles are retracted, and the diver experiences pressure and pain. At higher pressures the eustachian tube may become "locked" closed by the negative pressure in the middle ear. This can occur at about 3.9 feet of water. Further increases in pressure, at depths of only 4.3 to 17.4 feet of water, can cause the tympanic membrane to rupture.

Inner Ear: Inner ear injury during descent is directly related to impaired ability to equalize the middle ear pressure on the affected side. Sudden, large pressure changes in the middle ear can be transmitted to the inner ear, resulting in damage to the delicate mechanisms of the inner ear. This can cause severe vertigo and even deafness. Two mechanisms are theorized to explain inner ear barotrauma: the "implosive" and the "explosive" mechanisms.

The implosive mechanism theory involves clearing of the middle ear during descent. The pressure is transmitted from an inward bulging eardrum, causing the ossicles to be moved toward the inner ear at the oval window. This pressure wave is transmitted through the inner ear and causes an outward bulging of the other window, the round window membrane. If a diver performs a forceful Politzer maneuver and the eustachian tube suddenly opens, a rapid increase in middle ear pressure occurs. This causes the ossicles to suddenly return to their normal positions, causing the round window to implode.

The explosive theory suggests that when a diver attempts to clear a blocked middle ear space by performing a Politzer maneuver and the eustachian tube is blocked and locked, a dramatic increase in the intracranial pressure occurs. Since the fluids surrounding the brain communicate freely with the inner ear fluids, this pressure may be transmitted to the inner ear. A sudden rise in the inner ear pressure could then cause the round or oval window membrane to explode.

How is barotrauma diagnosed?

Diagnosis is initially based on careful history. If the history indicates ear pain or dizziness that occurs after diving or an airplane flight, barotrauma should be suspected. The diagnosis may be confirmed through ear examination, as well as hearing and vestibular testing.

How is barotrauma treated?

For outer ear barotrauma, the treatment consists of clearing the ear canal of the obstruction and restricting diving or flying until the blockage is corrected and the ear canal and drum return to normal.

55

For middle ear barotrauma, treatment consists of keeping the ear dry and free of contamination that could cause infection. Topical nasal steroids and decongestants may be started in an attempt to decongest the eustachian tube opening. The presence of pus may prompt the use of appropriate antibiotics. Most tympanic membrane perforations due to barotrauma will heal spontaneously. If the eustachian tube demonstrates chronic problems with middle ear equalization, the likelihood of recovery is drastically reduced.

For inner ear barotrauma, treatment consists of hospitalization and bed rest with the head elevated thirty to forty degrees. Controversy exists whether this type of injury needs immediate surgery. Once healed, a diver should not return to diving until hearing and balance function tests are normal.

How might barotrauma affect my life?

If barotrauma results from diving, you should not to return to diving until your ear examination is normal, including a hearing test and the demonstration that the middle ear can be autoinflated.

References

O'Reilly BJ, McRae A, Lupa H. The role of functional endoscopic sinus surgery in the management of recurrent sinus barotrauma. *Aviation, Space, and Environmental Medicine* 1995; 66(9): 876–79.

Stangerup SE, Tjernström Ø, Klokker M, et al. Point prevalence of barotitis in children and adults after flight, and the effects of autoinflation. *Aviation, Space, and Environmental Medicine* 1998; 69(1): 45–49.

Section 4.4

Ears and Altitude

Have you ever wondered why your ears pop when you fly on an airplane? Or why, when they fail to pop, you get an earache? Have you ever wondered why the babies on an airplane fuss and cry so much during descent?

Ear problems are the most common medical complaint of airplane travelers, and while they are usually simple, minor annoyances, they occasionally result in temporary pain and hearing loss.

How does air pressure affect the ear?

It is the middle ear that causes discomfort during air travel, because it is an air pocket inside the head that is vulnerable to changes in air pressure.

Normally, each time (or each second or third time) you swallow, your ears make a little click or popping sound. This occurs because a small bubble of air has entered your middle ear, up from the back of your nose. It passes through the eustachian tube, a membrane-lined tube about the size of a pencil lead that connects the back of the nose with the middle ear. The air in the middle ear is constantly being absorbed by its membranous lining and resupplied through the eustachian tube. In this manner, air pressure on both sides of the eardrum stays about equal. If and when the air pressure is not equal, the ear feels blocked.

What causes blocked ears and eustachian tubes?

The eustachian tube can be blocked, or obstructed, for a variety of reasons. When that occurs, the middle ear pressure cannot be equalized. The air already there is absorbed and a vacuum occurs, sucking the eardrum inward and stretching it. Such an eardrum cannot vibrate naturally, so sounds are muffled or blocked, and the stretching can be painful. If the tube remains blocked, fluid (like blood serum) will seep into the area from the membranes in an attempt to overcome the vacuum. This is called "fluid in the ear," serous otitis, or aero-otitis.

The most common cause for a blocked eustachian tube is the common cold. Sinus infections and nasal allergies (hay fever, etc.) are also causes. A stuffy nose leads to stuffy ears because the swollen membranes block the opening of the eustachian tube.

Children are especially vulnerable to blockages because their eustachian tubes are narrower than adults.

What are the three parts of the ear?

- **The outer ear:** the part that you can see on the side of the head plus the ear canal leading down to the eardrum.

- **The middle ear:** the eardrum and ear bones (ossicles), plus the air spaces behind the eardrum and in the mastoid cavities (vulnerable to air pressure).

- **The inner ear:** the area that contains the nerve endings for the organs of hearing and balance (equilibrium).

How can air travel cause ear problems?

Air travel is sometimes associated with rapid changes in air pressure. To maintain comfort, the eustachian tube must open frequently and wide enough to equalize the changes in pressure. This is especially true when the airplane is landing, going from low atmospheric pressure down closer to earth where the air pressure is higher.

Actually, any situation in which rapid altitude or pressure changes occur creates the problem. You may have experienced it when riding in elevators or when diving to the bottom of a swimming pool. Deep-sea divers are taught how to equalize their ear pressures; so are pilots. You can learn the tricks too.

How can a you unblock your ears?

Swallowing activates the muscle that opens the eustachian tube. You swallow more often when you chew gum or let mints melt in your mouth. These are good air travel practices, especially just before take-off and during descent. Yawning is even better. Avoid sleeping during descent, because you may not be swallowing often enough to keep up with the pressure changes. (The flight attendant will be happy to awaken you just before descent).

If yawning and swallowing are not effective, unblock your ears as follows:

- **Step 1:** Pinch your nostrils shut.
- **Step 2:** Take a mouthful of air.
- **Step 3:** Using your cheek and throat muscles, force the air into the back of your nose as if you were trying to blow your thumb and fingers off your nostrils.

When you hear a loud pop in your ears, you have succeeded. You may have to repeat this several times during descent.

What about babies' ears?

Babies cannot intentionally pop their ears, but popping may occur if they are sucking on a bottle or pacifier. Feed your baby during the flight, and do not allow him or her to sleep during descent.

What precautions should you take in unblocking your ears?

- When inflating your ears, you should not use force. The proper technique involves only pressure created by your check and throat muscles.
- If you have a cold, a sinus infection, or an allergy attack, it is best to postpone an airplane trip.
- If you recently have undergone ear surgery, consult with your surgeon on how soon you may safely fly.

What about decongestants and nose sprays?

Many experienced air travelers use a decongestant pill or nasal spray an hour or so before descent. This will shrink the membranes and help the ears pop more easily. Travelers with allergy problems should take their medication at the beginning of the flight for the same reason.

Decongestant tablets and sprays can be purchased without a prescription. However, they should be avoided by people with heart disease, high blood pressure, irregular heart rhythms, thyroid disease, or excessive nervousness. Such people should consult their physicians before using these medicines. Pregnant women should likewise consult their physicians first.

What should you do if your ears will not unblock?

Even after landing you can continue the pressure equalizing techniques, and you may find decongestants and nasal sprays to be helpful. (However, avoid making a habit of nasal sprays. After a few days, they may cause more congestion than they relieve). If your ears fail to open, or if pain persists, you will need to seek the help of a physician who has experience in the care of ear disorders. He or she may need to release the pressure or fluid with a small incision in the eardrum.

Section 4.5

Ear Emergencies

© 2006 A.D.A.M., Inc. Reprinted with permission.

Definition

Ear emergencies include objects stuck in the ear and ruptured eardrums.

Considerations

Children often stick objects into their ears. These objects can be difficult to remove because the ear canal is a tube of solid bone that is lined with thin, sensitive skin. Any object pressing against the skin can be very painful. In many cases, a doctor will need to use special instruments to examine the ear and safely remove the object.

Causes

Pain, hearing loss, dizziness, ringing in the ear, and ruptured eardrums can be caused by:

- Inserting cotton swabs, toothpicks, pins, pens, or other objects into the ear.

- Sudden changes in pressure, as from an explosion, blow to the head, flying, scuba diving, falling while water skiing, or being slapped on the head or ear.

- Loud percussions, such as a gun going off.

Symptoms

- Dizziness
- Loss of hearing
- Nausea and vomiting
- Noises in the ear
- Earache
- Bleeding from the ear
- Bruising or redness
- Swelling
- Object visible in the ear
- Sensations of an object in the ear
- Clear liquid coming out of the ear (brain fluid)

First Aid

Follow the steps below, depending on the type of ear emergency.

Object in the Ear

1. Calm and reassure the person.

2. If the object is sticking out and easy to remove, gently remove it by hand or with tweezers. Then, get medical help to make sure the entire object was removed.

3. If you think a small object may be lodged within the ear, but you cannot see it, **do not** reach inside the ear canal with tweezers. You can do more harm than good.

4. Try using gravity to get the object out by tilting the head to the affected side. **Do not** strike the person's head. Shake it gently in the direction of the ground to try to dislodge the object.

5. If the object doesn't come out, get medical help.

Insect in the Ear

1. **Do not** let the person put a finger in the ear, since this may make the insect sting.

2. Turn the person's head so that the affected side is up, and wait to see if the insect flies or crawls out.

3. If this doesn't work, try pouring mineral oil, olive oil, or baby oil into the ear. As you pour the oil, pull the ear lobe gently backward and upward for an adult, or backward and downward for a child. The insect should suffocate and may float out in the oil. **Avoid** using oil to remove any object other than an insect, since oil can cause other kinds of objects to swell.

Ruptured Eardrum

1. The person will have severe pain. Place sterile cotton gently in the outer ear canal to keep the inside of the ear clean.

2. Get medical help.

Cuts on the Outer Ear

1. Apply direct pressure until the bleeding stops.

2. Cover the injury with a sterile dressing shaped to the contour of the ear, and tape it loosely in place.

3. Apply cold compresses over the dressing to reduce pain and swelling.

4. If part of the ear has been cut off, keep the part. Get medical help immediately.

Drainage from Inside the Ear

1. Cover the outside of the ear with a sterile dressing shaped to the contour of the ear, and tape it loosely in place.

2. Have the person lie down on the side with the affected ear down so that it can drain. However, **do not** move the person if a neck or back injury is suspected.

3. Get medical help immediately.

Do Not

- **Do not** block any drainage coming from the ear.
- **Do not** try to clean or wash the inside of the ear.
- **Do not** attempt to remove the object by probing with a cotton swab, pin, or any other tool. To do so will risk pushing the object farther into the ear and damaging the middle ear.
- **Do not** reach inside the ear canal with tweezers.

Call Immediately for Emergency Medical Assistance If

The following symptoms, which may indicate significant trauma to the ear, should be evaluated by a physician:

- Pain in the ear
- Ringing sounds
- Dizziness (vertigo)
- Hearing loss
- Drainage or blood from the ear
- Recent blow to your ear or head

Prevention

- Never put anything in the ear canal without first consulting a physician.
- Never thump the head to try to correct an ear problem.
- Teach children not to put things in their ears.
- Avoid cleaning the ear canals altogether.
- Following an ear injury, avoid nose blowing and getting water in the injured ear.
- Treat ear infections promptly.

If you tend to feel pain and pressure when flying, drink lots of fluid before and during the flight. Avoid the use of alcohol, caffeine, or tobacco on the day of the flight. Chew gum, suck on a hard candy, or yawn during take-off and landing. Talk to your doctor about taking a decongestant or using a nasal spray before you fly.

References

Auerbach PS. *Wilderness Medicine*. 4th ed. St. Louis, MO: Mosby, 2001: 468–70.

DeLee JC, Drez, Jr., D, Miller MD, eds. *DeLee and Drez's Orthopaedic Sports Medicine*. 2nd ed. Philadelphia, PA: Saunders, 2003: 758.

Chapter 5

Ear Secretions and Growths

Chapter Contents

Section 5.1

Earwax (Cerumen)

What is earwax for?

Glands in the skin of the outer part of the ear canal make earwax (also called cerumen). The wax traps dust and small particles to keep the ear clean. It also helps keep water out of the ears.

How can I clean my ears?

The ears clean themselves of wax. You should not have to clean them. The wax builds up a little, then dries out and falls, or is wiped, out of the ear. Without wax, the ears become dry and itchy. A normal amount of earwax is healthy. Cotton swabs (such as Q-tips) are not recommended for cleaning. If you feel you must use cotton swabs, use them no more than once or twice a week. Use them gently. Do not push them into the ear. Use on the outer part of the ear.

What is earwax impaction?

Impaction means that several layers of earwax have been pushed together and may be stuck in the ear.

What causes it?

Normal wax builds up in the outer part of the ear canal, not near the eardrum. If a patient has build-up near the eardrum, it is usually because the wax has been pushed there. Patients who are trying to clean their ears with a cotton swab (Q-tip) or twisted tissue sometimes actually push the wax deeper into the ear. This not only can cause wax build-up, but it can injure the thin skin of the ear canal.

Who can get it?

Anyone can get impaction, but it tends to be more common in certain ethnic groups. People with narrow ear canals are more likely to get it. People who use cotton swabs in their ears are more likely to get it.

What are the signs and symptoms of it?

Ears feel plugged. There is a partial loss of hearing.

How is it treated?

You may try ear drops at home before calling a doctor. Eardrops soften the wax so it comes more easily out of the ear. Some drops can be found over-the-counter, such as Debrox or Murine Ear Drops. A mixture of one part hydrogen peroxide and one part water (or equal amounts) can also be used. You can use several drops twice a day. Tilt your head to one side and fill the ear canal using an eyedropper. Let soak in for a minute or two. Do this to the other ear if needed. Do this up to two times a day for three to four days. After three to four days, follow the same steps once a day. If impaction is a frequent problem, put two or three drops into each ear once a week. Stop using the drops if it causes any discomfort, dizziness, or drainage. If home treatment doesn't work, call the doctor. To clean out the wax, the doctor might wash it out, vacuum it out, or use special tools to get it out.

How long does it last?

If the impaction does not improve with home treatment after seven days, call the doctor.

When should I call the doctor?

If you or your child have tubes in the ears, call your doctor before using drops, oil, or peroxide to clean them out. If impaction is a frequent problem, ask the doctor to suggest ways you can prevent it. Call the doctor if impaction does not improve after seven days of home treatment. Call the doctor if you have questions or concerns.

Quick Answers

- Earwax (or cerumen) traps dust and small particles to keep the ears clean.

- The ears clean themselves of wax. You should not have to clean them. If you feel you must use cotton swabs, use them no more than once or twice a week.

- Impaction means that several layers of earwax have been pushed together.

- If a patient has build-up near the eardrum, it is usually because the wax has been pushed there with a cotton swab or twisted tissue.

- People who use cotton swabs in their ears are more likely to get it.

- If your ears feel plugged or if your hearing is muffled, it could be a sign of impaction.

- Eardrops soften the wax so it comes more easily out of the ear.

- If the impaction does not improve with home treatment after seven days, call the doctor.

- If impaction is a frequent problem, ask the doctor to suggest ways you can prevent it.

References

American Academy of Otolaryngology. *Earwax... and what to do about it.* 1995 (cited 2002 January 23). Available from: URL: http://www .sinuscarecenter.com/waxaao.html

Davidson TM. *Ambulatory Healthcare Pathways for Ear, nose, and Throat Disorders.* University of California San Diego. 2000 February 4 (cited 2002 January 23). Available from: URL: http://www.surgery .ucsd.edu/ent/davidson/pathway/earWax.htm

American Medical Association. *Atlas of the Body: The Ear.* Medem. 1999 (cited 2002 January 23). Available from: URL: http://www .medem.com/MedLB/article_detaillb.cfm?article_ID=ZZZYXNW 46JC&sub_cat=198

University of Florida. *Cerumen Impaction.* (cited 2002 January 23). Available from: URL: http://www.ent.health.ufl.edu/Patient%20Info/ cerumen.htm

Section 5.2

Benign Ear Cyst or Tumor

© 2006 A.D.A.M., Inc. Reprinted with permission.

Alternative Names

Osteomas; exostoses; tumor—ear; cysts—ear; ear cysts; ear tumors

Definition

Benign ear cysts are noncancerous lumps or growths within the canal of the ear, pinna, or other parts of the ear.

Causes, Incidence, and Risk Factors

Sebaceous cysts are the most common cysts seen in the ear. They are bulging, sac-like collections of dead skin cells and oils produced by oil glands in the skin.

They commonly occur behind the ear, within the ear canal, or on the scalp. The exact cause is unknown, but cysts may occur when oils are produced in a skin gland faster than they can be excreted out of the gland. If the cysts within the ear canal get infected, they are extremely painful.

Benign bony tumors of the ear canal (exostoses and osteomas) may be caused by an overgrowth of bone. Repeated exposure to cold water may increase the risk of benign tumors of the ear canal. Tumors may grow large enough to block the ear canal, trap wax in the canal, and interfere with hearing.

Symptoms

The symptoms of cysts include:

- small soft skin lumps on, behind, or in front of the ear that are usually not painful or tender (unless infected);

69

- cysts within the external ear canal that can be extremely painful.

The symptoms of benign tumors include:

- ear discomfort;
- gradual hearing loss in one ear (because the tumor blocks the external ear canal).

Note: There may be no symptoms.

Signs and Tests

Benign cysts and tumors are usually discovered during a routine ear examination. When looking into the ear, the doctor may see cysts or benign tumors that often appear as skin-covered mounds within the ear canal.

This disease may also alter the results of the following tests:

- Electronystagmography
- Caloric stimulation

Treatment

If the cyst or tumor is not painful and does not interfere with hearing, treatment is not necessary.

If a cyst becomes painful, it may be infected. Treatment may include antibiotics or removal of the cyst.

Benign bony tumors may progressively increase in size. If a benign tumor is painful or interferes with hearing, surgical removal of the tumor may be necessary.

Expectations (Prognosis)

Benign ear cysts and tumors are usually slow-growing and may disappear on their own.

Complications

- The cysts could become infected.
- Wax in the ear could become impacted.
- Hearing loss could occur if the tumor is large.

Calling Your Health Care Provider

Call for an appointment with a health care provider if you have symptoms of a benign ear cyst or tumor and there is discomfort, pain, or hearing loss.

Section 5.3

Otosclerosis

Reprinted from "Otosclerosis," National Institute on Deafness and Other Communication Disorders, National Institutes of Health, NIH Publication No. 99-4234, May 1999. Reviewed by David A. Cooke, M.D., on March 30, 2006.

What is otosclerosis?

Otosclerosis is the abnormal growth of bone of the middle ear. This bone prevents structures within the ear from working properly and causes hearing loss. For some people with otosclerosis, the hearing loss may become severe.

How do we hear?

Hearing is a series of events in which the ear converts sound waves into electrical signals and causes nerve impulses to be sent to the brain, where they are interpreted as sound. The ear has three main parts: the outer, middle, and inner ear. Sound waves enter through the outer ear and reach the middle ear, where they cause the eardrum to vibrate. The vibrations are transmitted through three tiny bones in the middle ear called the ossicles. These three bones are named the malleus, incus, and stapes (and are also known as the hammer, anvil, and stirrup). The eardrum and ossicles carry the vibrations to the inner ear. The stirrup transmits the vibrations through the oval window and into the fluid that fills the inner ear. The vibrations move through fluid in the snail-shaped hearing part of the inner ear (cochlea) that contains the hair cells. The fluid in the cochlea moves the top of the hair cells, which initiates the changes that lead to the production of the nerve

71

impulses. These nerve impulses are carried to the brain, where they are interpreted as sound. Different sounds stimulate different parts of the inner ear, allowing the brain to distinguish among various sounds, for example, different vowel and consonant sounds.

How does otosclerosis cause hearing impairment?

Otosclerosis can cause different types of hearing loss, depending on which structure within the ear is affected. Otosclerosis usually affects the last bone in the chain, the stapes, which rests in the entrance to the inner ear (the oval window). The abnormal bone fixates the stapes in the oval window and interferes with sound passing waves to the inner ear.

Otosclerosis usually causes a conductive hearing loss, a hearing loss caused by a problem in the outer or middle ear. Less frequently, otosclerosis may cause a sensorineural hearing loss (damaged sensory cells and/or nerve fibers of the inner ear), as well as a conductive hearing loss.

What causes otosclerosis?

The cause of otosclerosis is not fully understood, although research has shown that otosclerosis tends to run in families and may be hereditary, or passed down from parent to child. People who have a family

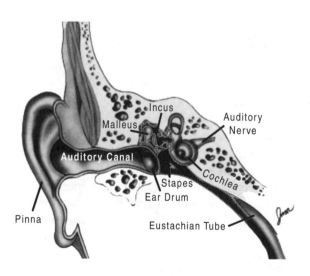

Figure 5.1. Anatomy of the ear

history of otosclerosis are more likely to develop the disorder. On average, a person who has one parent with otosclerosis has a 25 percent chance of developing the disorder. If both parents have otosclerosis, the risk goes up to 50 percent. Research shows that white, middle-aged women are most at risk.

Some research suggests a relationship between otosclerosis and the hormonal changes associated with pregnancy. While the exact cause remains unknown, there is some evidence associating viral infections (such as measles) and otosclerosis.

What are the symptoms of otosclerosis?

Hearing loss is the most frequent symptom of otosclerosis. The loss may appear very gradually. Many people with otosclerosis first notice that they cannot hear low-pitched sounds or that they can no longer hear a whisper.

In addition to hearing loss, some people with otosclerosis may experience dizziness, balance problems, or tinnitus. Tinnitus is a sensation of ringing, roaring, buzzing, or hissing in the ears or head that accompanies many forms of hearing loss.

How is otosclerosis diagnosed?

An examination by an otolaryngologist (ear, nose, and throat physician) or otologist (ear physician) is needed to rule out other diseases or health problems that may cause these same symptoms. An audiologist is a hearing health care professional who is trained to identify, measure, and rehabilitate hearing impairment and related disorders. An audiologist uses a variety of tests and procedures to assess hearing and balance function. The audiologist may produce an audiogram (a graph that shows a person's hearing sensitivity) and a tympanogram (a graph that shows how well the middle ear functions to conduct sound). Discuss these results with your audiologist/otologist.

How is otosclerosis treated?

In many cases surgery is an option for treatment of otosclerosis. In an operation called a stapedectomy, a surgeon (otolaryngologist or otologist) bypasses the diseased bone with a prosthetic device that allows sound waves to be passed to the inner ear. It is important to discuss the risks and possible complications of this procedure, as well as the benefits, with the surgeon. In rare cases, surgery can worsen the hearing loss.

73

If the hearing loss is mild, surgery may not be an option. Also, on occasion, some hearing loss persists after surgery. A properly fitted hearing aid may help some people with otosclerosis in situations that include persistent hearing loss. A hearing aid is designed to compensate for a hearing loss by amplifying sound. An audiologist can discuss the various types of hearing aids available and make a recommendation based on the specific needs of an individual.

What research is being done on otosclerosis?

Scientists are conducting research to improve understanding of otosclerosis. Genetic studies continue in order to identify the gene or genes that may lead to this disorder. Other researchers are studying the effectiveness of lasers currently used in surgery, of amplification devices, and of various stapes prostheses. Improved diagnostic techniques are also being examined and developed.

Section 5.4

Cholesteatoma

What is a cholesteatoma?

A cholesteatoma is a sac of skin that arises off the eardrum and erodes into the middle ear and mastoid bone. It is a benign growth or tumor that causes damage because as it grows, it erodes structures that fall in its path.

What structures can a cholesteatoma affect?

As the cholesteatoma grows into the middle ear it can erode the bones of hearing, causing a significant hearing loss. As it grows farther it can cause a facial paralysis as it erodes into the facial nerve that supplies the muscles of the face. It may also grow into the inner ear, causing spinning vertigo and inner ear or sensorineural hearing loss. If it is allowed to continue to grow it can erode into the brain cavity, causing infections such as meningitis or abscess. In addition, cholesteatoma may become infected, which will cause the ear to drain. Infections in the cholesteatoma cause them to grow more rapidly, thus increasing the damage that a cholesteatoma may cause.

What is the treatment of cholesteatoma?

For the vast majority of patients, the best treatment for cholesteatoma is surgery. This allows removal of the cholesteatoma and attempts to correct the damage the cholesteatoma has done. This surgery is called a mastoidectomy. At times this surgery may be accompanied by a tympanoplasty (repair of an eardrum) and an ossiculoplasty (repair of the bones of hearing).

How is a mastoidectomy performed?

That mastoid bone lies immediately behind the middle and external ears. If it is invaded by cholesteatoma, it must be opened up so that the cholesteatoma can be cleaned out. This is done using the microscope and high-speed drills. There are two basic types of mastoidectomies. In one type of surgery the back half of the external ear canal is removed, creating a common cavity between the external ear canal and the mastoid bone. This surgery, called a canal wall down mastoidectomy, offers excellent control of cholesteatoma. An alternative approach, in which the canal wall is not taken down, is termed a canal wall up mastoidectomy. The choice between performing a canal wall up and a canal wall down mastoidectomy is dependent on the degree of damage the cholesteatoma has done to the ear and mastoid bone and the condition of the ear and mastoid bone at the time of surgery. Your surgeon will suggest the best option for your particular cholesteatoma.

What are the advantages and disadvantages of the various types of mastoidectomy?

The main advantage of a canal wall down mastoidectomy is that it offers excellent control of the cholesteatoma. The main disadvantage to a canal wall down mastoidectomy is that it creates a cavity that can be visualized only by a physician looking in the ear. This cavity must be cleaned periodically (every six to twelve months). These cavities are more prone to infection, and particular care must be taken by the patient to keep the ear dry. The advantage of the canal wall up mastoidectomy is that the basic normal anatomy of the ear is maintained and, therefore, there is no cavity and no need for regular cleaning and special precautions with regard to water exposure. However, the disadvantage of the canal wall up mastoidectomy is that it has a lesser chance of clearing the cholesteatoma and a higher chance of recurrence of a cholesteatoma at a later date. Therefore, a patient with a canal wall up mastoidectomy must still be followed regularly by an ear specialist to ensure that no recurrence has occurred.

What can I expect after mastoidectomy surgery?

Mastoidectomy surgery can typically be performed as an outpatient procedure. If you are discharged from the hospital with a bandage over the ear, this dressing should be removed the morning after surgery. A cotton ball will be placed within the ear and this should be changed by the patient so as to keep it fresh and clean. A prescription for antibiotic ointment will be given to you that you are to use on the incision behind the ear two to three times per day. It is normal after mastoidectomy surgery for there to be some drainage from the ear for up to one week after surgery. Packing will be placed in the ear at the time of surgery and will be removed two to three weeks after the operation.

Please notify your doctor if you have any of the following symptoms:

- Increasing hearing loss
- Increasing pain
- Spinning vertigo
- Fever
- Increasing drainage from the ear

What are the possible complications of mastoidectomy surgery?

Most of the complications of mastoidectomy surgery have to do with the damage that the cholesteatoma has already caused to the ear. There is always a risk of inner ear damage when performing mastoidectomy surgery. The chances of inner ear damage are directly related to whether the cholesteatoma has already eroded into this structure. If the inner ear is damaged, the patient will have increasing hearing loss and spinning vertigo. The facial nerve, which supplies muscles to the face, runs through the middle ear. If the cholesteatoma has exposed this nerve there is risk of facial paralysis. Doctors utilize the microscope and special monitors to identify and protect this nerve. Using these techniques doctors are able to greatly minimize the risks to the facial nerve. The fine nerve that supplies taste to the anterior one-quarter of the tongue runs through the middle ear. This is frequently involved by the cholesteatoma and must be resected in order to completely remove the cholesteatoma. When this is done, the patient may experience a temporary alteration in taste.

What will my hearing be like after surgery?

The goals of mastoidectomy surgery are, in order of importance:

1. To create a safe ear (one that will not have complications);

2. To create a dry ear;

3. To improve hearing.

All attempts are made to provide the patient with the best hearing possible, given the amount of damage that has been done by the cholesteatoma.

Part Two

Hearing Disorders

Chapter 6

Hearing Loss: The Basics

Chapter Contents

Section 6.1

Types of Hearing Loss

Over twenty-five million Americans have some degree of hearing loss and, as the average age of the population increases, this number will rise. Hearing loss is characterized by:

- type of loss (conductive, sensory, neural);
- location of the problem (middle ear, cochlea, auditory nerve, central);
- degree of loss;
- the condition that causes it.

Conductive Hearing Loss

Conductive hearing loss results from external or middle ear problems, which are often mechanical in nature and often can be corrected by medicine or surgery. There are various causes for conductive hearing loss, including otitis media and otosclerosis.

Otitis Media

The most common cause of conductive hearing loss in children is otitis media infection in the middle ear cavity. The infection may start in the nose from a cold and spread to the middle ear via the eustachian tube. If the infection progresses, fluid forms in the middle ear, impeding transmission of sound, and can result in a mild, conductive hearing loss as long as the fluid persists. Chronic otitis media is a major cause of hearing loss in medically underserved areas worldwide.

Surgical treatment is usually necessary if the infection persists and, thanks to modern techniques, is highly successful. A perforated eardrum caused by otitis media or by physical tearing can be repaired in 95 percent of cases, restoring hearing to normal levels. Our knowledge of otitis media has dramatically increased over the past two decades and its treatment has had an important impact on children's health care. Antibiotic treatment, tympanostomy tubes, and adenoidectomy have been mainstays in treatment but development of vaccines against the most common bacteria is in progress. When perfected they should provide a major improvement in pediatric health care.

Otosclerosis

The most common cause of conductive hearing loss in adults is otosclerosis. About 10 percent of the entire population has otosclerosis but only 10 percent of those have hearing loss as a result. The loss results from fixation of the stapes (the third bone in the middle ear) so that sounds cannot be transported to the inner ear. Otosclerosis is thought to be an inherited condition. It usually begins in early adulthood and progresses slowly, typically causing up to a 60 dB loss in both ears. Surgical treatment is very effective, with over 90 percent of patients achieving normal hearing levels. Occasionally the otosclerotic bone will invade the cochlea to produce a sensory loss as well. Fortunately this is rare. Removal of the stapes (stapedectomy), which has been done for forty years, or the newer laser technique of partial removal (stapedotomy) followed by reconstruction with a small piston-like device result in better hearing with little risk to the inner ear or balance disturbance. This means patients return to work sooner after surgery and can expect significantly better hearing.

Sensory Hearing Loss

Sensory hearing losses are due to disorders in the inner ear, specifically, the cochlea. This type of loss may be present at birth (congenital hearing loss) resulting from abnormal cochlea development or inherited conditions, or the loss may be the result of an acquired condition, such as meningitis, an infection of the fluid around the brain often extending into the inner ear. Another example of a sensory hearing loss condition is Ménière disease.

Many hereditary conditions produce hearing loss at birth or later in life due to secondary degeneration of the inner ear structures. These usually occur as recessive conditions that often skip generations within a family. One of the most common of these conditions is Waardenburg syndrome. Affected people often have eyes of different color, a white forelock, wide-set eyes, and progressive hearing loss.

Usher syndrome (retinitis pigmentosa) and Alport syndrome (deafness and kidney disease) are other important genetic causes of deafness.

Ménière Disease

Ménière disease is a common condition caused by changes in the chemical composition and volume of fluid within the inner ear. The disease tends to affect only one ear and cause episodic spells of severe dizziness (vertigo) and hearing loss, which fluctuates but over time gradually deteriorates. The cause is unknown. Medical or, if necessary, surgical treatment usually controls the vertiginous spells. Medical therapy is directed toward salt restriction and fluid control and is successful in 70 percent of cases. For the remainder, surgical therapy is highly effective in relieving the spells of vertigo that often keep people with Ménière disease from working.

Noise-Induced Hearing Loss

We live in a very noisy world and it is clear that our hearing suffers as a result. Long-term overexposure to hazardous noise will produce a typical high-frequency sensory loss resulting from permanent damage of the cochlear outer hair cells. Hearing protection and noise-reduction techniques prevent this from happening. Gun-shooting and industrial noise are the most common causes of noise-induced hearing loss, and rock musicians often have hearing loss due to high sound levels of their amplified music.

Neural Hearing Loss

When a hearing loss results from a problem with the auditory nerve, it is referred to as a neural hearing loss. Its most important cause is the acoustic neuroma, a benign tumor that grows on the vestibular (balance) nerve and presses upon the auditory nerve. Early detection and prompt removal of the tumor is curative and may prevent future hearing loss.

The acoustic reflex is a way of testing for neural hearing loss. The stapedius is a small muscle attached to the stapes that contracts in response to any loud sound, thus protecting the ear. The level of sound required to elicit this acoustic reflex can be used as a rough measure of hearing sensitivity. If the middle ear is normal, absence of the acoustic reflex may indicate a neural type of hearing loss. Interestingly, the reflex will remain at normal levels even with severe cochlear hearing loss but tends to disappear with mild neural losses.

Neural hearing loss is also characterized by a greater loss of speech discrimination than experienced with sensory loss.

Central Auditory Dysfunction

Central auditory dysfunction refers to auditory impairment resulting from problems in the brain. Fortunately, central problems are uncommon. While they cause communication difficulties, they do not cause deafness because they usually affect only one side of the brain: both sides of the brain are involved in hearing. Central auditory dysfunction can result from aging, from Alzheimer disease, and from other uncommon problems.

Presbycusis

Age-related hearing loss is called presbycusis (presby = elder, cusis = hearing). Everyone who lives long enough will develop some degree of age-related hearing loss. Those who damage their ears through noise develop it sooner and people who live in noisy societies have more presbycusis than those who live in quiet environments.

Presbycusis is the most common form of hearing loss and is thought to be due to the combined effects of intrinsic aging of the peripheral or central auditory systems and the accumulated effects of wear and tear. Most cases of presbycusis include high-frequency sensitivity loss, which disrupts speech comprehension in proportion to the sensitivity loss. The condition worsens with age.

Two major forms of presbycusis are sensory and strial. The sensory form is due to loss of outer hair cells in the inner ear and is associated with high-frequency loss. Most people with sensory presbycusis can hear speech but have difficulty in understanding it. That is, their auditory sensitivity is satisfactory but speech discrimination (which depends upon high frequency hearing ability) is reduced. Fortunately, modern hearing aids can correct the high-frequency loss and provide great benefit to the wearer.

The strial or metabolic form of presbycusis is less common and affects both the low and high frequencies. This form of hearing loss is due to pathology of the stria vascularis, which, through its metabolism, is the source of electrical energy driving the cochlea. Recently, it has been shown that strial presbycusis, which is more common in women than in men, is associated with cardiovascular disease. Although

85

unproven as yet, it may be the case that measures to prevent cardio-vascular disease, such as fitness and exercise, weight reduction, lowering of high cholesterol levels, smoking cessation, and diet modification, may delay its onset. This appears to be a logical but untested hypothesis.

Tinnitus

Tinnitus, or ringing in the ears, is a very common problem. Tinnitus may be intermittent or constant in character, mild or severe in intensity, and vary from a low hiss to a high-pitched tinkling or ringing type of sound. It may be subjective (audible only to the patient) or objective (audible to others). Tinnitus is usually associated with hearing loss. In fact, in many cases, the first symptom of the hearing loss is tinnitus.

Section 6.2

Mechanism Underlying Stereocilia Self-Renewal Discovered

Reprinted from "Researchers Discover Mechanism Underlying Stereocilia Self-Renewal," National Institute on Deafness and Other Communication Disorders, National Institutes of Health, April 19, 2004.

Size is important. This is according to National Institute on Deafness and Other Communication Disorders (NIDCD) scientists investigating the internal mechanisms that underlie the hearing process and how the structures responsible for hearing rebuild themselves. This study is published in the March 15, 2004 issue of the *Journal of Cell Biology*.

Hearing happens at the level of the hair cells of the ear—the basic sensory elements of hearing—where sound energy is transformed into electrical energy by tiny hairlike projections jutting from the top of cells in bundles called stereocilia. The cells are called "hair cells" because of their appearance, and these structures can be seen only with powerful microscopes. Stereocilia are arranged in varying lengths, similar to a stack of soda straws graded in height forming a staircase-like bundle, to accommodate the different energies found in different frequencies of sound waves. When stimulated, the stereocilia bundle moves and the individual hair cells splay apart, which creates an electrical signal that travels to the brain by way of the auditory nerve, allowing hearing to take place. The bending action can cause damage to the stereocilia, but a delicate mechanism of turnover replaces the components of stereocilia in an orderly manner to minimize injury.

Researchers have looked at various factors that control and regulate the rate of repair or turnover that takes place in stereocilia. In this study, they found that the turnover rate is determined by size: longer stereocilia are replaced at a faster rate than shorter ones. The stereocilia, which are largely made up of the building block protein actin, rebuild themselves continuously, maintaining the overall structure. The scientists theorize that this activity may help maintain function over the course of a lifetime.

How this turnover mechanism is regulated remains unknown, but the researchers noted that the levels and activity of another protein, myosin, are correlated with stereocilia length in genetically altered mice. Mutations in the gene for myosin are known to prevent stereocilia elongation. The investigators say they will continue to look for other proteins in order to identify key players in the self-renewal mechanism and interactions between them. They believe that understanding how malfunctions occur in the ability of the hair cell bundles to make fine changes in their lengths may account for subtle changes in hearing. Moreover, long-term applications of this research may prove important in the development of treatments for temporary and permanent hearing loss due to stereocilia injury.

Section 6.3

Statistics about Hearing Disorders, Ear Infections, and Deafness

Excerpted from "Statistics about Hearing Disorders, Ear Infections, and Deafness," National Institute on Deafness and Other Communication Disorders, National Institutes of Health, June 18, 2004.

- Hearing loss is greater in men.

- Almost 12 percent of men who are sixty-five to seventy-four years of age are affected by tinnitus. Tinnitus is identified more frequently in white individuals, and the prevalence of tinnitus is almost twice as frequent in the South as in the Northeast.

- Approximately twenty-eight million Americans have a hearing impairment.

- Hearing loss affects approximately 17 in 1,000 children under age eighteen. Incidence increases with age: Approximately 314 in 1,000 people over age sixty-five have hearing loss and 40 to 50 percent of people seventy-five and older have a hearing loss.

- About 2 to 3 out of every 1,000 children in the United States are born deaf or hard-of-hearing. Nine out of every ten children who are born deaf are born to parents who can hear.

- Ten million Americans have suffered irreversible noise-induced hearing loss, and thirty million more are exposed to dangerous noise levels each day.

- Only one out of five people who could benefit from a hearing aid actually wears one.

- Three out of four children experience ear infection (otitis media) by the time they are three years old.

- At least twelve million Americans have tinnitus. Of these, at least one million experience it so severely that it interferes with their daily activities.

- Approximately 59,000 people worldwide have received cochlear implants. About 250,000 people would be good candidates for a cochlear implant. In the United States, about 13,000 adults and nearly 10,000 children have cochlear implants.

- Approximately four thousand new cases of sudden deafness occur each year in the United States. Hearing loss affects only one ear in nine out of ten people who experience sudden deafness. Only 10 to 15 percent of patients with sudden deafness know what caused their loss.

- Approximately 615,000 individuals have been diagnosed with Ménière disease in the United States. Another 45,500 are newly diagnosed each year.

- Approximately 3 to 6 percent of all deaf children and perhaps another 3 to 6 percent of hard-of-hearing children have Usher syndrome. In developed countries such as the United States, about 4 babies in every 100,000 births have Usher syndrome.

- One out of every 100,000 individuals per year develops an acoustic neurinoma (vestibular schwannoma).

Chapter 7

Diagnosing Hearing Loss

Chapter Contents

Section 7.1

Hearing Testing

Hearing Tests: An Overview

It's a common belief that hearing-impaired people just can't hear sounds loudly enough, but it's more complicated than that. The four main problems caused by hearing loss are:

- soft sounds can't be heard;
- key parts of particular speech sounds may not be heard;
- sounds are difficult to separate so voices become jumbled with background noise;
- a reduced range of hearing may make loud sounds intolerable.

Audiograms

Hearing tests measure what sounds you can and can't hear. Clinicians can use a variety of tests to find out about hearing. They will plot your test results on a graph called an audiogram. This graph shows how loud sounds need to be before you can hear them—called your hearing thresholds.

Hearing loss is measured in decibels (dB) and pitch in hertz (HZ). Decibels measure intensity, and hertz measures frequency. The results of a hearing test indicate the degree and type of hearing loss.

How Is Hearing Tested?

Children's and adults' hearing is tested differently. Hearing tests for young children will be addressed at the end of this section.

The most simple test of hearing ability is called pure tone audiometry, where you listen to a range of beeps and whistles, called pure tones, and indicate when you can hear them. The loudness of each tone is reduced until you can just hear the tone. The softest sounds you can hear are your hearing thresholds.

Your hearing may be tested with pure tones presented through headphones. This measurement is called air conduction. The sounds go via the air, down the ear canal, through the middle ear, and to the very delicate cochlea in the inner ear.

The sensitivity of the cochlea can also be tested by placing a small vibrator on the mastoid bone behind the ear. Sounds presented this way travel through the bones of the skull to the cochlea and hearing nerves, bypassing the middle ear. This type of testing is called bone conduction.

Interpreting the Results of Air and Bone Conduction Tests

Air conduction and bone conduction indicate to the clinician where the hearing problem is located. If the bone conduction hearing thresholds are the same as the air conduction thresholds, this indicates there is no blockage of sound in the outer or middle ear. The hearing loss may be caused by a loss of sensitivity in the cochlea or hearing nerve. This type of loss is called sensorineural hearing loss.

If the bone conduction hearing thresholds are normal, but there is a loss of hearing with air conduction, this indicates that the cochlea is normal and healthy, but there is some blockage to sound in the middle or outer ears. This is called a conductive hearing loss.

It is possible to have a sensorineural and conductive hearing loss—called a mixed hearing loss.

Tympanometry

Tympanometry is not a hearing test, but a test of how well the middle ear system is functioning and how well the eardrum can move. A small rubber tip is placed in the ear and a little air is pumped into the outer ear canal. If there is a problem in the middle ear, it may show up on this test. The results of tympanometry can indicate the location of a blockage that is causing the hearing loss and if medical treatment may help.

Speech Discrimination Tests

The ability to hear speech is a function of the ability to detect the sounds of speech, and the ability to understand speech. The range of audible sounds, not just the degree of hearing loss, can vary considerably from person to person.

93

Unfortunately, when hearing is damaged it is usually not just the volume or quantity of sound heard that is lost. Often the quality of the sound is also distorted. The amount of distortion can be measured using speech discrimination tests. Poor speech discrimination means that voices are distorted and not loud enough.

Hearing Tests for Young Children

The tests selected to assess hearing in infants and young children depend on the:

- child's age and ability to undertake the test;
- information that is needed about the child's hearing.

Most children will be assessed using a combination of behavioral and physiological tests.

Behavioral Tests

Behavioral tests are based on eliciting or observing a change in behavior in response to sound.

- *Behavioral observation audiometry (BOA)* noisemaker testing is carried out with infants younger than seven months of age and with older children who cannot respond when they hear a sound. Behavioral responses include startling to loud noises and stirring from sleep in response to a sound. An assortment of noisemakers, such as crunching cellophane, tiny bells, and chimes are used and most can be classified as low-, mid-, or high-frequency sounds.

- *Visual reinforcement orientation audiometry (VROA)* is used to test the hearing of children between seven months and three years of age. VROA involves the child turning toward the loudspeaker when a sound is presented. By altering the frequency and intensity of the sounds, it is possible to find out about the child's ability to hear sounds across a range of frequencies.

- *Play audiometry* is used to test the hearing of children from three years of age. This is also used to test the child's hearing when hearing devices are worn. Play audiometry works the same way as pure tone audiometry (person indicates when he or she can hear a tone), except when the child hears a tone, he or she puts a marble in a marble race, presses a computer key or puts a piece in a puzzle.

Electro-Physiological Tests

Physiological tests help determine which part of the auditory system is involved in the child's hearing loss. Physiological tests measure a physical response of a specific part of the auditory system and require little or no cooperation from the child.

- *Otoacoustic emission testing (OAE)* gives an idea about how hair cells in the cochlea are working. They respond to sound by producing a very soft sound of their own called an otoacoustic emission.

- *Brainstem evoked response audiometry (BERA)* provides information on electrical activity generated in response to sound along the nerve pathway, also called the brainstem, to the brain. It may be carried out while a baby is in natural sleep. If this is not possible, testing must be carried out in the hospital.

- *Electrocochleography (ECochG or EcoG)* is performed in the hospital, under anesthetic. It picks up the tiny electrical signals generated in the cochlea in response to sound. It provides information about the functioning of the cochlea and the start of the nerve pathway to the brain.

- *Tympanometry and acoustic reflex* give information about the middle ear, which is just behind the eardrum. A tympanogram, which shows if the eardrum is moving normally, may indicate a problem in the middle ear that can cause a conductive hearing loss. When a child has a normal tympanogram, it may be possible to test for the presence of a muscle reflex—acoustic reflex—in the middle ear. The absence of this reflex to different sounds gives information about the auditory system.

About Australian Hearing

Australian Hearing was established by the Australian government in 1947 to assist World War II veterans with ear damage and to care for Australian children who experienced hearing loss following the rubella epidemic of the late 1940s. It is one of the largest and most comprehensive providers of hearing services in the world. Australian Hearing is also home to the internationally renowned National Acoustic Laboratories, a leading research facility into hearing loss and treatment innovations. For more information visit our website at www.hearing.com.au.

Section 7.2

Newborn Hearing Screening

Speech, Language, and Hearing Skills

Here is a list of some things an infant with normal hearing should be able to do:

- Around two months of age
  - Startles to loud sound
  - Quiets to familiar voices
  - Makes vowel sounds like "ohh," "ahh"
- Around four months of age
  - Looks for sound sources
  - Starts babbling
  - Uses a variety of voice sounds, squeals, and chuckles
- Around six months of age
  - Turns head toward loud sound
  - Begins to imitate speech sound
  - Babbles ("baba," "mama," "gaga")
- Around nine months of age
  - Imitates speech sounds of others
  - Understands "no-no" or "bye-bye"
  - Turns head toward soft sounds
- Around twelve months of age
  - Correctly uses "mama" or "dada"
  - Gives toy when asked
  - Responds to singing or music
  - Readily turns toward all sounds

It Is Important to Have Your Baby's Hearing Checked

As many as three of every one thousand babies are born in the United States each year with hearing loss. Your baby can't tell you if he or she can't hear. Babies who do not hear your voice, a lullaby, or a nursery rhyme may have problems learning to talk.

It is vitally important to have your baby's hearing tested before you leave the hospital. Hearing problems need to be identified as early as possible so that you may take actions that give your baby the best chance to develop speech and language.

Babies can't tell us if they can't hear.

Why should my baby's hearing be screened?

Hearing loss is a hidden disability; that's why it is so important to have your baby's hearing evaluated. Each year, more than four thousand babies are born with hearing loss. Most babies born with hearing problems are otherwise healthy and have no family history of hearing loss.

It is important for you to be sure that your baby has normal hearing. It is unlikely that your baby will have a hearing loss; however, the only way to know is to have your baby's hearing tested as early as possible. The first year of life is critical to the development of normal speech and language.

How will my baby's screening test be done?

There are two types of hearing screening tests that may be used with your baby. Both tests are very safe and take only minutes to evaluate each ear. Most babies sleep through their hearing screening test.

1. *Auditory Brainstem Response (ABR)* tests the infant's ability to hear soft sounds through miniature earphones. Sensors measure your baby's brain waves to determine if soft sounds can be heard.

2. *Otoacoustic Emissions (OAE)* are measured directly with a miniature microphone and sent to a special computer to determine your baby's hearing status.

What if my baby does not pass the test?

There are many reasons your baby may not "pass" the first hearing test and require a second evaluation. Perhaps your baby was too active, too wide-awake, or you were discharged from the hospital before the hearing test was completed.

It is important that you follow through with any recommendations made by your audiologist, hospital staff member, or physician. Remember, your baby's hearing can be tested at any age.

If my baby passes the screening, do I need to have the hearing checked again?

Hearing screening tests can usually confirm that your baby has normal hearing. However, hearing problems in your baby can develop after you leave the hospital. If anyone in your family has hearing loss, your baby should be tested every year.

If you ever have concerns about your child's hearing, speech, or language, be sure to discuss them with your audiologist or physician.

The Joint Committee on Infant Hearing (JCIH) Year 2000 Position Statement

The American Academy of Audiology, the American Academy of Pediatrics, the American Speech-Language-Hearing Association, the Council on Education of the Deaf, and the Directors of Speech and Hearing Programs in State Health and Welfare Agencies have joined together to endorse universal detection of infants with hearing loss. The goal is that all infants with hearing loss will be identified before three months of age and receive intervention by six months of age.

Section 7.3

Hearing Loss Quick Test

Answer Yes, No, or Sometimes for each question.

1. Do you find it difficult to follow a conversation in a noisy restaurant or crowded room?

2. Do you sometimes feel that people are mumbling or not speaking clearly?

3. Do you experience difficulty following dialog in the theater?

4. Do you sometimes find it difficult to understand a speaker at a public meeting or a religious service?

5. Do you find yourself asking people to speak up or repeat themselves?

6. Do you find men's voices easier to understand than women's?

7. Do you experience difficulty understanding soft or whispered speech?

8. Do you sometimes have difficulty understanding speech on the telephone?

9. Does a hearing problem cause you to feel embarrassed when meeting new people?

10. Do you feel handicapped by a hearing problem?

11. Does a hearing problem cause you to visit friends, relatives or neighbors less often than you would like?

12. Do you experience ringing or noises in your ears?

13. Do you hear better with one ear than the other?

14. Have you had any significant noise exposure during work, recreation, or military service?

15.   Have any of your relatives (by birth) had a hearing loss?

To score the Hearing Health Quick Test, score 2 points for Yes, 1 point for Sometimes, and 0 points for No. Scores of 3 or more may mean that you have a hearing problem. Scores of 6 or more strongly suggest that a hearing check is warranted. In either case, ask your doctor to screen your hearing. Further testing by an audiologist may be recommended.

Chapter 8

Genetic and Congenital Deafness

Chapter Contents

Section 8.1

Congenital Deafness: An Overview

Reprinted from "Congenital Deafness," by Timothy C. Hain, M.D., last revised July 2001. Copyright © 2001 American Hearing Research Foundation. Reprinted with permission.

While acquired deafness associated with age or noise exposure is more common than genetic deafness by roughly two orders of magnitude, congenital deafness occurs in one out of every one thousand to two thousand births. Autosomal recessive inheritance is the most common form, accounting for more than 75 percent of all congenital deafness.

Non-inherited abnormalities of the inner ear, such as the Mondini malformation, account for roughly 20 percent of congenital sensorineural deafness. The bulk of the remaining (genetic) deafness is nonsyndromic, meaning that it does not have any obvious distinguishing features.

Nonsyndromic Deafness

Nonsyndromic means that deafness occurs in isolation, without other associated findings. About 80 percent of genetic hearing loss is nonsyndromic. Between 1992 and 2001, thirty-eight loci for autosomal dominant nonsyndromic deafness were mapped and eleven genes were cloned. Autosomal dominant loci are known as DFNA, autosomal recessive as DFNB, and X-linked as DFN.

Nonsyndromic deafness is highly heterogeneous, but mutations in the connexin-26 molecule (gap junction protein, gene GJB2) account for about 49 percent of patients with nonsyndromic deafness and about 37 percent of sporadic cases. About one in thirty-one individuals of European extraction are likely carriers. However, population analysis suggests that there are over one hundred genes involved in nonsyndromic hearing impairment (Morton, 1991). One mutation is particularly common, namely, the 30delG.

The following paragraphs describe the nomenclature for nonsyndromic deafness.

Autosomal Dominant (DFNA)

Autosomal dominant deafness is passed directly through generations. It is often possible to identify an autosomal dominant pattern through simple inspection of the family tree. An example of autosomal dominant deafness is the missense mutation in COL11A2 (DFNA13) (Leenheer et al, 2001). COL11A2 encodes a chain of type XI collagen.

Autosomal Recessive (DFNB)

Autosomal recessive disorders require a gene from both the mother and the father.

Syndromic Deafness

Syndromic deafness, which accounts for the remaining 20 percent of congenital deafness, comprises an immensely complicated interlinked set of disorders. The descriptions here are only to give the general flavor of the diseases and are not meant to include all features of the disorders. In most cases, an Online Mendelian Inheritance in Man (OMIM) database link to the main type of the genetic disorder is provided. This database is a catalog of human genes and genetic disorders.

Alport Syndrome

Alport syndrome is caused by mutations in COL4A3, COL4A4, or COL4A5. The classic phenotype is renal failure and progressive sensorineural deafness.

Branchiootorenal Syndrome

Branchiootorenal syndrome is caused by mutations in EYA1, a gene of 16 exons within a genomic interval of 156 kB. This syndrome is characterized by hearing disturbances and cataracts, branchial cleft fistulae, and preauricular pits. Mondini malformations and related dysplasias may occur.

X-linked Charcot-Marie-Tooth (CMT)

The dominant form of X-linked CMT is caused by a mutation in the connexin 32 gene mapped to the Xq13 locus. Usual clinical signs consist of a peripheral neuropathy combined with foot problems and "champagne bottle" calves. Sensorineural deafness occurs in some (Stojkovic and others, 1999).

As noted previously, the connexin gene is also associated with a large percentage of cases of nonsyndromic deafness. There are several other associated neuropathies and deafness syndromes. Autosomal recessive demyelinating neuropathy, autosomal dominant hereditary neuropathies type I and II, and X-linked hereditary axonal neuropathies with mental retardation are all associated with deafness (Stojkovic et al, 1999).

Goldenhar Syndrome

Oculoauriculovertebral dysplasia (OAVD) or Goldenhar syndrome was originally described in 1881. It includes a complex of features including hemifacial microtia, otomandibular dysostosis, epibulbar lipodermoids, coloboma, and vertebral anomalies that stem from developmental vascular and genetic field aberrations. It has diverse etiologies and is not attributed to a single genetic locus. The incidence is roughly one in forty-five thousand (Scholtz et al, 2001).

Jervell and Lange-Nielsen Syndrome

Jervell and Lange-Nielsen Syndrome is associated with cardiac arrhythmias. There is, by prolongation of the QT interval, torsade de pointe arrhythmias (turning of the points, in reference to the apparent alternating positive and negative QRS complexes), sudden syncopal episodes, and severe to profound sensorineural hearing loss.

Mohr-Tranebjaerg Syndrome (DFN-1)

Mohr-Tranebjaerg syndrome (DFN-1) is an X-linked recessive syndromic hearing loss characterized by postlingual sensorineural deafness in childhood, followed by progressive dystonia, spasticity, dysphagia, and optic atrophy. The syndrome is caused by a mutation thought to result in mitochondrial dysfunction. It resembles a spinocerebellar degeneration called Friedreich ataxia, which also may exhibit sensorineural hearing loss, ataxia, and optic atrophy. The cardiomyopathy characteristic of Friedreich ataxia is not seen in Mohr-Tranebjaerg syndrome.

Norrie Disease

Classic features of Norrie disease include specific ocular symptoms (pseudotumor of the retina, retinal hyperplasia, hypoplasia and necrosis of the inner layer of the retina, cataracts, phthisis bulbi), progressive sensorineural hearing loss, and mental disturbance, although less than one-half of patients are hearing impaired or mentally retarded.

Pendred Syndrome

Pendred syndrome is deafness associated with thyroid disease (goiter).

Stickler Syndrome

Stickler syndrome is caused by mutations in COL11. It is characterized by hearing impairment, midface hypoplasia, progressive myopia in the first year of life, and arthropathy.

Treacher Collins Syndrome

Treacher Collins syndrome (OMIM entry TCOF1) is characterized by coloboma of the lower eyelid (the upper eyelid is involved in Goldenhar syndrome), micrognathia, microtia, hypoplasia of the zygomatic arches, macrostomia, and inferior displacement of the lateral canthi with respect to the medial canthi.

Waardenburg Syndrome

The clinical symptoms of Waardenburg Syndrome (WS) type I and II include lateral displacement of the inner canthus of each eye; pigmentary abnormalities of hair, iris, and skin (often white forelock and heterochromia iridis); and sensorineural deafness. The combination of WS type I characteristics with upper limb abnormalities has been called Klein-Waardenburg syndrome or WS type III. The combination of recessively inherited WS type II characteristics with Hirschsprung disease has been called Waardenburg-Shah syndrome or WS type IV.

Usher Syndrome

Usher syndrome is characterized by hearing impairment and retinitis pigmentosa. Usher syndrome can be classified into three different types on the basis of clinical findings. In type I, there is both hearing impairment and vestibular impairment. In type II, there is hearing impairment without vestibular impairment. In type III, there is a variable amount of vestibular impairment.

Mitochondrial Disorders

Hearing loss is common in mitochondrial disorders, including MELAS (mitochondrial encephalomyopathy, lactic acidosis, and stroke like episodes), Kearns-Sayre syndrome, and MERRF (myoclonic epilepsy with ragged red fibers). These disorders are caused by mutations in mitochondrial DNA, and are characterized by muscular weakness, an abnormal muscle biopsy with "ragged red" fibers, and a variety of other findings that define the specific clinical phenotype. In MELAS, Sue et al recently reported that the hearing loss is caused by cochlear damage. It resembles presbyacusis in that it is generally symmetrical, gradual, and affects the higher frequencies first (Sue et al, 1998). Others have also reported hearing loss associated with mitochondrial mutations (Yamasoba et al, 1999). Mitochondrial DNA mutations accumulate naturally during life and are presently implicated as an important cause of normal aging. Mitochondrial defects have been reported to cause both unusual sensitivity to aminoglycosides as well as nonsyndromic sensorineural deafness (El-Schahawi et al, 1997—this paper reviews mitochondrial deafness).

Mohr-Tranebjaerg syndrome (DFN-1) is also thought to cause deafness via a mitochondrial disturbance.

Non-Inherited Congenital Deafness

These types of abnormalities account for roughly 20 percent of congenital deafness, the remainder being genetic in origin.

Mondini Dysplasia

The normal cochlea has two and one-half turns. A cochlear malformation consists of a membranous abnormality, a bony abnormality, or a combination of these two. If cochlear development is arrested in the embryo, a common cavity may occur instead of the snail-like cochlea. This is called the Mondini dysplasia or malformation.

Often accompanying the Mondini dysplasia is abnormal communication between the endolymphatic and perilymphatic spaces of the inner ear and subarachnoid space. It is usually caused by a defect in the cribriform area of the lateral end of the internal auditory canal. Presumably because of this abnormal channel, perilymphatic fistulae are more common in this disorder.

CT scans are not able to define abnormalities of the membranous labyrinth, but high-resolution MRI has been used to visualize these structures.

A related anomaly and more severe syndrome, the CHARGE association, consists of coloboma, heart disease, choanal atresia, retarded development, genital hypoplasia, ear anomalies including hypoplasia of the external ear and hearing loss. These individuals have a Mondini type deformity and absence of semicircular canals. A recent report documents that they have normal otolithic responses to off-vertical axis rotation (Wiener-Vacher et al, 1999).

Enlarged Vestibular Aqueduct Syndrome

First described by Valvassori, enlarged vestibular aqueduct syndrome is defined on the CT scan as a diameter greater than or equal to 1.5 mm measured midway between the operculum and the common crus. According to Murray et al (2000), coronal CT scan is the best view for evaluating it in children. Enlarged vestibular aqueducts can also be seen on high-resolution MRI. It may cause a fluctuating sensorineural hearing loss. Conservative management, including avoidance of head trauma and contact sports, has been the mainstay of treatment. Surgery to close the enlarged structure frequently results in significant hearing loss (Welling et al, 1999).

References

El-Schahawi M, and others. Two large Spanish pedigrees with nonsyndromic sensorineural deafness and the mtDNA mutation at nt 1555 in the 12S rRNA gene. Evidence of heteroplasmy. *Neurology* 1997; 48:453.

Leenheer and others. Autosomal dominant inherited hearing impairment caused by a missense mutation in COLA11A2 (DFNA13). *Arch Otolaryngol Head Neck Surg* 2001 Jan; 127(1):13–17.

Merchant SN and others. Temporal bone histopathologic and genetic studies in Mohr-Tranebjaerg Syndrome (DFN-1). *Otol Neurotol* 2001; 22:506–11.

Morton NE. 1991. Genetic epidemiology of hearing impairment. *Ann NYAS* 630:16–31.

Murray N, Tanaka J, Cameron D, Gianoli G. Coronal computed tomography of the normal vestibular aqueduct in children and young adults. *Arch Otolaryngol HNS* 2000; 126:1351–57.

Scholtz et al. Goldenhar's syndrome: congenital hearing deficit of conductive or sensorineural origin? *Otology Neurotol* 2001; 22:501–5.

Steel KP. A new era in the genetics of deafness. *NEJM* 1998.

Stojkovic and others. Sensorineural deafness in X-linked Charcot-Marie-Tooth disease with connexin 32 mutation (R142Q). *Neurology* 1999; 52:1010–14.

Strome SE, Baker KB, Langman AW. Imaging case of the month: Inner ear malformation. *American J. Otology* 1998; 19:396–97.

Sue CM and others. Cochlear origin of hearing loss in MELAS syndrome. *Ann Neurol* 1998; 43:350–59.

Welling B, and others. Sensorineural hearing loss after occlusion of the enlarged vestibular aqueduct. *Am J. Otol* 1999; 20:338–43.

Wiener-Vacher SR, Denise P, Narcey P, Manach Y. Vestibular function in children with the CHARGE association. *Arch Otolaryngol HNS* 1999; 125:342–34.

Yamasoba and others. Cochlear histopathology associated with mitochondrial transfer RNA (leu-UUR) gene mutation. *Neurology* 1999; 52:1705–7.

Section 8.2

Usher Syndrome

Reprinted from "Usher Syndrome," National Institute on Deafness and Other Communication Disorders, National Institutes of Health, NIH Publication No. 98-4291, July 2003.

What is Usher syndrome?

Usher syndrome is the most common condition that involves both hearing and vision problems. A syndrome is a disease or disorder that has more than one feature or symptom. The major symptoms of Usher syndrome are hearing impairment and retinitis pigmentosa, an eye disorder that causes a person's vision to worsen over time. Some people with Usher syndrome also have balance problems. There are three general types of Usher syndrome. Although the syndrome was first described by Albrecht Von Graefe in 1858, it was named for Charles Usher, a British eye doctor, who believed that the condition was inherited or passed from parents to their children.

Who is affected by Usher syndrome?

Approximately 3–6 percent of all deaf children and perhaps another 3-6 percent of hard-of-hearing children have Usher syndrome. In developed countries such as the United States, about 4 babies in every 100,000 births have Usher syndrome.

What causes Usher syndrome?

Usher syndrome is inherited or passed from parents to their children through genes. Genes are located in every cell of the body, except for red blood cells, which don't have a nucleus. Genes contain instructions that tell cells what to do. Some genes specify traits such as hair color. Other genes are involved in the development of body parts, such as the ear. Still others determine how parts of the body work. Each person inherits two copies of each gene, one from each parent.

Sometimes genes are altered or mutated. Mutated genes may cause cells to act differently than expected. Genes for Usher syndrome are autosomal recessive, a term meaning that 1) Usher genes are located on chromosomes other than the sex chromosomes, and 2) both parents must contribute the mutated gene to the child before the disorder is seen. Usually, parents are unaware that they have an Usher gene because they would need two of the mutated genes in order to show signs of Usher syndrome. A number of different genes have been found to cause the various types of Usher syndrome.

What are the types of Usher syndrome?

The three types of Usher syndrome are Usher syndrome type 1 (USH1), Usher syndrome type 2 (USH2), and Usher syndrome type 3 (USH3). USH1 and USH2 are the most common types. Together, they account for approximately 90–95 percent of all cases of children who have Usher syndrome.

What are the characteristics of the three types of Usher syndrome?

People with USH1 are profoundly deaf from birth and have severe balance problems. Many of these individuals obtain little or no benefit from hearing aids. Most use sign language as their primary means of communication. Because of the balance problems, children with USH1 are slow to sit without support and rarely learn to walk before they are eighteen months old. These children usually begin to develop vision problems by the time they are ten. Visual problems most often begin with difficulty seeing at night, but tend to progress rapidly until the individual is completely blind.

Individuals with USH2 are born with moderate to severe hearing impairment and normal balance. Although the severity of hearing impairment varies, most of these children perform well in regular classrooms and can benefit from hearing aids. These children most commonly use speech to communicate. The visual problems in USH2 tend to progress more slowly than the visual problems in USH1. USH2 is characterized by blind spots that begin to appear shortly after the teenage years. When an individual's vision deteriorates to blindness, his or her ability to speechread is lost.

Children born with USH3 have normal hearing and normal to near-normal balance. Hearing worsens over time. However, the rate at which hearing and sight are lost can vary between affected individuals, even within the same family. Children develop noticeable hearing problems by their teenage years and usually become deaf by mid- to late adulthood. Night blindness usually begins sometime during puberty. Blind spots appear by the late teenage years to early adulthood. By mid-adulthood, the individual is usually blind.

How is Usher syndrome diagnosed?

Hearing loss and retinitis pigmentosa are rarely found in combination. Therefore, most people who have retinitis pigmentosa and hearing loss probably have Usher syndrome. Special tests such as electronystagmography (ENG) to detect balance problems and electroretinography (ERG) to detect retinitis pigmentosa help doctors to detect Usher syndrome early. Early diagnosis is important in order to begin special educational training programs to help the individual manage the combined hearing and vision difficulties.

How is Usher syndrome treated?

Presently, there is no cure for Usher syndrome. The best treatment involves early identification in order to begin educational programs. The exact nature of these educational programs will depend on the severity of the hearing and vision impairments as well as the age and abilities of the individual. Typically, individuals will benefit from adjustment and career counseling; access to technology such as hearing aids, assistive listening devices, or cochlear implants; orientation and mobility training; and communication services and independent-living training that may include braille instruction, low-vision services, or auditory training.

What research is being conducted on Usher syndrome?

Researchers are currently trying to locate the genes that cause the syndrome and identify the function of those genes. This research will lead to improved genetic counseling and early diagnosis, and may eventually expand treatment options.

Scientists are also developing mice that have the same characteristics as humans who have the various types of Usher syndrome. Mouse models will make it easier to determine the function of the various genes involved in Usher syndrome. Research is also being conducted to improve the early identification of children with the syndrome. Treatment strategies such as the use of cochlear implants for hearing impairment and intervention strategies to alleviate retinitis pigmentosa are also being examined.

What are some of the latest research findings?

Currently, twelve loci have been found to cause Usher syndrome. A locus is a small segment of chromosome on which one or more genes are housed. For seven of the twelve loci, genes and the proteins that they encode have been identified. The genes that cause Usher syndrome are MY07A, USH1C, CDH23, PCDH15, and SANS, which cause USH1; USH2A, which causes USH2; and USH3A, which causes USH3. The resulting proteins that the genes encode help cells in the retina, the part of the eye that receives images of objects, and the cochlea to function.

In April 2003, National Institute on Deafness and Other Communication Disorders (NIDCD) researchers, along with their research collaborators from universities in New York, New York, and Tel Aviv, Israel, pinpointed a mutation, named R245X, of the PCDH15 gene that accounts for a large percentage of USH1 cases in today's Ashkenazi Jewish population. (The term Ashkenazi describes Jewish people who originate from Eastern Europe.) Because of this finding, researchers conclude that Ashkenazi Jewish infants with bilateral, profound hearing loss who lack another known mutation that causes hearing loss should be screened for the R245X mutation. If a child's USH1 is discovered early on, before he or she loses the ability to see, then that child is more likely to benefit from the full spectrum of intervention strategies that are available to help him or her communicate and participate in life's activities.

Section 8. 3

Waardenburg Syndrome

Reprinted from "Waardenburg Syndrome," National Institute on Deafness and Other Communication Disorders, National Institutes of Health, NIH Publication No. 91-3260, March 1999. Revised by David A. Cooke, M.D., on March 30, 2006.

Waardenburg syndrome (WS) is an inherited disorder often characterized by varying degrees of hearing loss and changes in skin and hair pigmentation. The syndrome got its name from a Dutch eye doctor named Petrus Johannes Waardenburg who first noticed that people with differently colored eyes often had a hearing impairment. He went on to study over a thousand individuals in deaf families and found that some of them had certain physical characteristics in common.

One commonly observed characteristic of Waardenburg syndrome is two differently colored eyes. One eye is usually brown and the other blue. Sometimes, one eye has two different colors. Other individuals with Waardenburg syndrome may have unusually brilliant blue eyes.

People with WS may also have distinctive hair coloring, such as a patch of white hair or premature gray hair as early as age twelve. Other possible physical features include a wide space between the inner corners of eyes called a broad nasal root. In addition, persons with WS may have low frontal hairline and their eyebrows may connect. The levels of hearing loss associated with the syndrome can vary from moderate to profound.

Individuals with Waardenburg syndrome may have some or all of the traits of the syndrome. For example, a person with WS may have a white forelock, a patch of white hair near the forehead, and no hearing impairment. Others may have white patches of skin and severe hearing impairment. The severity of the hearing impairment varies among individuals with WS, as do changes in the skin and hair.

On rare occasions, WS has been associated with other conditions that are present at birth, such as intestinal disorders, elevation of the shoulder blade, and disorders of the spine. A facial abnormality, known as cleft lip and/or palate, also has been associated with WS.

Types of Waardenburg Syndrome

There are at least six types of Waardenburg syndrome. The most common types of WS identified by scientists are Type 1 and Type 2. The different types of physical characteristics a person has determines the type of WS. Persons who have an unusually wide space between the inner corners of their eyes have WS Type 1. Hearing impairments occur in about 20 percent of individuals with this type of Waardenburg syndrome. Persons who do not have a wide space between the inner corners of their eyes, but who have many other WS characteristics are described as having WS Type 2. About 50 percent of persons with WS Type 2 have a hearing impairment or are deaf.

Cause

As a genetic disorder, Waardenburg syndrome is passed down from parent to child much like hair color, blood type, or other physical traits. A child receives genetic material from each parent. Because Waardenburg syndrome is usually a dominant condition, a child usually inherits the syndrome from just one parent who has the malfunctioning WS gene. WS Types I, II, and III are autosomal dominant disorders, which means there is a 50/50 chance that a child of an individual with these WS variants will also have the syndrome. WS Type IV is autosomal recessive, meaning two copies of the gene are required to have the disease. As a result, children of these individuals are far less likely to develop WS.

Research Studies

Scientists have identified and located six different genes for Waardenburg syndrome: PAX3, MITF, EDNRB, SLUG, SOX10, and EDN3. WS type 1 and type 3 have been associated with mutations in the PAX3 gene, WS type 2 with the MITF gene, and WS type 4 with the EDNRB and EDN3 genes. While scientists are studying all of these genes, currently, the most information is available on the PAX3 and MITF genes and their role in Waardenburg syndrome.

The PAX3 gene is located on chromosome 2 and controls some aspects of the development of the face and inner ear. The MITF gene is found on chromosome 3. It also controls the development of the ear and hearing. Scientists are now studying these genes to better understand how they operate in controlling the normal growth of the ear and the development of hearing. This information will help scientists understand why persons with WS sometimes develop hearing problems.

Section 8.4

Other Types of Syndromic Deafness

"Alström Syndrome," September 2005, "Jervell and Lange-Nielsen Syndrome," February 2005, "Pendred Syndrome," August 2005, "Stickler Syndrome," November 2004, and "Weissenbacher-Zweymüller Syndrome," November 2004, are reprinted from *Genetics Home Reference*, National Library of Medicine, National Institutes of Health.

Alström Syndrome

What is Alström syndrome?

Alström syndrome is a rare inherited condition that affects many body systems. Signs and symptoms of this condition begin in infancy or early childhood. Alström syndrome is characterized by progressive loss of vision and hearing, enlargement of the heart and weakening of cardiac muscle (cardiomyopathy), obesity, type 2 diabetes (the most common form of diabetes), and short stature. This disorder can also affect the liver, kidneys, bladder, and lungs. Some individuals with Alström syndrome have a skin condition called acanthosis nigricans, which causes the skin in body folds and creases to become thick, dark, and velvety. The signs and symptoms of Alström syndrome vary in severity, and affected individuals may not have all of the characteristic features of the disorder.

How common is Alström syndrome?

This condition is rare; only about 350 people are known to be affected worldwide.

What genes are related to Alström syndrome?

Mutations in the ALMS1 gene cause Alström syndrome.

The ALMS1 gene provides instructions for making a protein whose function is unknown. Mutations in the ALMS1 gene likely lead to an abnormally short, nonfunctional version of this protein. The ALMS1 protein is normally present at low levels in most tissues, so a lack of

115

this protein may help explain why the signs and symptoms of Alström syndrome affect many body systems.

How do people inherit Alström syndrome?

This condition is inherited in an autosomal recessive pattern, which means two copies of the gene in each cell are altered. The parents of an individual with Alström syndrome are carriers of one copy of the altered gene, but do not show signs and symptoms of the disorder.

Jervell and Lange-Nielsen Syndrome

What is Jervell and Lange-Nielsen syndrome?

Jervell and Lange-Nielsen syndrome is a condition that causes profound hearing loss and a disruption of the heart's normal rhythm. This disorder is a form of long QT syndrome, which is a heart condition that causes the cardiac muscle to take longer than usual to recharge between beats. If untreated, the irregular heartbeats can lead to fainting (syncope), seizures, or sudden death.

How common is Jervell and Lange-Nielsen syndrome?

Jervell and Lange-Nielsen syndrome is uncommon; it affects an estimated 1.6 to 6 in one million children. This disorder is responsible for less than 10 percent of all cases of long QT syndrome.

What genes are related to Jervell and Lange-Nielsen syndrome?

Mutations in the KCNE1 and KCNQ1 genes cause Jervell and Lange-Nielsen syndrome.

The proteins produced by these two genes work together to form a channel that transports positively charged potassium atoms (ions) out of cells. The movement of potassium ions through these channels is critical for maintaining the normal functions of the inner ear and cardiac muscle.

About 90 percent of cases of Jervell and Lange-Nielsen syndrome are caused by mutations in the KCNQ1 gene; KCNE1 mutations are responsible for the remaining 10 percent of cases. Mutations in these genes alter the usual structure and function of potassium channels or prevent the assembly of normal channels. These changes disrupt the flow of potassium ions in the inner ear and in cardiac muscle, leading to the hearing loss and irregular heart rhythm characteristic of Jervell and Lange-Nielsen syndrome.

How do people inherit Jervell and Lange-Nielsen syndrome?

This condition is inherited in an autosomal recessive pattern, which means two copies of the gene must be altered in each cell for a person to be affected by the disorder. Most often, the parents of a child with an autosomal recessive disorder are not affected but are carriers of one copy of the altered gene. Carriers of a KCNQ1 or KCNE1 mutation may have some signs and symptoms related to Jervell and Lange-Nielsen syndrome.

Pendred Syndrome

What is Pendred syndrome?

Pendred syndrome is a genetic condition typically associated with hearing loss and goiter, which is an enlargement of the thyroid gland (a butterfly-shaped organ at the base of the neck that produces hormones). Hearing loss is often evident at birth, but in some cases it does not develop until later in infancy or early childhood. Abnormalities of bones in the inner ear are also common in Pendred syndrome. If a goiter develops, it usually forms sometime after the onset of hearing loss, during late childhood, adolescence, or adulthood.

How common is Pendred syndrome?

This condition is one of the most common forms of syndromic deafness (hearing loss associated with a genetic syndrome). Pendred syndrome accounts for at least 5 percent of cases of profound hearing loss. Its exact incidence is unknown.

What genes are related to Pendred syndrome?

Mutations in the SLC26A4 gene cause Pendred syndrome.

The SLC26A4 gene produces a protein called pendrin. This protein transports negatively charged particles (anions), particularly chloride and iodide, into and out of cells. Although the exact function of pendrin is not fully understood, it appears to be important for normal thyroid function and inner ear development. Mutations in the

117

SLC26A4 gene likely impair pendrin activity, disrupting the transport of negatively charged particles. Disrupted transport in the thyroid and inner ear leads to the characteristic signs and symptoms of Pendred syndrome.

How do people inherit Pendred syndrome?

This condition is inherited in an autosomal recessive pattern, which means two copies of the gene in each cell are altered. Most often, the parents of an individual with an autosomal recessive disorder are carriers of one copy of the altered gene but do not show signs and symptoms of the disorder.

Stickler Syndrome

What is Stickler syndrome?

Stickler syndrome is a group of hereditary conditions character-ized by a distinctive facial appearance, eye abnormalities, hearing loss, and joint problems.

Genetic changes are related to the following types of Stickler syn-drome.

* Stickler syndrome, COL11A1

* Stickler syndrome, COL11A2

* Stickler syndrome, COL2A1

Stickler syndrome is a subtype of collagenopathy, types II and XI.

Whether there are two or three types of Stickler syndrome is con-troversial. Each type is presented here according to the gene involved. The classification of these conditions is changing as researchers learn more about the genetic causes.

Individuals with Stickler syndrome experience a range of signs and symptoms. Some people have almost no signs and symptoms; others have all of the features described below. In addition, each feature of this syndrome may vary from subtle to severe.

A characteristic feature of Stickler syndrome is a somewhat flat-tened facial appearance. This is caused by underdeveloped bones in the middle of the face, including the cheekbones and the bridge of the nose. A particular group of physical features, called Robin sequence, is common in children with Stickler syndrome. Robin sequence in-cludes a U-shaped cleft palate (an opening in the roof of the mouth) with a tongue that is too large for the space formed by the small lower jaw. Children with a cleft palate are also prone to frequent ear infections and swallowing difficulties.

Many people with Stickler syndrome are very nearsighted (described as having high myopia) because of the shape of the eye. People with eye involvement are prone to increased pressure within the eye (glaucoma) and tearing of the lining of the eye (retinal detachment). The jelly-like substance within the eye (the vitreous) has a distinctive appearance in the types of Stickler syndrome associated with the COL2A1 and COL11A1 genes. The type of Stickler syndrome associated with the COL11A2 gene does not affect the eye.

Another sign of Stickler syndrome is mild to severe hearing loss that, for some people, may be progressive. The joints of affected children and young adults may be very flexible (hypermobile). Arthritis often appears at an early age and worsens as a person gets older.

How common is Stickler syndrome?

Overall, the estimated prevalence of Stickler syndrome is about 1 in 10,000 people.

What genes are related to Stickler syndrome?

Mutations in the COL11A1, COL11A2, and COL2A1 genes cause Stickler syndrome.

These genes are involved in the production of type II and type XI collagen. Collagens are complex molecules that provide structure and strength to connective tissue (the tissue that supports the body's joints and organs). Mutations in any of these genes disrupt the production, processing, or assembly of type II or type XI collagen. Defective collagen molecules or reduced amounts of collagen affect the development of bones and other connective tissues, leading to the characteristic features of Stickler syndrome.

Other, as yet unknown, genes may also cause Stickler syndrome because not all individuals with the condition have mutations in one of the three identified genes.

How do people inherit Stickler syndrome?

This condition is inherited in an autosomal dominant pattern, which means one copy of the altered gene in each cell is sufficient to cause the disorder.

Weissenbacher-Zweymüller Syndrome

What is Weissenbacher-Zweymüller syndrome?

Weissenbacher-Zweymüller syndrome is an inherited disorder of bone growth. The condition is characterized by skeletal abnormalities that improve with age, hearing loss, and distinctive facial features. This condition has mild features that are similar to those of another skeletal disorder, otospondylomegaepiphyseal dysplasia (OSMED).

Weissenbacher-Zweymüller syndrome is a subtype of collagenopathy, types II and XI.

Infants born with this condition are smaller than average because the bones in their arms and legs are unusually short. The thigh and upper arm bones are shaped like dumbbells, and the bones of the spine (vertebrae) may also be abnormally shaped. High-tone hearing loss occurs in some cases. Distinctive facial features include wide-set, protruding eyes; a flat nasal bridge; a small, upturned nose; and a small lower jaw. Some affected infants are born with an opening in the roof of the mouth (a cleft palate). The skeletal signs of this condition tend to diminish during childhood, and jaw growth catches up with age. Most adults with Weissenbacher-Zweymüller syndrome are not unusually short.

How common is Weissenbacher-Zweymüller syndrome?

This condition is very rare; only a few families with the disorder have been reported worldwide.

What genes are related to Weissenbacher-Zweymüller syndrome?

Mutations in the COL11A2 gene cause Weissenbacher-Zweymüller syndrome.

The protein made by the COL11A2 gene is involved in the production of type XI collagen. This type of collagen is important for the normal development of bone and other connective tissues (tissues that form the body's supportive framework). At least one mutation in the COL11A2 gene is known to cause Weissenbacher-Zweymüller syndrome. This mutation disrupts type XI collagen, resulting in delayed bone development and the other features of the disorder.

How do people inherit Weissenbacher-Zweymüller syndrome?

Weissenbacher-Zweymüller syndrome is considered an autosomal dominant disorder because one copy of the altered gene is sufficient to cause the condition. This condition is caused by new mutations in the COL11A2 gene, meaning no other family members are affected.

Section 8.5

Otospondylomegaepiphyseal Dysplasia

Reprinted from *Genetics Home Reference*, National Library of Medicine, National Institutes of Health, November 2004.

What is otospondylomegaepiphyseal dysplasia?

Otospondylomegaepiphyseal dysplasia (OSMED) is an inherited disorder of bone growth that results in skeletal abnormalities, severe hearing loss, and distinctive facial features. The name of the condition indicates that it affects hearing (oto-) and the bones of the spine (spondylo-), and enlarges the ends of bones (megaepiphyses). The features of OSMED are similar to those of another skeletal disorder, Weissenbacher-Zweymüller syndrome.

Otospondylomegaepiphyseal dysplasia is a subtype of collagenopathy, types II and XI.

The distinctive characteristics of OSMED include severe bone and joint problems and very severe hearing loss. This disorder affects the epiphyses, the parts of the bone where growth occurs. People with the condition are often shorter than average because the bones in their arms and legs are unusually short. Other skeletal signs include enlarged joints, short hands and fingers, and flat bones of the spine (vertebrae). People with the disorder often experience back and joint pain, limited joint movement, and arthritis that begins early in life. Severe high-tone hearing loss is common. Typical facial features include protruding eyes; a sunken nasal bridge; an upturned nose with a large, rounded tip; and a small lower jaw. Some affected infants are born with an opening in the roof of the mouth, which is called a cleft palate.

How common is otospondylomegaepiphyseal dysplasia?

The frequency of this disorder is unknown, but it is very rare. Only a few families with the condition have been reported.

What genes are related to otospondylomegaepiphyseal dysplasia?

Mutations in the COL11A2 gene cause otospondylomegaepiphyseal dysplasia.

The protein made by the COL11A2 gene is involved in the production of type XI collagen. This type of collagen is important for the normal development of bone and other connective tissues (tissues that form the body's supportive framework). Mutations in the COL11A2 gene lead to a loss of function of this type of collagen, resulting in the signs and symptoms of OSMED.

How do people inherit otospondylomegaepiphyseal dysplasia?

OSMED is inherited in an autosomal recessive pattern, which means two copies of the gene must be altered for a person to be affected by the disorder. Most often, the parents of a child with an autosomal recessive disorder are not affected but are carriers of one copy of the altered gene. A recessive pattern of inheritance makes OSMED unique among the type II and type XI collagenopathies.

Section 8.6

Nonsyndromic Deafness

Reprinted from *Genetics Home Reference*, National
Library of Medicine, National Institutes of Health, August 2005.

What is nonsyndromic deafness?

Nonsyndromic deafness is hearing loss that is not associated with other signs and symptoms. In contrast, syndromic deafness involves hearing loss that occurs with abnormalities in other parts of the body.

Genetic changes are related to the following types of nonsyndromic deafness.

- nonsyndromic deafness, autosomal dominant
- nonsyndromic deafness, autosomal recessive
- nonsyndromic deafness, mitochondrial
- nonsyndromic deafness, X-linked

The different types of nonsyndromic deafness are named according to their inheritance patterns. Autosomal dominant forms are designated as DFNA, autosomal recessive forms as DFNB, and X-linked forms as DFN. Each type is also numbered in the order in which it was described. For example, DFNA1 was the first described autosomal dominant type of nonsyndromic deafness. Mitochondrial nonsyndromic deafness involves changes to the small amount of DNA found in mitochondria, the energy-producing centers within cells.

Most forms of nonsyndromic deafness are associated with permanent hearing loss caused by damage to structures in the inner ear. The inner ear consists of three parts: a snail-shaped structure called the cochlea that helps process sound, nerves that send information from the cochlea to the brain, and structures involved with balance. Loss of hearing caused by changes in the inner ear is called sensorineural deafness. Hearing loss that results from changes in the middle ear is called conductive hearing loss. The middle ear contains three tiny bones that help transfer sound from the eardrum to the inner ear. Some forms of nonsyndromic deafness involve changes in both the inner ear and the middle ear; this combination is called mixed hearing loss.

The severity of hearing loss varies and can change over time. It can affect one ear (unilateral) or both ears (bilateral). Degrees of hearing loss range from mild (difficulty understanding soft speech) to profound (inability to hear even very loud noises). The loss may be stable, or it may progress as a person gets older. Particular types of nonsyndromic deafness often show distinctive patterns of hearing loss. For example, the loss may be more pronounced at high, middle, or low tones.

Nonsyndromic deafness can occur at any age. Hearing loss that is present before a child learns to speak is classified as prelingual or congenital. Hearing loss that occurs after the development of speech is classified as postlingual.

How common is nonsyndromic deafness?

About 1 in 1,000 children in the United States is born with profound deafness. By age nine, about 3 in 1,000 children have hearing loss that affects the activities of daily living. More than half of these cases are caused by genetic factors. Most cases of genetic deafness (70 percent to 80 percent) are nonsyndromic; the remaining cases are caused by specific genetic syndromes. In adults, the chance of developing hearing loss increases with age; hearing loss affects half of all people older than 80 years.

What genes are related to nonsyndromic deafness?

Mutations in the ACTG1, CDH23, CLDN14, COCH, COL11A2, DFNA5, ESPN, EYA4, GJB2, GJB6, KCNQ4, MYO15A, MYO6, MYO7A, OTOF, PCDH15, POU3F4, SLC26A4, STRC, TECTA, TMC1, TMIE, TMPRSS3, USH1C, and WFS1 genes cause nonsyndromic deafness.

The GJB3 and MYO1A genes are associated with nonsyndromic deafness.

The causes of nonsyndromic deafness can be complex. Researchers have identified more than thirty genes that, when mutated, may cause nonsyndromic deafness; however, some of these genes have not been fully characterized. Many genes related to deafness are involved in the development and function of the inner ear. Gene mutations interfere with critical steps in processing sound, resulting in hearing loss. Different mutations in the same gene can cause different types of hearing loss, and some genes are associated with both syndromic and nonsyndromic deafness. In many families, the gene responsible for hearing loss has not been identified.

Deafness can also result from environmental factors or a combination of genetic and environmental factors. Environmental causes of hearing loss include certain medications, specific infections before or after birth, and exposure to loud noise over an extended period.

How do people inherit nonsyndromic deafness?

Nonsyndromic deafness can have different patterns of inheritance. Between 75 and 80 percent of cases are inherited in an autosomal recessive pattern, which means two copies of the gene in each cell are altered. Usually, each parent of an individual with autosomal recessive deafness is a carrier of one copy of the altered gene. These carriers do not have hearing loss.

Another 20 to 25 percent of nonsyndromic deafness cases are autosomal dominant, which means one copy of the altered gene in each cell is sufficient to result in hearing loss. People with autosomal dominant deafness most often inherit an altered copy of the gene from a parent who has hearing loss.

Between 1 and 2 percent of cases show an X-linked pattern of inheritance, which means the mutated gene responsible for the condition is located on the X chromosome. Males with X-linked nonsyndromic deafness tend to develop more severe hearing loss earlier in life than females who inherit a copy of the same gene mutation. A striking characteristic of X-linked inheritance is that fathers cannot pass X-linked traits to their sons.

Mitochondrial nonsyndromic deafness, which results from changes to the DNA in mitochondria, occurs in fewer than 1 percent of cases in the United States. The altered mitochondrial DNA is passed from a mother to her sons and daughters. This type of deafness is not inherited from fathers.

Section 8.7

Research Advances in Genetic Hearing Loss

"Gene that Blocks Regrowth of Hearing Cells Identified for the First Time" is reprinted from the National Institute on Deafness and Other Communication Disorders, National Institutes of Health, January 19, 2005. "Modifier Gene Makes Some Hearing Loss More Severe" is reprinted from the National Institute on Deafness and Other Communication Disorders, National Institutes of Health, April 13, 2005.

Gene that Blocks Regrowth of Hearing Cells Identified for the First Time

Researchers supported by the National Institute on Deafness and Other Communication Disorders (NIDCD) have come one step closer to understanding how hair cells regenerate, a finding that could lead to new treatments for restoring hearing. In the January 13, 2005, issue of *Science* magazine, scientists at the Massachusetts General Hospital in Boston, Massachusetts, report that they could cause hair cells to regrow by blocking the action of a single gene in mice.

Regeneration of hair cells is important because hair cells are the key links in the chain of signals that makes hearing possible. Hair cells are found in the cochlea, part of the inner ear that sends the electrical signal of sound to the brain. Vibrations from the eardrum and bones of the middle ear are relayed to the cochlea, where they stimulate the hair cells. This energy is converted to electrical signals that are carried by nerves to the brain and interpreted as sound.

In the current study, the researchers isolated a gene that was activated in the ear during the mouse life cycle. The gene, Rb1, encodes for the retinoblastoma protein, which has various functions throughout the body, including acting as a molecular switch to stop the growth of hair cells. Mice that were bred to be missing the retinoblastoma gene were found to have more hair cells than control mice. Mature hair cells grown in culture dishes also were able to regenerate when the retinoblastoma gene was blocked.

Dr. James Battey, director of NIDCD, has called this discovery "a very important first step toward learning" how to restore hearing in human patients. Hearing loss is one of the most common conditions affecting older adults.

Most deafness occurs because hair cells are damaged either by disease, injury, or aging. Humans are born with about fifty thousand inner ear hair cells, but the number gradually declines over time. Once these cells are lost, they cannot be restored.

Although the studies were done in mice, the mouse ear structure is very similar to that of humans. The next step will be to develop methods to reversibly block the Rb1 gene in inner ear hair cells to see if hair cells regenerate and hearing can be restored.

Modifier Gene Makes Some Hearing Loss More Severe

Scientists have identified a genetic mutation in humans that affects the severity of hearing loss caused by a mutation of another gene. National Institute on Deafness and Other Communication Disorders (NIDCD) scientists Drs. Julie Schultz and Andrew Griffith and co-authors at NIH and the Mayo Clinic Foundation reported their findings in the April 14, 2005, issue of the *New England Journal of Medicine*.

Genetic mutations are estimated to cause at least one half of all cases of congenital or childhood-onset hearing loss. Individual variations in the severity of hearing loss are common and typically attributed to environmental factors and modifier genes—genes that alter the clinical expression of a mutation in another gene.

In the current study, five adult siblings from the same family were found to possess a mutant form of the gene that encodes for the protein cadherin 23, which is required for the development of hair cells in the inner ear. However, the degree of hearing loss among the siblings varied. While three of the five individuals had severe to profound deafness, the other two had hearing loss only in the higher frequencies. This variability suggested the action of a modifier gene.

NIDCD scientists, led by Drs. Thomas Friedman and Konrad Noben-Trauth, had previously discovered that mutations of the cadherin 23 gene cause hearing loss in humans and mice. Dr. Noben-Trauth and his co-workers had also shown that alterations of another gene, ATP2B2, can affect the severity of hearing loss caused by a cadherin 23 mutant gene in mice. ATP2B2 encodes for a key cellular protein, known as a plasma-membrane calcium pump, that is thought to be important for regulating calcium concentrations both around and within hair bundles of hair cells. On the outside of the hair bundle, calcium is required to maintain the correct structure of the hair bundles, and on the inside it may act as an important signaling or regulatory molecule.

In this study, Dr. Schultz and her co-workers found that a mutant form of the human ATP2B2 gene, called V586M, accounted for the more severe hearing loss in the siblings who were profoundly deaf. The two siblings with better hearing were found to have normal copies of the gene. About one in twenty Caucasians are carriers of V568M.

Although V568M does not cause hearing loss, the current findings suggest that V568M may exacerbate hearing loss caused by environmental factors or other genetic influences. Further research is needed to determine the role of V568M and other mutations of the calcium pump in hearing loss associated with advanced age, exposure to loud noise, and mutations in other deafness genes.

Chapter 9

Sensorineural Hearing Disorders

Chapter Contents

Section 9.1

Auditory Neuropathy

Reprinted from "Auditory Neuropathy," National Institute on Deafness
and Other Communication Disorders, National Institutes of Health,
NIH Publication No. 03-5343, March 2003.

What is auditory neuropathy?

Auditory neuropathy is a hearing disorder in which sound enters the inner ear normally but the transmission of signals from the inner ear to the brain is impaired. It can affect people of all ages, from infancy through adulthood. The number of people affected by auditory neuropathy is not known, but the condition affects a relatively small percentage of people who are deaf or hearing-impaired.

People with auditory neuropathy may have normal hearing, or hearing loss ranging from mild to severe; they always have poor speech-perception abilities, meaning they have trouble understanding speech clearly. Often, speech perception is worse than would be predicted by the degree of hearing loss. For example, a person with auditory neuropathy may be able to hear sounds, but would still have difficulty recognizing spoken words. Sounds may fade in and out for these individuals and seem out of sync.

What causes auditory neuropathy?

Although auditory neuropathy is not yet fully understood, scientists believe the condition probably has more than one cause. In some cases, it may involve damage to the inner hair cells—specialized sensory cells in the inner ear that transmit information about sounds through the nervous system to the brain. Other causes may include faulty connections between the inner hair cells and the nerve leading from the inner ear to the brain, or damage to the nerve itself. A combination of these problems may occur in some cases. Although outer hair cells—hair cells adjacent to and more numerous than the inner hair cells—are generally more prone to damage than inner hair cells, outer hair cells seem to function normally in people with auditory neuropathy.

What are the roles of the outer and inner hair cells?

Outer hair cells help amplify sound vibrations entering the inner ear from the middle ear. When hearing is working normally, the inner hair cells convert these vibrations into electrical signals that travel as nerve impulses to the brain, where the impulses are interpreted as sound.

Are there risk factors for auditory neuropathy?

Several factors have been linked to auditory neuropathy in children. However, a clear cause and effect relationship has not been proven. Some children who have been diagnosed with auditory neuropathy experienced certain health problems as newborns, or during or shortly before birth. These problems include jaundice, premature birth, low birth weight, and an inadequate supply of oxygen to the unborn baby. In addition, some drugs that have been used to treat medical complications in pregnant women or newborns may damage the inner hair cells in the baby's ears, causing auditory neuropathy.

Auditory neuropathy runs in some families, which suggests that genetic factors may be involved in some cases. Some people with auditory neuropathy have neurological disorders that also cause problems outside of the hearing system. Examples of such disorders are Charcot-Marie-Tooth syndrome and Friedreich ataxia.

How is auditory neuropathy diagnosed?

Health professionals, including otolaryngologists (ear, nose, and throat doctors), pediatricians, and audiologists, use a combination of methods to diagnose auditory neuropathy. These include tests of auditory brainstem response (ABR) and otoacoustic emissions (OAE). The hallmark of auditory neuropathy is a negligible or very abnormal ABR reading together with a normal OAE reading. A normal OAE reading is a sign that the outer hair cells are working normally.

An ABR test monitors brain wave activity in response to sound using electrodes that are placed on the person's head and ears. An OAE test uses a small, very sensitive microphone inserted into the ear canal to monitor the faint sounds produced by the outer hair cells in response to stimulation by a series of clicks. ABR and OAE testing are painless and can be used for newborn babies and infants as well as older children and adults. Other tests may also be used as part of a more comprehensive evaluation of an individual's hearing and speech-perception abilities.

131

Does auditory neuropathy ever get better or worse?

Some newborn babies who have been diagnosed with auditory neuropathy improve and start to hear and speak within a year or two. Other infants stay the same, while some get worse and show signs that the outer hair cells no longer function (otoacoustic emissions). In adults with auditory neuropathy, hearing can remain stable, fluctuate up and down, or progressively worsen, depending on the underlying cause.

What treatments, devices, and other approaches can help people with auditory neuropathy to communicate?

Researchers are still seeking effective treatments for people with auditory neuropathy. Meanwhile, professionals in the hearing field differ in their opinions about the potential benefits of hearing aids, cochlear implants, and other technologies for people with auditory neuropathy. Some professionals report that hearing aids and personal listening devices such as frequency modulation (FM) systems are helpful for some children and adults with auditory neuropathy. Cochlear implants (electronic devices that compensate for damaged or nonworking parts of the inner ear) may also help some people with auditory neuropathy. However, no tests are currently available to determine whether an individual with auditory neuropathy might benefit from a hearing aid or cochlear implant.

Debate also continues about the best ways to educate and provide communication skills for children who have hearing impairments such as auditory neuropathy. However, most hearing health experts agree that parents should work with a team of professionals who consider the situation and options for each child as well as the child's family members and caregivers. Most also agree that parents and caregivers should interact often with infants who have auditory neuropathy by holding, facing, smiling at, and responding to the child.

There are two main philosophies of how to teach infants and children with auditory neuropathy how to communicate. One philosophy favors using sign language as the child's first language. The second philosophy encourages the use of listening skills and skills in spoken English together with technologies such as hearing aids and cochlear implants. A combination of these two approaches can also be used. Some health professionals believe it may be especially difficult for children with auditory neuropathy to learn to communicate only through spoken language because their ability to understand speech is often greatly impaired. Adults with auditory neuropathy and older children who have already developed spoken language may benefit from learning how to speechread (also known as lip reading).

What research is being done for auditory neuropathy?

Scientists are working to understand the causes of auditory neuropathy, and are searching for genes that may be involved in causing this condition. Researchers are also continuing to investigate the potential benefits of cochlear implants for children with auditory neuropathy, and are examining why cochlear implants may benefit some people with the condition but not others.

Section 9.2

Autoimmune Inner Ear Disease

Copyright © 2003 League for the Hard of Hearing. All rights reserved.
Reprinted with permission.

What is autoimmune inner ear disease?

Autoimmune inner ear disease (AIED) is a poorly understood syndrome of potentially reversible progressive sensorineural hearing loss with or without dizziness. The classic clinical presentation of this disease is with bilateral fluctuating progressive sensorineural hearing loss occurring over several months. Tinnitus (noises in the ear) and aural fullness, "pressure," may also occur as well as dizziness or vertigo.

It is felt that this clinical syndrome of potentially reversible sensorineural hearing loss is caused by autoimmune dysfunction. Autoimmune diseases are set off when an out of control immune system causes the body to attack its own tissues by failing to distinguish the body's own cells from invaders such as bacteria or viruses or cells from other organisms. Autoimmune disease forms a large family of disorders, which, according to the National Institute of Allergy and Infectious Diseases, strike an estimated fourteen to fifty million Americans.

AIED can also be seen in people with other autoimmune diseases. New research has pointed out that many people with one autoimmune disease can have more than one type of autoimmune disease.

How often does AIED occur?

AIED is uncommon, probably accounting for less than one percent of all cases of sensorineural hearing loss or dizziness. The exact incidence is unknown partially because this disease is in the process of being defined and identified. It is felt that a significant percentage of patients with Ménière Disease, especially those with bilateral symptoms, may be due to autoimmune inner ear dysfunction.

How is the diagnosis of AIED made?

Your physician can make the diagnosis based upon your history, physical examination findings, blood tests, and results of hearing and vestibular tests. A fairly specific test, Western Blot immunoassay for Heat Shock Protein-70 antibodies, correlates with active disease and potential steroid responsiveness in patients with bilateral rapidly progressive sensorineural hearing loss. However this laboratory test does not demonstrate correlation in all cases. Therefore a therapeutic trial of medication should be undertaken as directed by your physician for this potentially reversible sensorineural hearing loss.

Is there any way we can find out more about AIED, and why is this important?

Physician scientists are actively investigating the cause and treatment of AIED. Because of its unique potential reversibility, intensive study of this sensorineural hearing loss may provide leads for understanding other forms of sensorineural hearing loss.

There is a multicenter clinical trial funded by the National Institute of Deafness and Communication Disorders (NIDCD) to study the cause of AIED and to evaluate a response to Prednisone and an alternative drug, Methotrexate. These drugs have a long track record for treatment of other autoimmune diseases. Since the number of patients with AIED are few, it is imperative that this scarce population and its treatment be thoroughly investigated in centers involved with the clinical trial.

Section 9.3

Presbycusis:
Age-Related Hearing Loss

Over twenty-five million Americans have some degree of hearing loss, and this number is increasing as the average age of the population increases. As we get older, our hearing begins to lose some of its sharpness and clarity. This process of age-related hearing loss is known as presbycusis (presby = elder, cusis = hearing).

Presbycusis is the most common form of hearing loss. Everyone who lives long enough will develop some degree of presbycusis, some sooner than others. Those who damage their ears from loud noise exposure will develop it sooner.

Most people with presbycusis can learn to communicate effectively through the use of such common-sense techniques as looking at the talker, turning off background noise, and using hearing aids as necessary. Presbycusis seldom causes total deafness, but many people experience considerable difficulty in their later years. Hearing loss impairs communication, subtly at first and increasing with the magnitude of the loss. Unfortunately, many people try to hide their hearing loss instead of accepting it as another of life's challenges. Those who do so risk becoming isolated from those close to them. When family and friends understand that it is hearing loss and not an attitude problem that has created the difficulties and the misunderstandings that arise from hearing loss, and when all concerned work together to improve communication, hearing losses need not become a barrier to healthy human relations.

Normal Ear Function

The ear has three parts:

• The outer ear collects sound waves.

135

- The middle ear increases the sound energy and transmits the sound to the inner ear.

- The inner ear transforms the sound waves into nerve impulses that are interpreted by the brain.

Sound waves normally pass through the ear canal, causing the eardrum to vibrate. This motion is transmitted by three small bones that increase the sound energy—the malleus (hammer), the incus (anvil), and the stapes (stirrup). The stapes fits into the oval window and is held in place by a ligament permitting it to move in and out of the window, much like a speaker cone in a radio or stereo set. These vibrations cause movement of the hair cells in the cochlea, and are transformed into electrical impulses. These impulses are carried by the hearing nerve to the brain, where they are interpreted as sound.

Causes

Presbycusis is caused by a combination of factors. The two most important are the aging process in the auditory system and wear and tear from a lifetime of noise exposure. Other factors, such as age-related diseases, possible toxic effects of drugs, chemicals, heredity, and even diet may play a role for some people. Presbycusis tends to run in families, and some develop hearing loss earlier and to a greater degree than others. Most people with presbycusis lose hearing in the high frequencies, which impairs understanding of speech more than the hearing of it. Many people refer to this by the outdated term, nerve deafness, when, in fact, true nerve deafness is very rare.

The most common type of presbycusis is sensory. Sensory hearing losses are caused by loss of outer hair cells in the inner ear (cochlea), and usually begin in the high frequencies. Some forms of presbycusis are associated with cardiovascular disease in women. Although unproven as yet, it may be the case that measures to prevent cardiovascular disease, such as fitness and exercise, weight reduction, lowering of high cholesterol levels, smoking cessation, and diet modification, may delay the onset of presbycusis.

One of the main contributors to presbycusis is noise. We live in a very noisy world and it is clear that our hearing suffers as a result. Long-term exposure to loud noise will produce a typical high-frequency sensory hearing loss that is similar to the loss due to aging. Hearing protection devices and noise-reduction techniques prevent this from happening. Gun-shooting and industrial noise are the most common causes of noise-induced hearing loss. People who live in quiet parts of the world have less presbycusis than those who live in modern industrialized cities, thus, measures to reduce our exposure to noise are likely to help us keep our ears young(er).

Effects of Presbycusis

Presbycusis affects our ability to hear speech in two ways: detecting sounds (sensitivity) and understanding sounds (word discrimination). Speech sounds cover a wide range of frequencies so that both the type and degree of hearing loss determine its impact. Sensory presbycusis begins in the highest frequencies, actually above the speech range at first. This may result in tinnitus—a ringing sound in the ears—before there is any serious loss of speech understanding. Tinnitus annoys some people, but most accept the ringing as a normal part of presbycusis. Fortunately, the ringing comes and goes and is easily masked by background sounds.

As the loss extends into the speech range (500–3000 Hz), the common complaint is "I can hear but I can't understand." Background noise adds to the problem. The louder and lower frequency segments of speech, such as the vowels, can be heard; however, the high-pitched consonants, such as t, p, k, f, s, and ch, are not heard due to the high frequency sensitivity loss. One then confuses and misinterprets what is being spoken ("Did you say mash, math, map, or mat?"). With some forms of presbycusis, all frequencies are affected so that people complain of not being able to hear the speaker but are able to understand if the speech is made louder.

The difficulties in speech understanding due to presbycusis may be compounded by aging in the brain, which is evident mainly from a slowing of speech processing. Seniors often note more difficulty in speech understanding than younger persons with the same degree of hearing loss. In difficult listening situations, such as in noisy halls or rooms with an echo, or with rapid speech and foreign accents, the older listeners' difficulties increase more than younger listeners'. People with central hearing difficulties need more than hearing aids to communicate: they need slower speakers, quieter rooms, and face-to-face conversation.

Diagnosis

The diagnosis of presbycusis involves a physical examination and medical history to rule out other common causes of hearing loss, such as fluid in the ear or a wax obstruction, and an audiogram (hearing test) done in a sound-treated room by a audiologist. In some cases, lab tests and imaging studies are recommended to rule out treatable causes of sensory hearing loss.

The typical types of audiograms seen in people with presbycusis are shown below.

Treatment

Less than 5 percent of patients with inner ear hearing loss can be helped medically. Consequently, hearing aids are the main resource for improving communication and reducing hearing handicaps in persons with sensory hearing loss. Unfortunately, only 10 percent of people who might benefit from an aid actually own one, which indicates a substantial under service. Of these, about half do not use their aid(s) regularly, which prevents full adaptation to the devices.

Hearing Aids

A hearing aid is a miniature, personal loudspeaker system designed to increase the intensity of sound and deliver it to the ear with as little distortion as possible. Significant improvements in hearing aid design have allowed greater choices in selecting and fitting hearing aids. Many technological innovations in the past ten years have increased the number and types of hearing aids, both in physical size and in sophistication. Current hearing aids include devices that fit behind the ear, in the ear, in the canal, and most recently, completely in the canal. Unfortunately, many people associate hearing loss with the "stigma" of aging. Introduction of the smaller devices that fit entirely in the ear canal has been met with obvious appeal. However, people with dexterity or vision problems are often unable to insert and adjust the smaller aids properly and are better served with larger hearing aids. A hearing aid dispenser reviews such issues with the patient during the pre-fitting session.

Hearing aids now offer a wide variety of amplification options. They no longer merely provide simple amplification, but may include circuitry to reduce the gain for loud sounds, automatic loudness adjusting circuits that automatically decrease sound levels of continuous background noise, and controls that automatically increase the loudness of soft sounds while decreasing loud sounds. There are also aids with several programs that the listener picks for different listening situations: wide frequency amplification for quiet places, reduced low frequencies in noisy situations, and a telephone program for phone use. These hearing aids are digitally programmed by an external programmer device. Individual programming of the hearing aid enables the dispenser to make significant modifications for an individual wearer's needs. Such multi-memory hearing aids typically include a user-operated remote control with which to make program and volume changes.

Some hearing aids now have multiple microphones, one to improve directionality in background noise situations, and another for places where a broad range of sound input is desired. The most recent introduction in hearing aid technology is the fully digital instrument that has the processing power of a desktop personal computer and fits into the small, canal-sized instruments. These aids have many features not available in conventional hearing aids, and will undoubtedly provide improved hearing in future years.

The new hearing aid systems require a higher level of training and sophistication on the part of the user and the fitter. In addition, these new systems are considerably more expensive than conventional hearing aids. Currently, the digital in-the-canal aid costs approximately $2,500 for one aid. Usually an aid for each ear is most beneficial. Neither Medicare nor most insurance carriers provide financial coverage for hearing aids. The specific hearing needs, lifestyle, and adaptability of the hearing aid wearer must be taken into account during the pre-fitting process.

Hearing Aid Candidacy

After the necessary interview and evaluation, an audiologist will recommend the type of hearing aid, specify the acoustical requirements of the aids, and provide training in the use of them. The potential advantages and limitations of hearing aids will be reviewed, and follow-up is provided during the initial trial as well as after the purchase. It is mandatory to provide patients with a free or low-cost thirty-day hearing aid trial period prior to purchasing the aid(s). This trial period enables patients the opportunity to wear the aid(s) in their own home and social environment to determine their satisfaction.

Adaptation to hearing aid use takes time and requires a significant adjustment. It may take several months, during which time the brain adapts to the new way things sound. Some people become frustrated during this time but should be encouraged to continue. Using the aid only part of the day delays adaptation.

Many people resist amplification because of the social stigma associated with hearing loss. Since our culture unfortunately views hearing loss as a consequence of aging, resistance to a hearing aid is inevitable. Factors of motivation, personal adjustment, and family support are vital factors in hearing aid satisfaction.

Assistive Listening Devices

Although substantial improvements have been achieved in hearing aid design and application, few people with severe hearing impairment can ever come close to achieving normal hearing with the use of a aid alone. The physiological realities of age-related hearing loss, coupled with the electronic constraints of hearing aids, renders normal hearing impossible, especially considering the levels of noise and background interference found in most public places. The amplification of unwanted sounds (e.g., multiple speakers in groups, background noise, ventilation) by hearing aids often obscures the speaker's message.

Assistive listening devices (ALDs) are situation-specific amplification systems designed for use in difficult listening environments. ALDs commonly use a microphone placed close to the desired sound source (e.g., a television, theater stage, or speaker's podium) so that sound is transmitted directly to the listener. Transmission methods include infrared, audio loop, FM radio, or direct audio input. These methods improve the signal-to-noise ratio. That is, the desired sounds are enhanced while competing noises are decreased, allowing for improved understanding. ALDs are becoming more available in churches, theaters, and classrooms, enabling hearing-impaired people to avoid the isolation imposed by the inability to hear a sermon, play, or public address.

Amplified telephones, low-frequency doorbells, amplified ringers, and closed-captioned TV decoders are just a few examples of the number of devices currently available for everyday use. In addition, flashing alarm clocks, alarm bed vibrators, and flashing smoke detectors provide valuable help for severely hearing-impaired individuals.

Cochlear Implants

A small percentage of people have a progressive hearing loss that leads to total or near-total deafness. As the loss progresses, these people no longer benefit from standard hearing aids. While some can get by at times by lip reading and guessing, most find that additional help is needed. Fortunately, the implantable cochlear device known as a cochlear implant is very effective for people with recent onset deafness. During outpatient surgery, the device is implanted into the inner ear. Four to six weeks later the speech processor is hooked up and programmed. At first, speech sounds very mechanical and different. However, in a few weeks to months, the brain is able to make sense out of these sounds and most people are not only able to "hear" the ordinary sounds of the world around them, but are able to understand speech well with the combination of the implant and lip reading. Some are able to talk on the telephone.

Medical Therapy

Once thought to be untreatable, some inner ear hearing losses are now responding to medical therapy. About one-third of people with sudden hearing loss recover hearing. The majority of people with autoimmune hearing loss recover substantial amounts of the loss with corticosteroid and other anti-immune treatments. However, for the vast majority of people with presbycusis, definitive treatment must await the results of our ongoing research programs in hair cell regeneration. It is impossible to predict when this research will provide help for people with presbycusis. However, it is likely that within the next decade we will be better able to know if and when this research may be applied to people with hearing loss.

Prevention

While some degree of presbycusis is inevitable, it may be prevented in part by avoiding hazardous noise exposure. If noise cannot be avoided, use of suitable hearing protection is essential. Insert ear plugs reduce noise by about 15 to 25 decibels (dB) and may permit people to work in otherwise hazardous areas with less risk of hearing damage. Remember that the effects of noise accumulate over a lifetime and that the gun shooting and loud music exposure during adolescence will contribute to communication difficulties during the senior years.

Ototoxic drugs such as cisplatin for cancer chemotherapy and some antibiotics may cause a mild high-frequency loss indistinguishable from sensory presbycusis, to profound hearing loss and deafness. While the search for protective agents continues, diligent monitoring provides the best method for early detection and the opportunity to modify the treatment plan.

Risk factors for cardiovascular disease as well as the disease itself affect hearing to some extent. Hypertension, hyperlipidemia, and diabetes mellitus have all been associated with excessive hearing loss. Therefore, it is logical that good general health would lower the risk of hearing loss due to disease. In addition, high-lipid diets are associated with poorer hearing.

Summary

Presbycusis refers to the hearing loss that people experience as they grow older. It is due to a variety of causes including aging, noise exposure, diseases, and toxins. Presbycusis may cause communication difficulties. However, in a few weeks to months, the brain is able to make sense out of these sounds and most people are not only able to "hear" the ordinary sounds of the world around them, but are able to understand speech well. Most are able to talk on the telephone.

Section 9.4

Hyperacusis

Reprinted with permission from the Royal National Institute for Deaf People (RNID), © 2005. For additional information, contact the RNID Information Line, 19-23 Featherstone Street, London EC1Y 8SL, Telephone: 0808 808 0123, Textphone: 0808 808 9000, Fax: 020 7296 8199, E-mail: informationline@rnid.org.uk, or visit their website at http://www.rnid.org.uk.

What is hyperacusis?

If you have hyperacusis you will have an increased sensitivity to the sounds that most people are able to tolerate. People with hyperacusis are not all affected by the same type of sounds.

You can get hyperacusis on its own or with a range of other conditions such as depression, migraine, Ménière disease, chronic fatigue syndrome, and visual oversensitivity. If you have hyperacusis you may also have tinnitus. This is the word for noises that some people hear

"in the ears" or "in the head," such as buzzing, ringing, wh[...]
ing, and other sounds. You may also find that the area [...]
ear is painful or aches.

What is obscure auditory dysfunction?

If you have hyperacusis you are likely to have normal hearing; however, you may have difficulty understanding speech in noisy places, such as a train station. This is a mild difficulty sometimes known as "obscure auditory dysfunction" or "auditory processing difficulty."

What are the effects of hyperacusis?

If you have hyperacusis it might feel painful or startling. It may make you feel angry, distressed, or anxious. You may find yourself panicking when you try to get away from the sound.

You may find that after being exposed to an uncomfortable sound the discomfort continues for a period of time afterward and becomes worse if you hear the sound again.

Your reaction to an uncomfortable sound may be made worse if you are in an environment where you expect to hear the sound. When you are afraid of hearing a sound you may become anxious, which increases your discomfort, and when you are afraid or stressed the brain produces substances that increase the sensitivity to sound. However, everyone reacts differently to hyperacusis.

What causes hyperacusis?

There are probably a number of different causes of hyperacusis but researchers don't really have a clear understanding of why some people have it. It is possible that some functions of the hearing system, which normally "balance" sounds and protect the system, may be affected.

However, we do know that some people first develop it after sudden exposure to very high levels of sound or after a head injury. This may damage delicate structures within the inner ear and the brain, which leads to hyperacusis. When you are in a noisy environment your brain sends information about loud noise back to the inner ear, so that the "volume" can be turned down and the inner ear can be protected. It is thought that damage to this feedback mechanism may be an underlying cause of hyperacusis.

Our brain also plays a vital role in processing the sound signals it receives from the inner ear. Problems in the way these signals are processed could be another cause of hyperacusis.

How can a person get treatment for hyperacusis?

If you think you have hyperacusis you should visit your doctor. He or she may refer you to a specialist in audiology or audiological medicine, or to the ear, nose, and throat (ENT) department in your local hospital. They will be able to investigate your hearing system to try to find a cause for your hyperacusis and to advise you on the most appropriate treatment.

You may need specialized hearing therapy, usually from a hearing therapist. And you may also be referred to a clinical psychologist or behavioral therapist to help you manage the anxiety, phobia, stress, and avoidance that are associated with hyperacusis and may make it worse.

What is auditory desensitization?

As part of your treatment you may be offered auditory desensitization as part of an auditory retraining program. This should be available through an audiology department and is usually carried out by an audiologist or hearing therapist.

It aims to help improve the level of noise you can tolerate and involves listening to different types of sound known as "white," "broadband," or "pink" noise on a daily basis. This noise is played through small noise generators that you wear in your ear canal. You start by listening to a very low level of noise for a very short time. The level and length of time is gradually increased. Some people may find this gives them initial relief, but auditory desensitization is usually a long process and you may need to follow this treatment for at least twelve months in order to achieve a long-term positive effect.

How does a behavior modification program help?

An auditory desensitization program will be more effective if you follow a behavior modification program at the same time. A clinical psychologist can help design an individual program for you. This aims to break down any routines that you may have developed to avoid noisy situations. It should also help you control the anxiety patterns that you may have developed because of the pain and distress caused by certain sounds.

How can you help yourself?

If you have hyperacusis there are several ways you can help yourself:

- Try not to wear earmuffs or earplugs unless you really need to, and then only for short periods of time.

- Try not to avoid situations where you might hear sounds that will cause you discomfort.

- Try to avoid being in a completely quiet environment. It is important to try and listen to everyday sounds, as a quiet environment tends to make hyperacusis worse.

Is it a good idea to use earplugs or earmuffs?

Some people with hyperacusis tend to use devices such as earplugs or earmuffs to block out sound. Your audiology specialist may refer to these as "attenuators." Although these may provide temporary relief, in the long term they can undo any progress you are making to adapt to sound and they may even make hyperacusis worse.

However, if you are exposed to loud sounds for a long time, for example in your job, this can make hyperacusis worse. Therefore, you may find it helps to wear special "active" electronic sound attenuators and musicians' earplugs if you work in a noisy place. Your audiology department may be able to provide these.

Section 9.5

Sudden Deafness

Reprinted from "Sudden Deafness," National Institute on Deafness
and Other Communication Disorders, National Institutes of Health,
NIH Publication No. 00-4757, March 2003.

Sudden sensorineural hearing loss (SSHL), or sudden deafness, is a rapid loss of hearing. SSHL can happen to a person all at once or over a period of up to three days. It should be considered a medical emergency. A person who experiences SSHL should visit a doctor immediately.

A doctor can determine whether a person has experienced SSHL by conducting a normal hearing test. If a loss of at least 30 decibels in three connected frequencies is discovered, it is diagnosed as SSHL. A decibel is a measure of sound. A decibel level of 30 is half as loud as a normal conversation. A frequency is another way of measuring sound. Frequencies measure sound waves and help to determine what makes one sound different from another sound.

Hearing loss affects only one ear in nine out of ten people who experience SSHL. Many people notice it when they wake up in the morning. Others first notice it when they try to use the deafened ear, such as when they make a phone call. Still others notice a loud, alarming "pop" just before their hearing disappears. People with SSHL often experience dizziness or a ringing in their ears (tinnitus), or both.

Some patients recover completely without medical intervention, often within the first three days. This is called a spontaneous recovery. Others get better slowly over a one- or two-week period. Although a good to excellent recovery is likely, 15 percent of those with SSHL experience a hearing loss that gets worse over time.

Approximately four thousand new cases of SSHL occur each year in the United States. It can affect anyone, but for unknown reasons it happens most often to people between the ages of thirty and sixty.

Causes/Diagnosis

Though there are more than one hundred possible causes of sudden deafness, it is rare for a specific cause to be precisely identified.

Only 10 to 15 percent of patients with SSHL know what caused their loss. Normally, diagnosis is based on the patient's medical history. Possible causes include the following:

- Infectious diseases
- Trauma, such as a head injury
- Abnormal tissue growth
- Immunologic diseases such as Cogan syndrome
- Toxic causes, such as snakebites
- Ototoxic drugs (drugs that harm the ear)
- Circulatory problems
- Neurologic causes such as multiple sclerosis
- Relation to disorders such as Ménière disease

Treatment

People who experience SSHL should see a physician immediately. Doctors believe that finding medical help fast increases the chances for recovery. Several treatments are used for SSHL, but researchers are not yet certain which is the best for any one cause. If a specific cause is identified, a doctor may prescribe antibiotics for the patient. Or, a doctor may advise a patient to stop taking any medicine that can irritate or damage the ear.

The most common therapy for SSHL, especially in cases with an unknown cause, is treatment with steroids. Steroids are used to treat many different disorders and usually work to reduce inflammation, decrease swelling, and help the body fight illness. Steroid treatment helps some SSHL patients who also have conditions that affect the immune system, which is the body's defense against disease.

Another common method that may help some patients is a diet low in salt. Researchers believe that this method aids people with SSHL who also have Ménière disease, a hearing and balance disorder.

Research

Two factors that help hearing function properly are good air and blood flow inside the ear. Many researchers now think that SSHL happens when important parts of the inner ear do not receive enough oxygen. A common treatment for this possible cause is called carbogen inhalation. Carbogen is a mixture of oxygen and carbon dioxide that seems to help air and blood flow better inside the ear. Like steroid therapy, carbogen inhalation does not help every patient, but some SSHL patients taking carbogen have recovered over a period of time.

Chapter 10

Ototoxicity

Ototoxicity ("ear poisoning") is due to drugs or chemicals that damage the inner ear or the vestibulo-cochlear nerve, which sends balance and hearing information from the inner ear to the brain. Ototoxicity can result in temporary or permanent disturbances of hearing, balance, or both.

Many chemicals have ototoxic potential, including over-the-counter drugs, prescription medications, and environmental chemicals. If you are taking any drugs on the advice of your physician, do not stop taking them just because you see them listed in the following. Speak with your doctor or other health care advisor about your concerns.

Substances that may cause ototoxicity include:

- **Aminoglycoside antibiotics**, including gentamicin, streptomycin, kanamycin, tobramycin, neomycin, amikacin, netilmicin, dihydro-streptomycin, and ribostamycin. All members of this family are well known for their potential to cause permanent ototoxicity. They can enter the inner ear through the blood system, through inhalation, or via diffusion from the middle ear into the inner ear. They enter the blood stream in largest amounts when given intravenously (by IV).

- **Anti-neoplastics (anti-cancer drugs).** Cisplatin is well known to cause hearing loss that is many times massive and permanent. Carboplatin has been implicated as well.

The information in this chapter is reprinted with permission form the Vestibular Disorders Association (VEDA), http://www.vestibular.org. © 2006 VEDA. All rights reserved.

149

- **Environmental chemicals**, including butyl nitrite, mercury, carbon disulfide, styrene, carbon monoxide, tin, hexane, toluene, lead, trichloroethylene, manganese, and xylene. Most are associated with hearing disturbances that may be permanent; mercury has also been linked to permanent balance problems.

- **Loop diuretics**, including bumetanide (Bumex), ethacrynic acid (Edecrin), furosemide (Lasix), and torsemide (Demadex). These drugs cause ringing in the ears or decreased hearing that reverses when the drug is stopped. Note: Hydrochlorothiazide (HCTZ) and Maxzide, diuretics commonly prescribed to people with Ménière's disease or other forms of endolymphatic hydrops, are not loop diuretics.

- **Aspirin and quinine products.** These may cause temporary ototoxicity, particularly tinnitus, but may also reduce hearing.

Symptoms of ototoxicity vary considerably from drug to drug and person to person. They range from mild imbalance to total incapacitation, and from tinnitus to total hearing loss.

A bilateral (two-sided) vestibular loss usually doesn't produce intense vertigo, vomiting, and nystagmus but instead a headache, a feeling of ear fullness, imbalance to the point of being unable to walk, and a bouncing and blurring of vision (oscillopsia). It also produces inability to tolerate head movement, a wide-based gait (walking with the legs farther apart than usual), difficulty walking in the dark, a feeling of unsteadiness and actual unsteadiness while moving, lightheadedness, and severe fatigue. If the damage is severe, symptoms such as oscillopsia and problems with walking in the dark or with the eyes closed are not going to go away.

The diagnosis of ototoxicity is based upon the patient's history, symptoms, and test results. There is no specific test; this makes a positive history for ototoxin exposure crucial to the diagnosis.

At present, there are no treatments that can reverse the damage. Currently available treatments are aimed at reducing the effect of the damage and rehabilitating function. Individuals with hearing loss may be helped with hearing aids, and those with profound bilateral losses have benefited from cochlear implants. In the case of lost balance function, physical therapy is of great value for many individuals. The aim is to help the brain become accustomed to the changed information from the inner ear and to assist the individual in developing other ways to maintain balance.

Chapter 11

Tinnitus

Chapter Contents

Section 11.1

Facts about Tinnitus

Reprinted from "The Noise in Your Ears: Facts about Tinnitus," National Institute on Deafness and Communication Disorders, National Institutes of Health, NIH Publication No. 00-4896, February 2001.

Do you hear a ringing, roaring, clicking, or hissing sound in your ears? Do you hear this sound often or all the time? Does the sound bother you a lot? If you answer yes to these questions, you may have tinnitus (tin-NY-tus).

Tinnitus is a symptom associated with many forms of hearing loss. It can also be a symptom of other health problems. According to estimates by the American Tinnitus Association, at least twelve million Americans have tinnitus. Of these, at least one million experience it so severely that it interferes with their daily activities. People with severe cases of tinnitus may find it difficult to hear, work, or even sleep.

What causes tinnitus?

- **Hearing loss:** Doctors and scientists have discovered that people with different kinds of hearing loss also have tinnitus.

- **Loud noise:** Too much exposure to loud noise can cause noise-induced hearing loss and tinnitus.

- **Medicine:** More than two hundred medicines can cause tinnitus. If you have tinnitus and you take medicine, ask your doctor or pharmacist whether your medicine could be involved.

- **Other health problems:** Allergies, tumors, and problems in the heart and blood vessels, jaws, and neck can cause tinnitus.

What should I do if I have tinnitus?

The most important thing you can do is to go see your doctor. Your doctor can try to determine what is causing your tinnitus. He or she can check to see if it is related to blood pressure, kidney function, diet, or allergies. Your doctor can also determine whether your tinnitus is related to any medicine you are taking.

To learn more about what is causing your tinnitus, your doctor may refer you to an otolaryngologist, an ear, nose, and throat doctor. He or she will examine your ears and your hearing to try to find out why you have tinnitus. Another hearing professional, an audiologist, can measure your hearing. If you need a hearing aid, an audiologist can fit you with one that meets your needs.

How will hearing experts treat my tinnitus?

Although there is no cure for tinnitus, scientists and doctors have discovered several treatments that may give you some relief. Not every treatment works for everyone, so you may need to try several to find the ones that help.

Treatments can include:

- **Hearing aids:** Many people with tinnitus also have a hearing loss. Wearing a hearing aid makes it easier for some people to hear the sounds they need to hear by making them louder. The better you hear other people talking or the music you like, the less you notice your tinnitus.

- **Maskers:** Maskers are small electronic devices that use sound to make tinnitus less noticeable. Maskers do not make tinnitus go away, but they make the ringing or roaring seem softer. For some people, maskers hide their tinnitus so well that they can barely hear it. Some people sleep better when they use maskers. Listening to static at a low volume on the radio or using bedside maskers can help. These are devices you can put by your bed instead of behind your ear. They can help you ignore your tinnitus and fall asleep.

- **Medicine or drug therapy:** Some medicines may ease tinnitus. If your doctor prescribes medicine to treat your tinnitus, he or she can tell you whether the medicine has any side effects.

- **Tinnitus retraining therapy:** This treatment uses a combination of counseling and maskers. Otolaryngologists and audiologists help you learn how to deal with your tinnitus better. You may also use maskers to make your tinnitus less noticeable. After a while, some people learn how to avoid thinking about their tinnitus. It takes time for this treatment to work, but it can be very helpful.

153

- **Counseling:** People with tinnitus may become depressed. Talking with a counselor or people in tinnitus support groups may be helpful.

- **Relaxing:** Learning how to relax is very helpful if the noise in your ears frustrates you. Stress makes tinnitus seem worse. By relaxing, you have a chance to rest and better deal with the sound.

What can I do to help myself?

Think about things that will help you cope. Many people find listening to music very helpful. Focusing on music might help you forget about your tinnitus for a while. It can also help mask the sound. Other people like to listen to recorded nature sounds, like ocean waves, the wind, or even crickets.

Avoid anything that can make your tinnitus worse. This includes smoking, alcohol, and loud noise. If you are a construction worker, an airport worker, or a hunter, or if you are regularly exposed to loud noise at home or at work, wear earplugs or special earmuffs to protect your hearing and keep your tinnitus from getting worse.

If it is hard for you to hear over your tinnitus, ask your friends and family to face you when they talk so you can see their faces. Seeing their expressions may help you understand them better. Ask people to speak louder, but not shout. Also, tell them they do not have to talk slowly, just more clearly.

Section 11.2

Tinnitus Research

Reprinted from "Tinnitus Research," National Institute on Deafness
and Other Communication Disorders, National Institutes of Health,
December 2001.

For the first time, scientists have located an area in the brain involved in the production of tinnitus. Tinnitus is a ringing, roaring, buzzing, or clicking sound that occurs inside the head. These findings are in a study by Alan H. Lockwood, M.D., of the State University of New York in Buffalo and his colleagues, in the January 22, 1998, issue of *Neurology*.

Using positron-emission tomography (PET), Dr. Lockwood's group was able to map brain regions of individuals who had tinnitus in only one ear. These individuals also had the ability to change the loudness of their tinnitus by performing special movements of their face and mouth. Cerebral blood flow, an indication of increased brain activity, was measured while these individuals were at rest, while they performed the movements that affected their tinnitus, and while they listened to loud beeps or pure tones that were presented using ear phones. The PET scan detected changes in the auditory cortex, that part of the brain that processes sounds, on the side of the brain opposite the tinnitus. In contrast, the auditory cortex on both sides of the brain reacted to pure tones presented to one ear at a time. Since external tones presented to one ear affect both sides of the brain, the fact that the internal tones of tinnitus affect only one side of brain indicates that tinnitus may be initiated by brain activity rather than by the ear.

"This work represents a breakthrough and moves us a step closer to understanding the phenomenon of tinnitus. We feel certain that this study will lead to further research that will ultimately translate into treatment options for the millions of people who suffer with this difficult condition," said James F. Battey, M.D., Ph.D., director, National

Institute on Deafness and Other Communication Disorders (NIDCD), which funded the study.

The authors suggest that this study may improve knowledge of how tinnitus occurs and may lead to finding treatments. "Without objective information on how and where the condition originates, developing effective treatments has been difficult. We have taken a critical step down the road toward a cure for this disabling condition," said Lockwood. Ultimately, this study opens the door to further research such as the development of drugs to change the brain activity in the involved areas. Dr. Lockwood's colleagues are R. J. Salvi, Ph.D., M. L. Coad, B.A., M. L. Towsley, M.A., D. S. Wack, M.A., and B. W. Murphy, M.S., from the VA Western New York Health Care System and State University of New York, both in Buffalo.

Tinnitus is a symptom that accompanies many kinds of hearing loss. The phenomenon of tinnitus presents so many issues to address because there are many different experiences of tinnitus with many different causes. The mechanisms that produce tinnitus are not fully known and are associated with nearly all diseases and disorders of the ear that cause hearing loss. Controlling these mechanisms, therefore, may alleviate the tinnitus. As it is a symptom, tinnitus is difficult for the scientists to address. The NIDCD is supporting several biomedical research projects that cover a variety of aspects of the condition which will provide necessary data: developing a comprehensive database and an understanding of the phenomenon of tinnitus that accompanies sensorineural hearing loss; tinnitus and masking devices; the role of calcium imbalance in inducing cochlear tinnitus; and otoacoustic emissions and cochlear function. The NIDCD is also supporting several noninvasive imaging studies that will hopefully differentiate the various kinds of tinnitus.

As the nation's focal point for research in human communication, the NIDCD conducts and supports biomedical and behavioral research and research training on normal mechanisms as well as diseases and disorders of hearing, balance, smell, taste, voice, speech and language that affect forty-six million Americans. The NIDCD is one of the institutes of the National Institutes of Health, the nation's lead agency for biomedical and behavioral health research.

Chapter 12

Noise-Induced Hearing Loss

Chapter Contents

Section 12.1

Noise-Induced Hearing Loss: An Overview

Reprinted from "Noise-Induced Hearing Loss," National Institute on
Deafness and Other Communication Disorders, National Institutes of
Health, NIH Publication No. 97-4233, September 2002.

Every day we experience sound in our environment such as the television, radio, washing machine, automobiles, buses, and trucks. But when an individual is exposed to harmful sounds—sounds that are too loud or loud sounds over a long time—sensitive structures of the inner ear can be damaged, causing noise-induced hearing loss (NIHL).

How do we hear?

Hearing is a series of events in which the ear converts sound waves into electrical signals that are sent to the brain and interpreted as sound. The ear has three main parts: the outer, middle, and inner ear. Sound waves enter through the outer ear and reach the middle ear, where they cause the eardrum to vibrate.

The vibrations are transmitted through three tiny bones in the middle ear, called the ossicles. These three bones are named the malleus, incus, and stapes (and are also known as the hammer, anvil, and stirrup). The eardrum and ossicles amplify the vibrations and carry them to the inner ear. The stirrup transmits the amplified vibrations through the oval window and into the fluid that fills the inner ear. The vibrations move through fluid in the snail-shaped hearing part of the inner ear (cochlea) that contains the hair cells. The fluid in the cochlea moves the top portion of the hair cells, called the hair bundle, which initiates the changes that lead to the production of nerve impulses. These nerve impulses are carried to the brain, where they are interpreted as sound. Different sounds move the hair bundles in different ways, thus allowing the brain to distinguish one sound from another, such as vowels from consonants.

What sounds cause NIHL?

NIHL can be caused by a one-time exposure to loud sound as well as by repeated exposure to sounds at various loudness levels over an extended period of time. The loudness of sound is measured in units called decibels. For example, normal conversation is approximately 60 decibels, the humming of a refrigerator is 40 decibels, and city traffic noise can be 80 decibels. Examples of sources of loud noises that cause NIHL are motorcycles, firecrackers, and firearms, all emitting sounds from 120 to 140 decibels. Sounds of less than 80 decibels, even after long exposure, are unlikely to cause hearing loss.

Exposure to harmful sounds causes damage to the sensitive hair cells of the inner ear as well as the hearing nerve. These structures can be injured by two kinds of noise: loud impulse noise, such as an explosion, or loud continuous noise, such as that generated in a wood-working shop.

What are the effects of NIHL?

Impulse sound can result in immediate hearing loss that may be permanent. The structures of the inner ear may be severely damaged. This kind of hearing loss may be accompanied by tinnitus, a ringing, buzzing, or roaring in the ears or head, which may subside over time. Hearing loss and tinnitus may be experienced in one or both ears, and tinnitus may continue constantly or occasionally throughout a life-time.

Continuous exposure to loud noise also can damage the structure of the hair cells, resulting in hearing loss and tinnitus. Exposure to impulse and continuous noise may cause only a temporary hearing loss. If the hearing recovers, the temporary hearing loss is called a temporary threshold shift. The temporary threshold shift largely disappears sixteen to forty-eight hours after exposure to loud noise.

Both forms of NIHL can be prevented by the regular use of hearing protectors such as earplugs or earmuffs.

What are the symptoms of NIHL?

The symptoms of NIHL increase gradually over a period of continuous exposure. Sounds may become distorted or muffled, and it may be difficult for the person to understand speech. The individual may not be aware of the loss, but it can be detected with a hearing test.

Who is affected by NIHL?

More than thirty million Americans are exposed to hazardous sound levels on a regular basis. Individuals of all ages, including children, adolescents, young adults, and older people, can develop NIHL.

Exposure occurs in the workplace, in recreational settings, and at home. Noisy recreational activities include target shooting and hunting, snowmobiling, riding go-carts, woodworking and other noisy hobbies, and playing with power horns, cap guns, and model airplanes. Harmful noises at home include vacuum cleaners, garbage disposals, gas-powered lawn mowers, leaf blowers, and shop tools. And it makes no difference where a person lives—both urban and rural settings offer their own brands of noisy devices on a daily basis. Of the twenty-eight million Americans who have some degree of hearing loss, about one-third can attribute their hearing loss, at least in part, to noise.

Can NIHL be prevented?

NIHL is preventable. All individuals should understand the hazards of noise and how to practice good health in everyday life.

- Know which noises can cause damage (those above 90 decibels).

- Wear earplugs or other hearing protective devices when involved in a loud activity (special earplugs and earmuffs are available at hardware stores and sporting good stores).

- Be alert to hazardous noise in the environment.

- Protect children who are too young to protect themselves.

- Make family, friends, and colleagues aware of the hazards of noise.

- Have a medical examination by an otolaryngologist, a physician who specializes in diseases of the ears, nose, throat, head, and neck, and a hearing test by an audiologist, a health professional trained to identify and measure hearing loss and to rehabilitate persons with hearing impairments.

What research is being done for NIHL?

Scientists are studying the internal workings of the ear and the mechanisms that cause NIHL so that better prevention and treatment strategies can be developed. For example, scientists have discovered that damage to the structure of the hair bundle is related to temporary and permanent loss of hearing. When the hair bundle is exposed to prolonged periods of damaging sound, the basic structure of the hair bundle is destroyed and the important connections among hair cells are disrupted. These structural changes lead directly to hearing loss.

Recent NIDCD Research: Recent findings by National Institute on Deafness and Other Communication Disorders (NIDCD) researchers show that hair bundles are capable of rebuilding their structure from top to bottom over a forty-eight-hour period (the common duration of temporary hearing loss). Researchers suggest that permanent hearing loss may occur when damage is so severe that it overwhelms the self-repair mechanism.[1]

Drug Therapies: Other studies involve potential drug therapies for NIHL. For example, scientists are studying how changes in blood flow in the cochlea affect hair cells. When a person is exposed to loud noise, blood flow in the cochlea drops. However, a drug that is used to treat peripheral vascular disease (any abnormal condition in blood vessels outside the heart) maintains circulation in the cochlea during exposure to noise. These findings may lead to the development of treatment strategies to reduce NIHL.

Continuing efforts will provide opportunities that can aid research on NIHL as well as other diseases and disorders that cause hearing loss.

Notes

1. Schneider M.E., Belyantseva I.A., Azevedo R.B., Kachar B. Rapid renewal of auditory hair bundles. *Nature*. 22 Aug 2002. 418(6900): 837–38.

Section 12.2

Frequently Asked Questions about Noise and Hearing Loss Prevention

Reprinted from "Noise and Hearing Loss Prevention: Frequently Asked Questions," Centers for Disease Control, National Institute for Occupational Safety and Health. The text of this document is available online at http://www.cdc.gov/niosh/topics/noise/faq/faq.html#losehearing; accessed September 6, 2005.

Don't we lose our hearing as we age?

It's true that most people's hearing test gets worse as they get older. But for the average person, aging does not cause impaired hearing before at least the age of sixty. People who are not exposed to noise and are otherwise healthy keep their hearing for many years. People who are exposed to noise and do not protect their hearing begin to lose their hearing at an early age. For example, by age twenty-five the average carpenter has "fifty-year-old" ears! That is, by age twenty-five, the average carpenter has the same hearing as someone who is fifty years old and has worked in a quiet job.

Can you poke out your eardrums with earplugs?

That is unlikely for two reasons. First, the average ear canal is about 1 1/4 inches long. The typical earplug is between 1/2 and 3/4 of an inch long. So even if you inserted the entire earplug, it would still not touch the eardrum. Second, the path from the opening of the ear canal to the eardrum is not straight. In fact, it is quite irregular. This prevents you from poking objects into the eardrum.

We work in a dusty, dirty place. Should I worry that our ears will get infected by using earplugs?

Using earplugs will not cause an infection. But use common sense. Have clean hands when using earplugs that need to be rolled or formed with your fingers in order for you to insert them. If this is inconvenient, there are plenty of earplugs that are pre-molded or that have stems so that you can insert them without having to touch the part that goes into the ear canal.

Can you hear warning sounds, such as backup beeps, when wearing hearing protectors?

The fact is that there are fatal injuries because people do not hear warning sounds. However, this is usually because the background noise was too high or because the person had severe hearing loss, not because someone was wearing hearing protectors. Using hearing protectors will bring both the noise and the warning sound down equally. So if the warning sound is audible without the hearing protector, it will usually be audible when wearing the hearing protector. For the unusual situations where this is not the case, the solution may be as simple as using a different hearing protector. Also, many warning systems can be adjusted or changed so warning signals are easier to detect.

Won't hearing protectors interfere with our ability to hear important sounds our machinery and equipment make?

Hearing protectors will lower the noise level of your equipment; it won't eliminate it. However, some hearing protectors will reduce certain frequencies more than others; so wearing them can make noises sound different. In cases where it's important that the sound just be quieter without any other changes, there are hearing protectors that can provide flat attenuation.

There are also noise-activated hearing protectors that allow normal sounds to pass through the ear and only "turn-on" when the noise reaches hazardous levels. There are even protectors that professional concert musicians use that can lower the sound level while retaining sound fidelity.

Will we be able to hear each other talk when wearing hearing protectors?

Some people find they can wear hearing protectors and still understand speech. Others will have trouble hearing speech while wearing hearing protectors. Being able to hear what other people say depends on many things: distance from the speaker, ability to see the speaker's face, general familiarity with the topic, level of background noise, and whether or not one has an existing hearing impairment. In some cases, wearing hearing protectors can make it easier to understand speech.

In other instances, people may be using hearing protectors to keep out too much sound. You may need a protector that reduces the sound enough to be safe without reducing the sound too much to hear speech at a comfortably loud level. For those people who work in noise and must communicate, it may also be necessary to use communication headsets. Allow your employees to try different protectors. Some will work better than others at helping them to hear speech, and different protectors may work better for different people.

How long does it take to get used to hearing protectors?

Think about getting a new pair of shoes. Some shoes take no time to get used to. Others—even though they are the right size—can take a while to get used to. Hearing protectors are no different from other safety equipment in terms of getting used to them. But if hearing protectors are the wrong size, or are worn out, they will not be comfortable. Also, workers may need more than one kind of protector at their job. For example, no one would wear golf shoes to go bowling. If hearing protectors are not suitable for the work being done, they probably won't feel comfortable.

How long can someone be in a loud noise before it's hazardous?

The degree of hearing hazard is related to both the level of the noise and the duration of the exposure. But this question is like asking how long people can look at the sun without damaging their eyes. The safest thing to do is to ensure workers always protect their ears by wearing hearing protectors anytime they are around loud noise.

How can I tell if a noise situation is too loud?

There are two rules: First, if you have to raise your voice to talk to someone who is an arm's length away, then the noise is likely to be hazardous. Second, if your ears are ringing or sounds seem dull or flat after leaving a noisy place, then you probably were exposed to hazardous noise.

How often should your hearing be tested?

Anyone regularly exposed to hazardous noise should have an annual hearing test. Also, anyone who notices a change in his or her hearing (or who develops tinnitus) should have his or her ears checked.

People who have healthy ears and who are not exposed to hazardous noise should get a hearing test every three years.

Since I already have hearing loss and wear a hearing aid, hearing prevention programs don't apply to me, right?

If you have hearing loss, it's important to protect the hearing that you have left. Loud noises can continue to damage your hearing, making it even more difficult to communicate at work and with your family and friends.

Section 12.3

Hearing Protection

Reprinted from "Choose the Hearing Protection that's Right for You," Centers for Disease Control, National Institute for Occupational Safety and Health. The text of this document is available online at http://www.cdc.gov/niosh/topics/noise/abouthlp/chooseprotection.html; accessed October 11, 2005.

There are many types of hearing protection on the market today. The following descriptions will help you to choose the hearing protection that is right for you.

Expandable Foam Plugs

These plugs are made of a formable material designed to expand and conform to the shape of each person's ear canal. Roll the expandable plugs into a thin, crease-free cylinder. Whether you roll plugs with thumb and fingers or across your palm doesn't matter. What's critical is the final result—a smooth tube thin enough that about half the length will fit easily into your ear canal. Some individuals, especially women with small ear canals, have difficulty rolling typical plugs small enough to make them fit. A few manufacturers now offer a small size expandable plug.

Pre-Molded, Reusable Plugs

Pre-molded plugs are made from silicone, plastic, or rubber and are either manufactured as "one-size-fits-most" or available in several sizes. Many pre-molded plugs are available in sizes for small, medium, or large ear canals.

A critical tip about pre-molded plugs is that a person may need a different size plug for each ear. The plugs should seal the ear canal without being uncomfortable. This takes trial and error of the various sizes. Directions for fitting each model of pre-molded plug may differ slightly depending on how many flanges they have and how the tip is shaped. Insert this type of plug by reaching over your head with one hand to pull up on your ear. Then use your other hand to insert the plug with a gentle rocking motion until you have sealed the ear canal.

Advantages of pre-molded plugs are that they are relatively inexpensive, reusable, washable, convenient to carry, and come in a variety of sizes. Nearly everyone can find a plug that will be comfortable and effective. In dirty or dusty environments, you don't need to handle or roll the tips.

Canal Caps

Canal caps often resemble earplugs on a flexible plastic or metal band. The earplug tips of a canal cap may be a formable or pre-molded material. Some have headbands that can be worn over the head, behind the neck, or under the chin. Newer models have jointed bands increasing the ability to properly seal the earplug.

The main advantage canal caps offer is convenience. When it's quiet, employees can leave the band hanging around their necks. They can quickly insert the plug tips when hazardous noise starts again. Some people find the pressure from the bands uncomfortable. Not all canal caps have tips that adequately block all types of noise. Generally, the canal caps tips that resemble stand-alone earplugs seem to block the most noise.

Earmuffs

Earmuffs come in many models designed to fit most people. They work to block out noise by completely covering the outer ear. Muffs can be "low profile," with small ear cups, or large enough to hold extra materials for use in extreme noise. Some muffs also include electronic components to help users communicate or to block impulsive noises.

Workers who have heavy beards or sideburns or who wear glasses may find it difficult to get good protection from earmuffs. The hair and the temples of the glasses break the seal that the earmuff cushions make around the ear. For these workers, earplugs are best. Other potential drawbacks of earmuffs are that some people feel they can be hot and heavy in some environments.

Miscellaneous Devices

Manufacturers are receptive to comments from hearing protection users. This has led to the development of new devices that are hybrids of the traditional types of hearing protectors. Because many people like the comfort of foam plugs, but don't want to roll them in dirty environments, a plug is now available that is essentially a foam tip on a stem. You insert this plug much like a pre-molded plug without rolling the foam.

Scientists are developing earmuffs using high-tech materials to reduce weight and bulk, but still effectively block noise. On the horizon may be earplugs with built in two-way communication capability.

Still, the best hearing protector is the one that is comfortable and convenient and that you will wear every time you are in an environment with hazardous noise.

Section 12.4

Risk to Hearing from Personal Stereo Systems

Warning: Personal Stereo Systems May Be More Than Just Music To Your Ears

Personal stereo systems with headphones ("Walkman-type") have become an almost required accessory for today's teenagers. Commuters, joggers, health club patrons, factory workers, and office workers are also seen using these systems. Several studies have looked at the maximum output levels of personal stereo systems with headphones and have found that these levels pose a risk to the listener's hearing (Clark, 1991).

How Loud Is Too Loud?

To know if a sound is loud enough to cause a damage to your ears, it is important to know both the level of intensity (measured in decibels, dBA) and the length of exposure to the sound. In general, the louder the sound, the less time required before hearing will be affected. Experts agree that continued exposure to noise above 85 dBA (approximately the level of a city street), over time, will eventually harm your hearing.

Personal Stereo Systems: The Facts

Personal stereo systems with headphones produce sounds as loud as 105–120 dBA if turned up to maximum levels. Some studies concluded that in the majority of cases, unless the exposure time continued for several hours a day, over several years, the risk may be minimal (Findlay, 1974). More recent studies concluded that personal stereo systems present a hazard to hearing for a substantial portion of listeners (Catalano and Levin, 1985). In 1998, the League for the Hard of Hearing conducted a pilot study in conjunction with the City University of New York and found the maximum output level of personal stereo systems to be 112 dBA. Although subjects interviewed set the systems at safe listening levels in quiet settings, they reported increasing the volume to hazardous levels while riding the subway, exercising, or walking to and from work. Although guidelines in the workplace have been established to protect a worker's hearing, the same protection is not available for the use of personal stereo systems with headphones. The consumer must, therefore, take full responsibility for preserving hearing.

Steps to Protect Your Hearing While Listening to Personal Stereo Systems

To determine if you are at risk for a noise-induced hearing loss from wearing your personal stereo system, it would be necessary to know how loud your particular system is and how long you use it each day. Since systems vary in output, it is important to follow these simple steps to protect yourself from a permanent noise-induced hearing loss due to personal stereo system use:

- Look for a personal stereo system with an "automatic volume limiter," which limits the output of the system to safe levels. Sony Walkman and Sony Sport both include an automatic volume limiter and limit the output at 85 dBA.

- Set your system at a comfortable level in a quiet room. Do not turn it up when you are in a noisy setting to "block out" the noise. This will only add to the noise and increase the risk to your hearing.

- Limit the amount of time you use the personal stereo system with headphones.

- Do not interchange headsets with systems. The League for the Hard of Hearing has found that this will increase output and risk to hearing.

- Follow this simple rule of thumb: If you cannot hear other people talking when you are wearing headphones or if other people have to shout to you to be heard at three feet away while the headphones are on, it is too loud and could be damaging to your hearing.

- If you notice any ringing in your ears, or that speech sounds are muffled after wearing a personal stereo system, discontinue its use and have your hearing checked by a qualified audiologist.

Chapter 13

Bone Disorders Can Lead to Hearing Loss

For people with metabolic bone disorders such as Paget disease of bone or osteogenesis imperfecta, hearing loss is an often overlooked yet serious handicap. To understand the nature of hearing loss in individuals with metabolic bone disorders, it is important to first understand the basic mechanism of hearing.

Anatomy of the Ear

The ear is divided into three sections: the external, middle, and inner ear. The external ear includes the outer ear and the ear canal, at the end of which is the eardrum. Behind the eardrum is a small chamber called the middle ear. The middle ear contains three tiny bones (the incus, the malleus, and the stapes) that connect the eardrum and the inner ear; they act in series to transmit airborne sound through the middle ear to the cochlea in the inner ear. Once the sound (or vibration) reaches the cochlea, it is converted into nerve impulses and transmitted by the auditory nerve to the brain, where it is interpreted. A person with a hearing impairment might have a problem in the middle ear, inner ear, auditory nerve, brain, or more than one of these areas.

Reprinted from "Hearing Loss and Bone Disorders," National Institutes of Health Osteoporosis and Related Bone Diseases National Resource Center, November 2000.

Types of Hearing Loss

The three primary types of hearing impairment are: conductive, sensorineural, or mixed. When hearing loss is caused by a physical problem in the external ear or in the middle ear, it is referred to as a conductive hearing loss. Sensorineural hearing loss occurs when a sound is conducted normally from the exterior ear through the eardrum to the middle ear, but the inner ear does not transmit the sound normally to the brain. When the middle ear and the inner ear are involved, the hearing loss is referred to as a mixed hearing loss. Hearing loss is also classified according to degree of severity—mild, moderate, severe, or profound—and according to whether the hearing loss affects low, high, or all frequencies of sound.

Hearing Loss in Osteogenesis Imperfecta

As many as 50 percent of people with osteogenesis imperfecta (OI) experience hearing loss beginning early in adulthood. It generally appears as a conductive loss in the late teens or twenties due to problems with the small bones in the middle ear. They may be fragile or malformed, or the footplate of the stapes may become fixed and rigid and no longer capable of transmitting sound effectively to the inner ear. Changes can also be observed in other areas of the middle and inner ear. A sensorineural (nerve) loss may also develop. There is much variation in the severity of the hearing loss; some people may be deaf in old age, while others may be hard of hearing. Some people with OI never develop significant hearing problems.

Management

It is recommended that any child with OI, and especially those who demonstrate speech problems, speech delay, or recurrent ear infections, should undergo a formal audiologic assessment. Young adults should have baseline assessment for later comparison, and adults experiencing tinnitus (ringing), often an early symptom of a fixed stapes, should undergo audiologic assessment. For either conductive, sensorineural, or mixed hearing loss, hearing aids that provide adequate amplification can help individuals of all ages.

Individuals with conductive loss that is severe and progressive may be helped with a surgical procedure known as a stapedectomy. In this procedure, the fixed foot process of the stapes is replaced by a prosthesis that allows for the normal propagation of sound waves to the inner ear. It should be noted, however, that this surgery should not be considered routine in OI because of tissue fragility. There are also many other pre- and postoperative issues that need to be assessed, discussed, and clarified before any individual with OI may be considered a "good candidate" for surgery. As a general rule, patients should seek treatment centers where the otologists (doctors with a subspecialty in ear disorders) have considerable experience with stapes surgery.

Hearing Loss in Paget Disease of Bone

Although many people lose some degree of hearing as part of the aging process, individuals with Paget disease are more likely than other people the same age to have a hearing loss. Research studies have shown that Paget disease causes hearing loss when the temporal bone is involved (i.e., the bone surrounding the inner ear), and this hearing loss is usually not due to compression or other effects on the auditory nerve. Paget disease affects the cochlea, the coiled structure of the inner ear that converts sound vibration into nerve impulses. A change in the bone density of the cochlear capsule has also been observed in patients with Paget disease who have a hearing loss, and this change may be associated with hearing loss in Paget disease. When the temporal bone is involved, a more severe and progressive hearing loss may occur that may involve both sides or one side predominantly.

The type of hearing loss in Paget disease may be conductive, sensorineural, or both. Some causes of the conductive component of the hearing loss may be correctable through surgery; however, this type of surgery has been found overall to be less effective than it is when the cause is other than Paget disease.

Management

If a hearing loss is progressive and is due to Paget disease, treating the underlying Paget disease may slow the progression of the hearing loss. Any loss of hearing should be investigated as a medical condition because it may be due to serious or correctable problems such as perforation of the eardrum, infection, or even tumor in rare cases. It is especially important to investigate the cause of hearing loss when it involves one side more than the other because the presence of a tumor is more likely.

It is recommended that persons with Paget disease and hearing loss, or with Paget disease involving the skull, undergo a baseline hearing test and evaluation by an ear, nose, and throat specialist or an otologist. The doctor may also want to study the temporal bone with special tests to determine whether Paget disease is present in the ear.

Hearing loss can cause individuals to miss important communications and to withdraw from full participation in life. Even if hearing loss cannot be corrected with medication or surgery, most hearing loss can be overcome with a hearing aid. Other devices maybe used along with hearing aids and are available through hearing aid specialists and ear, nose, and throat doctors.

Chapter 14

Electronic Hearing Devices

Chapter Contents

Section 14.1

Hearing Aids

Excerpted from "Hearing Aids," National Institute on Deafness and Other Communication Disorders, National Institutes of Health, NIH Publication No. 99-4340, February 2001.

What is a hearing aid?

A hearing aid is an electronic, battery-operated device that amplifies and changes sound to allow for improved communication. Hearing aids receive sound through a microphone, which then converts the sound waves to electrical signals. The amplifier increases the loudness of the signals and then sends the sound to the ear through a speaker.

How common is hearing loss and what causes it?

Approximately twenty-eight million Americans have a hearing impairment. Hearing loss is one of the most prevalent chronic health conditions in the United States, affecting people of all ages, in all segments of the population, and across all socioeconomic levels. Hearing loss affects approximately 17 in 1,000 children under age eighteen. Incidence increases with age: approximately 314 in 1,000 people over age sixty-five have hearing loss. Hearing loss can be hereditary, or it can result from disease, trauma, or long-term exposure to damaging noise or medications. Hearing loss can vary from a mild but important loss of sensitivity, to a total loss of hearing.

There are different types of hearing loss. Conductive hearing loss occurs when sound waves are prevented from passing to the inner ear. This can be caused by a variety of problems including buildup of earwax (cerumen), infection, fluid in the middle ear (ear infection or otitis media), or a punctured eardrum. Sensorineural (nerve) hearing loss develops when the auditory nerve or hair cells in the inner ear are damaged by aging, noise, illness, injury, infection, head trauma, toxic medications, or an inherited condition. Mixed hearing loss is a combination of both conductive and sensorineural hearing loss. A conductive hearing loss can often be corrected with medical or surgical treatment, while sensorineural hearing loss usually cannot be reversed.

People with hearing loss may experience some or all of the following problems:

- Difficulty hearing conversations, especially when there is background noise.
- Hissing, roaring, or ringing in the ears (tinnitus).
- Difficulty hearing the television or radio at a normal volume.
- Fatigue and irritation caused by the effort to hear.
- Dizziness or problems with balance.

How can I find out if I have hearing loss?

If you think you might have hearing loss, visit your physician, who may refer you to an otolaryngologist or audiologist. An otolaryngologist is a physician who specializes in ear, nose, and throat disorders, and will investigate the cause of the hearing loss. An audiologist is a hearing health professional who identifies and measures hearing loss and will perform a hearing test to assess the type and degree of loss.

How can hearing aids help?

On the basis of the hearing test results, the audiologist can determine whether hearing aids will help. Hearing aids are particularly useful in improving the hearing and speech comprehension of people with sensorineural hearing loss. When choosing a hearing aid, the audiologist will consider your hearing ability, work and home activities, physical limitations, medical conditions, and cosmetic preferences. For many people, cost is also an important factor. You and your audiologist must decide whether one or two hearing aids will be best for you. Wearing two hearing aids may help balance sounds, improve your understanding of words in noisy situations, and make it easier to locate the source of sounds.

What are the different kinds of hearing aids?

There are several types of hearing aids. Each type offers different advantages, depending on its design, levels of amplification, and size. Before purchasing any hearing aid, ask whether it has a warranty that will allow you to try it out. Most manufacturers allow a thirty- to sixty-day trial period during which aids can be returned for a refund.

There are four basic styles of hearing aids for people with sensorineural hearing loss:

- **In-the-ear (ITE) hearing aids** fit completely in the outer ear and are used for mild to severe hearing loss. The case, which holds the components, is made of hard plastic. ITE aids can accommodate added technical mechanisms such as a telecoil, a small magnetic coil contained in the hearing aid that improves sound transmission during telephone calls. ITE aids can be damaged by earwax and ear drainage, and their small size can cause adjustment problems and feedback. They are not usually worn by children because the casings need to be replaced as the ear grows.

- **Behind-the-ear (BTE) hearing aids** are worn behind the ear and are connected to a plastic ear mold that fits inside the outer ear. The components are held in a case behind the ear. Sound travels through the ear mold into the ear. BTE aids are used by people of all ages for mild to profound hearing loss. Poorly fitting BTE ear molds may cause feedback, a whistle sound caused by the fit of the hearing aid or by buildup of earwax or fluid.

- **Canal aids** fit into the ear canal and are available in two sizes. The in-the-canal (ITC) hearing aid is customized to fit the size and shape of the ear canal and is used for mild or moderately severe hearing loss. A completely-in-canal (CIC) hearing aid is largely concealed in the ear canal and is used for mild to moderately severe hearing loss. Because of their small size, canal aids may be difficult for the user to adjust and remove, and may not be able to hold additional devices, such as a telecoil. Canal aids can also be damaged by earwax and ear drainage. They are not typically recommended for children.

- **Body aids** are used by people with profound hearing loss. The aid is attached to a belt or a pocket and connected to the ear by a wire. Because of its large size, it is able to incorporate many signal processing options, but it is usually used only when other types of aids cannot be used.

Do all hearing aids work the same way?

The inside mechanisms of hearing aids vary among devices, even if they are the same style. Three types of circuitry, or electronics, are used:

- **Analog/adjustable:** The audiologist determines the volume and other specifications you need in your hearing aid, and then a laboratory builds the aid to meet those specifications. The audiologist retains some flexibility to make adjustments. This type of circuitry is generally the least expensive.

- **Analog/programmable:** The audiologist uses a computer to program your hearing aid. The circuitry of analog/programmable hearing aids will accommodate more than one program or setting. If the aid is equipped with a remote control device, the wearer can change the program to accommodate a given listening environment. Analog/programmable circuitry can be used in all types of hearing aids.

- **Digital/programmable:** The audiologist programs the hearing aid with a computer and can adjust the sound quality and response time on an individual basis. Digital hearing aids use a microphone, receiver, battery, and computer chip. Digital circuitry provides the most flexibility for the audiologist to make adjustments for the hearing aid. Digital circuitry can be used in all types of hearing aids and is typically the most expensive.

What can I expect from my hearing aids?

Using hearing aids successfully takes time and patience. Hearing aids will not restore normal hearing or eliminate background noise. Adjusting to a hearing aid is a gradual process that involves learning to listen in a variety of environments and becoming accustomed to hearing different sounds. Try to become familiar with hearing aids under nonstressful circumstances a few hours at a time. Programs are available to help users master new listening techniques and develop skills to manage hearing loss. Contact your audiologist for further information about programs that may suit your individual needs.

What questions should I ask before buying hearing aids?

Before you buy a hearing aid, ask your audiologist these important questions:

- Are there any medical or surgical considerations or corrections for my hearing loss?
- Which design is best for my hearing loss?
- What is the total cost of the hearing aid?

- Is there a trial period to test the hearing aids? What fees are nonrefundable if they are returned after the trial period?

- How long is the warranty? Can it be extended?

- Does the warranty cover future maintenance and repairs?

- Can the audiologist make adjustments and provide servicing and minor repairs? Will loaner aids be provided when repairs are needed?

- What instruction does the audiologist provide?

- Can assistive devices such as a telecoil be used with the hearing aids?

What problems might I experience while adjusting to my hearing aids?

Become familiar with your hearing aid. Your audiologist will teach you to use and care for your hearing aids. Also, be sure to practice putting in and taking out the aids, adjusting volume control, cleaning, identifying right and left aids, and replacing the batteries with the audiologist present.

The hearing aids may be uncomfortable. Ask the audiologist how long you should wear your hearing aids during the adjustment period. Also, ask how to test them in situations where you have problems hearing, and how to adjust the volume or program for sounds that are too loud or too soft.

Your own voice may sound too loud. This is called the occlusion effect and is very common for new hearing aid users. Your audiologist may or may not be able to correct this problem; however, most people get used to it over time.

Your hearing aid may "whistle." When this happens, you are experiencing feedback, which is caused by the fit of the hearing aid or by the buildup of earwax or fluid. See your audiologist for adjustments.

You may hear background noise. Keep in mind that a hearing aid does not completely separate the sounds you want to hear from the ones you do not want to hear, but there may also be a problem with the hearing aid. Discuss this with your audiologist.

What are some tips for taking care of my hearing aids?

The following suggestions will help you care for your hearing aids:

- Keep hearing aids away from heat and moisture.

- Replace dead batteries immediately.
- Clean hearing aids as instructed.
- Do not use hairspray or other hair care products while wearing hearing aids.
- Turn off hearing aids when they are not in use.
- Keep replacement batteries and small aids away from children and pets.

What research is being done on hearing aids?

The National Institute on Deafness and Other Communication Disorders (NIDCD) supports more than thirty grants for scientists to conduct studies on hearing aid research and development. These studies cover areas such as the application of new signal processing strategies and ways to improve sound transmission and reduce noise interference, as well as psychophysical studies of the impact of abnormal hearing function on speech recognition. Other studies focus on the best way to select and fit hearing aids in children and other difficult-to-test populations, and on reducing bothersome aspects such as feedback and the occlusion effect. Further research will determine the best ways to manipulate speech signals in order to enhance understanding.

To improve hearing aid performance, especially in noisy situations, NIDCD has entered into two collaborative ventures. The first was formed between NIDCD and the Department of Veterans Affairs (VA) to expand and intensify hearing aid research and development. The program includes a contract for the development of hearing aids as well as clinical trials. The knowledge gained will be used to help people choose the best hearing aid for their particular type of hearing impairment.

In the second collaboration, the National Aeronautics and Space Administration (NASA) and the VA have joined NIDCD in surveying all federal laboratories for acoustic and electronic technologies that might improve hearing aids. The most promising technologies have been presented to auditory scientists and hearing aid manufacturers in the hope of forming research partnerships that will lead to commercial application of these technologies.

Ear, Nose, and Throat Disorders Sourcebook, Second Edition

Section 14.2

Bone-Anchored Hearing Aids

Reprinted with permission of the University of
Maryland Medical Center, www.umm.edu, © 2004.

What is a bone-anchored hearing aid (BAHA)?

The BAHA is a surgically implantable system for treatment of
hearing loss that works through direct bone conduction. It has been
used since 1977, and was cleared by the FDA in 1996 as a treatment
for conductive and mixed hearing losses in the United States. In 2002,
the FDA approved its use for the treatment of unilateral sensorineural hearing loss.

BAHA is used to help people with chronic ear infections, congenital external auditory canal atresia, and single-sided deafness who
cannot benefit from conventional hearing aids. The system is surgically implanted and allows sound to be conducted through the bone
rather than via the middle ear—a process known as direct bone conduction.

How does a BAHA work?

The BAHA consists of three parts: a titanium implant, an external abutment, and a sound processor. The system works by enhanc-
ing natural bone transmission as a pathway for sound to travel to the
inner ear, bypassing the external auditory canal and middle ear. The
titanium implant is placed during a short surgical procedure and over
time naturally integrates with the skull bone. For hearing, the sound
processor transmits sound vibrations through the external abutment
to the titanium implant. The vibrating implant sets up vibrations
within the skull and inner ear that finally stimulate the nerve fibers
of the inner ear, allowing hearing.

Who is a candidate for the BAHA system?

The BAHA is used to rehabilitate people with conductive and mixed
loss hearing impairment. This includes people with chronic infection

of the ear canal, people with absence of or a very narrow ear canal as a result of a congenital ear malformation, infection, or surgery, and people with a single-sided hearing loss as a result of surgery for a vestibular schwannoma (a tumor of the balance and hearing nerves).

Chronic Ear Infection: Treatment for hearing losses with the BAHA is suitable for people with a conductive or mixed hearing impairment caused by a chronic infection of the middle or outer ear that results in a persistent and unpleasant discharge. The first goal, of course, is to manage the infection. In rare cases, chronic infections fail to respond to treatment, but are determined to be nonthreatening. In other cases, infections respond to treatment, but recur with use of a conventional in-the-canal hearing aid. When a hearing aid is placed in a susceptible ear canal, a chronic or recurrent infection may be aggravated by the obstruction of the canal and the resulting excessive humidity and lack of drainage. In these cases, the BAHA may be a good solution for hearing rehabilitation.

The BAHA sound processor transmits sound directly to the hearing nerve without involving the ear canal. With BAHA there is no occlusion of the ear canal to aggravate infection. A BAHA sound processor offers sound quality at least as good as a conventional air conduction device. For those who need high levels of amplification, problems related to feedback and discomfort are usually resolved.

Congenital Hearing Loss: Congenital conductive hearing loss caused by a malformation of the middle or external ear resulting in a missing or incomplete ear canal (external auditory canal atresia) is effectively managed with a BAHA. Traditionally people with this type of hearing loss have been offered an old-fashioned bone-conducting hearing aid. These are either held on the head using a steel spring headband or included in the frame of a pair of glasses. Traditional bone conductors have several disadvantages. The sound quality is poor, as the skin acts as a barrier for the sound to travel to the inner ear. They are uncomfortable—patients complain of pain and headaches due to the constant pressure of the headband. They are also cumbersome, obtrusive, and insecure.

The BAHA system can be a real solution for people with this type of impairment. The BAHA sound processor is directly integrated to the skull bone. Because of this direct interface, the BAHA offers significantly better sound quality than that of a traditional bone conductor. The BAHA sound processor works without pressure on the skin, avoiding the headaches and soreness associated with the conventional bone conductor. BAHA offers excellent wearing comfort and a better aesthetic result.

BAHA for Unilateral Deafness: One ear does not provide adequate hearing in many situations. Patients with severe hearing loss on one side, but normal hearing in the other ear have difficulty understanding speech in background noise (such as group conversations and restaurants) and determining which direction sound comes from. Unilateral deafness can result from viral infections, trauma, acoustic neuromas and other ear tumors, and ear surgery.

Until recently, the best available approach for providing help in this situation has been the CROS (contralateral routing of offside signal) hearing aid. This technique utilized hearing aid microphones worn in both ears and routed sound from the deaf ear to the hearing ear. Unfortunately, most patients were unsatisfied with this system. Common complaints included the cosmetic appearance and discomfort of the headband, and the use of a hearing aid mold in the good ear. Most patients felt the benefit from the device was not worth the disadvantages.

The BAHA, now an FDA-cleared solution for unilateral deafness, provides a completely unique benefit. The BAHA device is placed on the side of the deaf ear, transfers sound through bone conduction, and stimulates the cochlea of the normal hearing ear. The BAHA effectively transmits sounds from the bad side to the normal ear and ultimately results in a sensation of hearing from a deaf ear. Stereo hearing results in improved understanding of speech, especially in background noise, and aids in the localization of sound.

The BAHA offers significant advantages to the traditional CROS hearing aid. The device is placed behind the ear, leaving the canal open. It is worn under the hair and is not perceptible to others. Because it is held in place by a clip and directly integrated with the skull bone, there is no need for a head band and pressure against the skin of the head. In recent clinical trials patients preferred the sound and speech clarity achieved with the BAHA verses the CROS and verses the unaided condition.

Section 14.3

Cochlear Implants

Reprinted from the U.S. Food and Drug Administration,
October 26, 2004.

Cochlear Implants: An Overview

What is a cochlear implant?

A cochlear implant is an implanted electronic hearing device, designed to produce useful hearing sensations to a person with severe
to profound nerve deafness by electrically stimulating nerves inside
the inner ear.

These implants usually consist of two main components:

*   The externally worn microphone, sound processor, and trans-
    mitter system.

*   The implanted receiver and electrode system, which contains
    the electronic circuits that receive signals from the external sys-
    tem and send electrical currents to the inner ear.

Current devices have a magnet that holds the external system in
place next to the implanted internal system. The external system may
be worn entirely behind the ear or its parts may be worn in a pocket,
belt pouch, or harness.

Who uses cochlear implants?

Cochlear implants are designed to help severely to profoundly deaf
adults and children who get little or no benefit from hearing aids. Even
individuals with severe or profound "nerve deafness" may be able to
benefit from cochlear implants.

What determines the success of cochlear implants?

Many things determine the success of implantation. Some of them
are:

- how long the patient has been deaf—as a group, patients who have been deaf for a short time do better than those who have been deaf a long time;

- how old they were when they became deaf—whether they were deaf before they could speak;

- how old they were when they got the cochlear implant—younger patients, as a group, do better than older patients who have been deaf for a long time;

- how long they have used the implant;

- how quickly they learn;

- how good and dedicated their learning support structure is;

- the health and structure of their cochlea—number of nerve (spiral ganglion) cells that they have;

- implanting variables, such as the depth and type of implanted electrode and signal processing technique;

- intelligence and communicativeness of patient.

How does a cochlear implant work?

A cochlear implant receives sound from the outside environment, processes it, and sends small electric currents near the auditory nerve. These electric currents activate the nerve, which then sends a signal to the brain. The brain learns to recognize this signal and the person experiences this as "hearing."

The cochlear implant somewhat simulates natural hearing, where sound creates an electric current that stimulates the auditory nerve. However, the result is not the same as normal hearing.

Why are there different kinds of implants?

Current thinking is that the inner ear responds to sound by at least two separate ways.

One theory, the place theory, says the cochlea responds greater to a simple tone at one place along its length. Another theory is that the ear responds to the timing of the sound.

Researchers, following the place theory, devised implants that separated the sound into groups. For example, they sent the lower pitches to the area of the cochlea where it seemed more responsive to lower pitches. And they sent higher pitches to the area more responsive to high pitches. Thus, they used several channels and electrodes spaced out inside the cochlea. Since there were also timing theories, researchers devised implants that made the sound signals into pulses to see if the cochlea would respond better to various kinds of pulses.

Most modern cochlear implants are versatile, in that they are somewhat capable of being adjusted to respond to sound in various ways. Audiologists try a variety of adjustments to see what works best with a particular patient.

How long have cochlear implants been available?

The first commercial devices were approved by the FDA in the mid-1980s. However, research with this device began in the 1950s.

Benefits and Risks of Cochlear Implants

What are the benefits of cochlear implants?

People with implants may experience the following:

- Hearing ranges from near normal ability to understand speech to no hearing benefit at all.

- Adults often benefit immediately and continue to improve for about three months after the initial tuning sessions. Then, although performance continues to improve, improvements are slower. Cochlear implant users' performances may continue to improve for several years.

- Children may improve at a slower pace. A lot of training is needed after implantation to help the child use the new "hearing" he or she now experiences.

- Most perceive loud, medium, and soft sounds. People report that they can perceive different types of sounds, such as footsteps, slamming of doors, sounds of engines, ringing of the telephone, barking of dogs, whistling of the tea kettle, rustling of leaves, the sound of a light switch being switched on and off, and so on.

- Many understand speech without lip-reading. However, even if this is not possible, using the implant helps lip-reading.

- Many can make telephone calls and understand familiar voices over the telephone. Some good performers can make normal telephone calls and even understand an unfamiliar speaker. However, not all people who have implants are able to use the phone.

- Many can watch TV more easily, especially when they can also see the speaker's face. However, listening to the radio is often more difficult as there are no visual cues available.

- Some can enjoy music. Some enjoy the sound of certain instruments (piano or guitar, for example) and certain voices. Others do not hear well enough to enjoy music.

What are the risks of cochlear implants?

General Anesthesia Risks

- General anesthesia is drug-induced sleep. The drugs, such as anesthetic gases and injected drugs, may affect people differently. For most people, the risk of general anesthesia is very low. However, for some people with certain medical conditions, it is more risky.

Risks from the Surgical Implant Procedure

- Injury to the facial nerve: this nerve goes through the middle ear to give movement to the muscles of the face. It lies close to where the surgeon needs to place the implant, and thus it can be injured during the surgery. An injury can cause a temporary or permanent weakening or full paralysis on the same side of the face as the implant.

- Meningitis: this is an infection of the lining of the surface of the brain. People who have abnormally formed inner ear structures appear to be at greater risk of this rare, but serious complication. For further information on the risk of meningitis in cochlear recipients, please refer to the following section in this chapter.

- Cerebrospinal fluid leakage: the brain is surrounded by fluid that may leak from a hole created in the inner ear or elsewhere from a hole in the covering of the brain as a result of the surgical procedure.

- Perilymph fluid leak: the inner ear or cochlea contains fluid. This fluid can leak through the hole that was created to place the implant.

- Infection of the skin wound.

- Blood or fluid collection at the site of surgery.

- Attacks of dizziness or vertigo.

- Tinnitus, which is a ringing or buzzing sound in the ear.

- Taste disturbances: the nerve that gives taste sensation to the tongue also goes through the middle ear and might be injured during the surgery.

- Numbness around the ear.

- Reparative granuloma: this is the result of localized inflammation that can occur if the body rejects the implant.

- There may be other unforeseen complications that could occur with long term implantation that we cannot now predict.

Other Risks Associated with the Use of Cochlear Implants

People with a cochlear implant may experience the following risks:

- May hear sounds differently. Sound impressions from an implant differ from normal hearing, according to people who could hear before they became deaf. At first, users describe the sound as "mechanical," "technical," or "synthetic." This perception changes over time, and most users do not notice this artificial sound quality after a few weeks of cochlear implant use.

- May lose residual hearing. The implant may destroy any remaining hearing in the implanted ear.

- May have unknown and uncertain effects. The cochlear implant stimulates the nerves directly with electrical currents. Although this stimulation appears to be safe, the long-term effect of these electrical currents on the nerves is unknown.

- May not hear as well as others who have had successful outcomes with their implants.

- May not be able to understand language well. There is no test a person can take before surgery that will predict how well he or she will understand language after surgery.

- May have to have it removed temporarily or permanently if an infection develops after the implant surgery. However, this is a rare complication.

- May have their implant fail. In this situation, a person with an implant would need to have additional surgery to resolve this problem and would be exposed to the risks of surgery again.

- May not be able to upgrade their implant when new external components become available. Implanted parts are usually compatible with improved external parts. That way, as advances in technology develop, a person can upgrade his or her implant by changing only its external parts. In some cases, though, this won't work and the implant will need changing.

- May not be able to have some medical examinations and treatments. These treatments include the following:

  - MRI imaging: MRI is becoming a more routine diagnostic method for early detection of medical problems. Even being close to an MRI imaging unit will be dangerous because it may dislodge the implant or demagnetize its internal magnet. The FDA has approved some implants, however, for some types of MRI studies done under controlled conditions.

  - neurostimulation

  - electrical surgery

  - electroconvulsive therapy

  - ionic radiation therapy

- Will depend on batteries for hearing. For some devices new or recharged batteries are needed every day.

- May damage their implant. Contact sports, automobile accidents, slips and falls, or other impacts near the ear can damage the implant. This may mean needing a new implant and more surgery. It is unknown whether a new implant will work as well as the old one.

- May find them expensive. Replacing damaged or lost parts may be expensive.

- Will have to use it for the rest of life. During a person's lifetime, the manufacturer of the cochlear implant could go out of business. Whether a person will be able to get replacement parts or other customer service in the future is uncertain.

- May have lifestyle changes because their implant will interact with the electronic environment. An implant may do the following:

  - set off theft detection systems

  - set off metal detectors or other security systems

  - be affected by cellular phone users or other radio transmitters

- have to be turned off during takeoffs and landings in aircraft
- interact in unpredictable ways with other computer systems

- Will have to be careful of static electricity. Static electricity may temporarily or permanently damage a cochlear implant. It may be good practice to remove the processor and headset before contact with static-generating materials such as children's plastic play equipment, TV screens, computer monitors, or synthetic fabric. For more details regarding how to deal with static electricity, contact the manufacturer or implant center.

- Have less ability to hear both soft sounds and loud sounds without changing the sensitivity of the implant. The sensitivity of normal hearing is adjusted continuously by the brain, but the design of cochlear implants requires that a person manually change the sensitivity setting of the device as the sound environment changes.

- May develop irritation where the external part rubs on the skin and have to remove it for a while.

- Can't let the external parts get wet. Damage from water may be expensive to repair and the person may be without hearing until the implant is repaired. Thus, the person will need to remove the external parts of the device when bathing, showering, swimming, or participating in water sports.

- May hear strange sounds caused by its interaction with magnetic fields, like those near airport passenger screening machines.

Frequently Asked Questions

How is the external transmitter held in place correctly?

Usually, the transmitter and receiver contain magnets, which attract each other to stay aligned.

Can the sound processor be removed at night?

Yes. But you should turn it off to save the battery. Some users wear the sound processor all night so they can hear.

Can I use the implant while playing sports?

Probably. Most implants are durable enough to allow playing sports. However, the external parts of most are not waterproof, so you would have to remove them before swimming or other water sports. Deep water diving may harm the internal implant due to the high water pressure.

How long does it take me to get maximum benefit from a cochlear implant?

It depends a lot on you and your rehabilitation group. It depends on how long you have been without hearing. It depends on whether you could speak well before you lost your hearing. Usually, there is a rapid rise in your ability to interpret the sounds after receiving an implant. This rapid rise slows after about three months but continues.

What sounds can be heard with a cochlear implant?

You will probably hear most sounds of medium to high loudness. Patients often report that they can hear footsteps, slamming of doors, ringing telephones, car engines, barking dogs, lawn mowers, and various other environmental sounds. You may hear some softer sounds too.

Will the cochlear implant help me control the loudness of my voice?

Yes. The cochlear implant usually helps you control the loudness of your voice because you can hear your voice in relation to background sounds.

Do those who have an implant system use it?

Yes. Most people use their processors routinely from morning to night. Adults who have never been able to hear have the most difficult time learning spoken language and dealing with the sensation of hearing. Some of these adults may give up and stop using their implant.

Insurance Questions

Do insurance companies pay for cochlear implants?

Because cochlear implants are recognized as standard treatment for severe to profound nerve deafness, most insurance companies cover them. Medicare, Medicaid, the Veteran's Administration, and other public health care plans cover cochlear implants. More than 90 percent of all commercial health plans cover cochlear implants. Cochlear implant centers usually take the responsibility of obtaining prior authorization from the appropriate insurance company before proceeding with surgery.

Do I pay for the repairs?

Maybe. You will not have to pay for repairs if they are covered by a warranty or if you have insurance that covers repairs. Many health plans do not include specific benefits to cover repairs and replacement of parts for cochlear implants. However, the policy may have durable medical equipment (DME) benefits that can be applied. Read your benefits booklet for DME or prosthetic repair benefits, or check with the health plan.

My health plan has denied coverage for a cochlear implant. How can I appeal?

First, determine specifically why the cochlear implant was denied. Make sure you have the denial in writing. If you do not receive a written denial, ask for one. An appeal is most effective when structured in response to the specific reason for denial of coverage. If a specific denial reason is not provided, contact the plan and ask for clarification. Second, contact your cochlear implant center and advocacy groups and ask for help.

My health plan informs me that I have exhausted my rehabilitation benefits. How can I appeal this decision and obtain coverage for additional audiology or speech therapy services?

Many health plans have limited rehabilitation services. They have a predetermined cut-off point for postoperative cochlear implant services. However, you may be able to get extended medical benefits based on your need for more services by having your clinician argue your case. You may have an easier case if your child is the implant user. The manufacturer of your implant may help your clinician develop the case.

How can I insure my external parts against theft, damage, or loss?

External parts, if purchased new, probably carry a warranty from the manufacturer against defects and materials. Usually, under such warranties, equipment lost, damaged beyond repair, or stolen will be replaced one time at no cost.

After the warranty expires, you may have some options, such as:

- buying a service contract from the implant manufacturer;

- getting repair and replacement coverage through your health plan;

- getting coverage through your personal home property and casualty or homeowner's policy.

What Educators Need to Know about Their Students with Cochlear Implants

- Cochlear implants do not make hearing normal.

- Benefit of an implant depends, in part, on the:
  - type of communication training (total communication, auditory-oral communication, cued speech, etc.) a student used before the implant;
  - type of communication the student uses after the implant.

- To get maximum benefit from a cochlear implant, a student will need individual training, such as:
  - speech training;
  - lip reading training;
  - auditory training.

- To progress with their classmates, students with cochlear implants may still need special accommodation in the classroom:
  - preferential seating
  - a note taker
  - a quiet environment, away from air handlers and other noise
  - a sign-language interpreter or cued speech interpreter

- Students need time to adjust and accommodate to their cochlear implants. The amount of time they need varies. During the accommodation period, students need language input from all sources they used before their implants.

- Educators should treat their students with cochlear implants as individuals, each having particular communication needs. Students don't get equal benefits from cochlear implants.

- Students with cochlear implants may find it harder to:
  - digest new and difficult subject matter;
  - interact in unfamiliar and complex social situations.
- Educators should be aware that frequent changes to educational programs involving students with cochlear implants (program hopping) may impede learning.
- Educators can help their students in other ways to achieve full benefits from cochlear implants:
  - intervening early when there appears to be a problem
  - promoting family counseling
  - promoting specialized speech and language therapies
  - explaining to families that speech and language are not the same thing, and that education is based on language development
  - getting more information and support from local and national organizations of teachers of the hearing impaired
- To assure that students with cochlear implants don't fall behind their classmates, educators should frequently evaluate them and their educational settings.
- Particularly for their younger students, educators need to assure that external cochlear implant components are securely attached or removed during active school events. The components are expensive and are easily lost or damaged.
- Students will often need extra batteries, either new or recharged, for their implants to work.
- Students with cochlear implants are usually not able to interpret complex auditory signals, such as those in music.

Before, During, and After Implant Surgery

What happens before surgery?

Primary care doctors usually refer patients to ear, nose, and throat doctors (ENT doctors or otolaryngologists) to test them to see if they are candidates for cochlear implants.

Tests often done include the following:

- examination of external, middle, and inner ear for signs of infection or abnormality

- various tests of hearing, such as an audiogram
- a trial of hearing aid use to assess its potential benefit
- exams to evaluate middle and inner ear structures:
    - CT (computerized tomography) scan. This type of x-ray helps the doctor see if the cochlea has a normal shape. This scan is especially important if the patient has a history of meningitis because it helps see if there is new bone growth in the cochlea that could interfere with the insertion of the implant. This scan also may indicate which ear should be implanted.
    - MRI (magnetic resonance imaging) scan
- psychological examination to see if the patient can cope with the implant
- physical exam to prepare for general anesthesia

What happens during surgery?

The doctor or other hospital staff may:

- insert some intravenous (i.v.) lines;
- shave or clean the scalp around the site of the implant;
- attach cables, monitors, and patches to the patient's skin to monitor vital signs;
- put a mask on the patient's face to provide oxygen and anesthetic gas;
- administer drugs through the i.v. and the face mask to cause sleep and general anesthesia;
- awaken the patient in the operating room and take him or her to a recovery room until all the anesthesia is gone.

What happens after surgery?

Immediately after waking, a patient may feel:

- pressure or discomfort over his (or her) implanted ear;
- dizziness;
- queasiness (have nausea);
- disoriented or confused for a while;
- soreness in the throat for a while from the breathing tube used during general anesthesia.

Then, a patient can expect to:

- keep the bandages on for a while;
- have the bandages be stained with some blood or fluid;
- go home in about a day after surgery;
- have stitches for a while;
- get instructions about caring for the stitches, washing the head, showering, and general care and diet;
- have an appointment in about a week to have the stitches removed and have the implant site examined;
- have the implant "turned on" (activated) about three to six weeks later;

Can a patient hear immediately after the operation?

No. Without the external transmitter part of the implant a patient cannot hear. The clinic will give the patient the external components about a month after the implant surgery in the first programming session.

Why is it necessary to wait three to six weeks after the operation before receiving the external transmitter and sound processor?

The waiting period provides time for the operative incision to heal completely. This usually takes three to six weeks. After the swelling is gone, your clinician can do the first fitting and programming.

What happens during the initial programming session?

An audiologist adjusts the sound processor to fit the implanted patient, tests the patient to ensure that the adjustments are correct, determines what sounds the patient hears, and gives information on the proper care and use of the device.

Is it beneficial if a family member participates in the training program?

Yes! A family member should be included in the training program whenever possible to provide assistance. The family member should know how to manage the operations of the sound processor.

Do patients have more than one implant?

Usually, patients have only one ear implanted, though a few patients have implants in both ears.

How can I help my child receive the most benefit from his or her cochlear implant?

- Try to make hearing and listening as interesting and fun as possible.

- Encourage your child to make noises.

- Talk about things you do as you do them.

- Show your child that he or she can consciously use and evaluate the sounds he or she receives from his or her cochlear implant.

- Realize that the more committed you, your child's teachers, and your health professionals are to helping your child, the more successful he or she will be.

What can I expect a cochlear implant to achieve in my child?

As a group, children are more adaptable and better able to learn than adults. Thus, they can benefit more from a cochlear implant. Significant hearing loss slows a child's ability to learn to talk and affects overall language development. The vocal quality and intelligibility of speech from children using cochlear implants seems to be better than from children who have only acoustic hearing aids.

How important is the active cooperation of the patient?

Extremely important. The patient's willingness to experience new acoustic sounds and cooperate in an auditory training program are critical to the degree of success with the implant. The duration and complexity of the training varies from patient to patient.

Section 14.4

Risk of Bacterial Meningitis in Children with Cochlear Implants

Reprinted from "Risk of Bacterial Meningitis in Children with Cochlear Implants" and "Risk of Bacterial Meningitis in Children with Cochlear Implants: Questions and Answers," Centers for Disease Control and Prevention, Early Hearing Detection and Intervention Program, March 22, 2005.

Background

In summer 2002, the U.S. Food and Drug Administration (FDA) began receiving reports of bacterial meningitis occurring among people who had cochlear implants. In response, the Centers for Disease Control and Prevention (CDC), with the FDA and the health departments of thirty-six states, the District of Columbia, Chicago, and New York City, began an investigation.

Conducting the Study

The purposes of the study were (1) to find out how many children who had cochlear implants got bacterial meningitis afterwards and (2) to find out what factors might make it more likely that someone would get meningitis after getting a cochlear implant. The study was limited to children who were six years of age or younger when they got their implant because the majority of cases reported were in children in this age group, and because children in this age group will receive most implants in the future. Children who had received their implant during the period from January 1, 1997, through August 6, 2002 were included. Potential cases of bacterial meningitis were identified from reports to implant manufacturers, the FDA Adverse Events Reporting System, and CDC and state and local health department tracking systems. In addition, study researchers contacted the parents of all the children in this group to ask them if their child had been seriously ill since getting the implant.

Some Basic Facts about the Study

A total of 4,262 children six years of age or younger received a cochlear implant during the period from January 1, 1997, through August 6, 2002. This large study group was used to estimate how many of the children with cochlear implants got bacterial meningitis. This number was then compared with the number of children of this age in the general population who got bacterial meningitis.

A smaller study group was used to find what factors made it more likely for someone with an implant to get meningitis. This smaller study was made up of all twenty-six children with confirmed bacterial meningitis and a random sample of two hundred children with implants who did not get bacterial meningitis after receiving the implant.

Detailed interviews of parents were done only for the small study group. A review of medical records was also done.

The study was limited to children who received their cochlear implants in the United States.

Study Findings and Conclusions

The study found that:

- Bacterial meningitis occurred more often in children with all types of cochlear implants than in children of the same age group in the general population.

- The majority of cases of meningitis were caused by *S. pneumoniae*, a type of bacteria.

- Children with an implant with a positioner were much more likely to get bacterial meningitis than children with other types of cochlear implants. (The implant with a positioner was voluntarily taken off the market by the manufacturer in July 2002.)

- Because the study was not able to find out how the positioner increased the risk for bacterial meningitis, it was not clear whether removing the implant would lower the risk and we cannot make recommendations about that. The removal procedure could place the child at risk for meningitis or other related complications following surgery.

- Children with a cochlear implant who had inner ear malformations and cerebrospinal fluid leaks were at increased risk for bacterial meningitis.

Recommendations

- Children should be up-to-date on vaccines at least two weeks before having a cochlear implant if they are not already up-to-date on these vaccinations.

- Parents of children who have already received an implant should check with their child's doctor to ensure that their child is up-to-date on all vaccinations.

- Doctors and other health care providers should review vaccination records of their patients who are cochlear implant recipients or candidates to ensure that they have received pneumococcal vaccinations based on the age-appropriate schedules for high-risk people and that they have received age-appropriate Hib vaccinations.

- Parents of children with cochlear implants should be watchful for possible signs and symptoms of meningitis and seek prompt attention for any bacterial infection their child might have. Any questions parents have about their child's health should be discussed with the child's doctor.

- Parents of children with cochlear implants should also be watchful for signs and symptoms of an ear infection, which can include ear pain, fever, and decreased appetite.

- Parents should seek prompt medical attention for any possible ear infections.

- Parents should talk about the risks and benefits of cochlear implants with their child's doctor and should discuss whether their child has certain medical conditions that might make him or her more likely to get meningitis.

Questions and Answers

What is meningitis and what are its signs and symptoms?

Meningitis is an infection in the fluid that is around the brain and spinal cord. There are two types of meningitis—viral and bacterial. Bacterial is the more serious of the two and is the type that has been reported in people with cochlear implants. Signs and symptoms of meningitis are high fever, headache, stiff neck, nausea or vomiting, discomfort looking into bright lights, and sleepiness or confusion. A young child or infant with meningitis might be sleepy, cranky, or eat less.

What should be done if someone has signs or symptoms of meningitis?

Any person who is showing signs or symptoms of meningitis should seek immediate medical care by contacting his or her doctor or going to a clinic or emergency room. If that person has a cochlear implant, the doctor or other health care provider should be told. The doctor can look at and examine the person and do others tests as needed.

Why wasn't the risk of meningitis for children with an implant compared with the risk for children with severe to profound hearing loss but with no implant?

Children with cochlear implants were not compared with children without implants because the information that would have allowed such a comparison was not available during this study. However, scientists in Denmark, sponsored by CDC, do have access to the needed data and are now working on a joint project that could make such a comparison possible.

Can vaccinations protect children with cochlear implants from getting meningitis?

Some vaccines are very good at preventing meningitis. However, as good as they are, vaccines can't prevent all types of meningitis. Current vaccines protect against the most common strains of bacteria causing meningitis, but they do not protect against all strains.

Are any changes being made to meningitis immunization recommendations for people with cochlear implants?

Before the cochlear implant and meningitis study began, there were no special immunization recommendations for people with cochlear implants. However, in October 2002 (before study results were available), researchers saw that people with cochlear implants might be more likely to get bacterial meningitis, especially pneumococcal meningitis. Because there are two vaccines that can prevent pneumococcal meningitis, CDC recommended that people with cochlear implants get the vaccine using the schedule for people who are at high risk. The findings made in this study agree with that decision and led the Advisory Committee for Immunization Practices to adopt these recommendations on June 19, 2003. Recommendations for the timing and type of pneumococcal vaccination vary with age and each person's vaccination history. The following immunization schedule provides age-specific information. However, any immunization decisions should be talked over with a health care provider.

Use of Pneumococcal Vaccinations for People with Cochlear Implants

- Children younger than two years of age who have cochlear implants should get pneumococcal conjugate vaccine (Prevnar®) according to the routine pneumococcal conjugate vaccination schedule for this age group.

- Children who have cochlear implants, who are two years of age or older, and who have completed the pneumococcal conjugate vaccine (Prevnar®) series should have one dose of the pneumococcal polysaccharide vaccine (Pneumovax® 23). If they have just gotten the pneumococcal conjugate vaccine, they should wait at least two months following the last dose before getting the pneumococcal polysaccharide vaccine.

- Children who have cochlear implants, who are twenty-four through fifty-nine months of age, and who have never had either the pneumococcal conjugate vaccine or the pneumococcal polysaccharide vaccine should get a total of two doses of the pneumococcal conjugate vaccine two or more months apart and then, at least two months later, should get one dose of the pneumococcal polysaccharide vaccine.

- People who have cochlear implants and who are five years of age or older should get one dose of pneumococcal polysaccharide vaccine.

What can parents of children with cochlear implants do to reduce their child's risk of getting meningitis?

First of all, parents need to watch their child for any of the possible signs and symptoms of meningitis, and to get prompt medical attention if the child develops these symptoms. Parents should also seek prompt medical attention if they think their child might have an ear infection or any other bacterial infection. Second, parents should be sure that all of the child's immunizations are up-to-date. In addition, like all children, children with cochlear implants should not be near tobacco smoke because it has been shown to increase the risk for bacterial infections.

Can someone who has lost his or her hearing as a result of having meningitis still get meningitis again?

Yes, anyone who has had bacterial meningitis can get it again. This is true whether or not the first meningitis caused a loss of hearing. A person who gets some kinds of bacterial meningitis might be more likely to get it again.

Have more cases of bacterial meningitis occurred in children with cochlear implants in recent months?

Yes. The study included only the twenty-six children with confirmed bacterial meningitis that occurred before September 15, 2002. In the months since that date, six additional cases of meningitis have occurred in the group of children who received their implant when they were six years of age or younger. Any additional cases of bacterial meningitis in cochlear implant recipients should be reported to CDC's Early Hearing Detection and Intervention Program by calling 1-877-232-4327 (voice), 1-877-232-7672 (TTY).

Chapter 15

Communicating with the Deaf and Hard of Hearing

Chapter Contents

Section 15.1

American Sign Language

Reprinted from "American Sign Language," National Institute on Deafness and Other Communication Disorders, National Institutes of Health, NIH Publication No. 00-4756, February 2000.

What is American Sign Language?

American Sign Language (ASL) is a complete, complex language that employs signs made with the hands and other movements, including facial expressions and postures of the body. It is the first language of many deaf North Americans, and one of several communication options available to deaf people. ASL is said to be the fourth most commonly used language in the United States.

Is sign language the same around the globe?

No one form of sign language is universal. For example, British Sign Language (BSL) differs notably from ASL. Different sign languages are used in different countries or regions.

Where did ASL originate?

The exact beginnings of ASL are not clear. Many people believe that ASL came mostly from French Sign Language (FSL). Others claim that the foundation for ASL existed before FSL was introduced in America in 1817. It was in that year that a French teacher named Laurent Clerc, brought to the United States by Thomas Gallaudet, founded the first school for the deaf in Hartford, Connecticut. Clerc began teaching FSL to Americans, though many of his students were already fluent in their own forms of local, natural sign language. Today's ASL likely contains some of this early American signing. Which language had more to do with the formation of modern ASL is difficult to prove. Modern ASL and FSL share some elements, including a substantial amount of vocabulary. However, they are not mutually comprehensible.

How does ASL compare with spoken language?

In spoken language, the different sounds created by words and tones of voice (intonation) are the most important devices used to communicate. Sign language is based on the idea that sight is the most useful tool a deaf person has to communicate and receive information. Thus, ASL uses hand shape, position, and movement; body movements; gestures; facial expressions; and other visual cues to form its words. Like any other language, fluency in ASL happens only after a long period of study and practice.

Even though ASL is used in America, it is a language completely separate from English. It contains all the fundamental features a language needs to function on its own—it has its own rules for grammar, punctuation, and sentence order. ASL evolves as its users do, and it also allows for regional usage and jargon. Every language expresses its features differently; ASL is no exception. Whereas English speakers often signal a question by using a particular tone of voice, ASL users do so by raising the eyebrows and widening the eyes. Sometimes, ASL users may ask a question by tilting their bodies forward while signaling with their eyes and eyebrows.

Just as with other languages, specific ways of expressing ideas in ASL vary as much as ASL users themselves do. ASL users may choose from synonyms to express common words. ASL also changes regionally, just as certain English words are spoken differently in different parts of the country. Ethnicity, age, and gender are a few more factors that affect ASL usage and contribute to its variety.

Why does ASL become a first language for many deaf people?

Parents are often the source of a child's early acquisition of language. A deaf child who is born to deaf parents who already use ASL will begin to acquire ASL as naturally as a hearing child picks up spoken language from hearing parents. However, language is acquired differently by a deaf child with hearing parents who have no prior experience with ASL. Some hearing parents choose to introduce sign language to their deaf children. Hearing parents who choose to learn sign language often learn it along with their child. Nine out of every ten children who are born deaf are born to parents who hear. Other communication models, based in spoken English, exist apart from ASL, including oral, auditory-verbal, and cued speech. As with any language, interaction with other children and adults is also a significant factor in acquisition.

207

Why emphasize early language learning?

Parents should introduce deaf children to language as early as possible. The earlier any child is exposed to and begins to acquire language, the better that child's communication skills will become. Research suggests that the first six months are the most crucial to a child's development of language skills. All newborns should be screened for deafness or hearing loss before they leave the hospital or within the first month of life. Very early discovery of a child's hearing loss or deafness provides parents with an opportunity to learn about communication options. Parents can then start their child's language learning process during this important stage of development.

What does recent research say about ASL and other sign languages?

Some studies focus on the age of ASL acquisition. Age is a critical issue for people who acquire ASL, whether it is a first or second language. For a person to become fully competent in any language, exposure must begin as early as possible, preferably before school age. Other studies compare the skills of native signers and non-native signers to determine differences in language processing ability. Native signers of ASL consistently display more accomplished sign language ability than non-native signers, again emphasizing the importance of early exposure and acquisition.

Other studies focus on different ASL processing skills. Users of ASL have shown ability to process visual mental images differently than hearing users of English. Though English speakers possess the skills needed to process visual imagery, ASL users demonstrate faster processing ability—suggesting that sign language enhances certain processing functions of the human brain.

Section 15.2

Assistive Listening Devices

Why do we need assistive listening devices?

While the efficacy of modern hearing aids has long been established, many hearing aid users will still experience difficulty hearing in various situations. For these individuals as well as for individuals who do not wear hearing aids, the properly chosen assistive listening device (ALD) can prove invaluable in helping to alleviate these difficulties.

What types of ALDs are there?

ALDs can be divided into two basic categories, alerting devices and communication devices. An alerting (or alarm) device would indicate that something important is occurring, whereas a communication device would facilitate the reception and understanding of spoken material.

What types of things can an alerting device tell us?

An alerting device can tell us that it's time to wake up, there is someone at the door, the telephone is ringing, the baby is crying, or a smoke alarm has gone off.

What are the different ways an alerting device can tell us something important is happening?

An alerting device can indicate that something important is happening by producing sound, extra loud sound, light, vibration, or a combination of some or all of these.

I have trouble hearing my doorbell but live in an apartment and don't want to get an extra loud bell because this might disturb my neighbors. What can I do?

A common problem with doorbells is that the bell cannot be heard in a distant room. There are wireless doorbell systems in which the sound-producing element (or receiver) can be placed at a location far away from the pushbutton (or transmitter), such as a bedroom, basement, or attic. In addition, it is possible to use multiple receivers that can produce sound in more than one location at the same time, which can make it possible to hear the doorbell in different locations within the same house or apartment.

The small battery-operated alarm clocks are just not loud enough for me to hear. What can I do?

Some people use a radio clock set to a loud volume and tuned to a news station. There are still mechanical alarm clocks available which some people find easier to hear. There are also extra loud alarm clocks that can also be used with a flashing light and/or a bed shaker. In addition, there is a small battery-operated vibrating alarm clock that can be placed under the pillow and is especially useful for people who travel.

If I use a flashing light for the doorbell, what happens if I'm in another room when the doorbell rings?

Many flashing light ALDs can also be used with remote receivers. These receivers can be plugged into other outlets in the house or apartment and have an outlet into which a lamp or light bulb can be plugged. When the main unit is activated, the remote units will also be activated, causing the lights that are plugged into them to flash. The main unit communicates with the remote units by sending a high-frequency signal over the house AC wiring so that no additional wiring is required. You can have as many remote units as you need.

If I want to have a remote unit flash a light when the phone or doorbell rings and the light flashes, how do I tell whether the my phone is ringing or there is someone at the door?

The rhythm of the flashing will be very different depending on whether the telephone is ringing or there is someone at the door so that it is very easy to tell them apart.

Are there alarm devices that can be used with body worn receivers?

Body worn receivers are available that will vibrate and indicate the nature of the alarm condition. In addition, there are units specially designed to be used by people that are deaf-blind.

What are some smoke alarm ALD issues?

Individuals with normal hearing can usually hear a smoke alarm even when it has gone off in another room or area of the house so that there is no problem with using separate and independent smoke alarms. Using separate and independent smoke alarms that have flashing lights may present a problem if the individual is in another room and does not see the flashing light. The best type of separate flashing smoke alarms to use in this case would be those units that have the capability of being wired in tandem so that if one of them goes off, all of them will go off so that the flashing can easily be observed no matter where one happens to be within the house or apartment.

In addition to flashing lights, there are also smoke detectors with a built-in radio transmitter that will cause a receiver unit to activate a bed shaker, causing it to vibrate. With this type of system, it is possible to use more than one smoke detector/transmitter so that smoke detection is available at more than one location.

What types of communication ALDs are there?

Basically, communication ALDs are used for the telephone, TV, the movies, theater, lectures, and noisy situations.

I'd like to get a louder telephone—what's out there?

There are a number of possibilities—you may be able to make your present telephone louder (described below). There are also complete telephones available with built-in amplification. These usually have other useful features as well such as a tone control, an extra loud ring, and a flashing light.

What exactly is a T coil?

A telephone coil is a small coil of wire within the hearing aid, activated by a switch on the hearing aid, which allows the hearing aid to pick up the phone signal directly. It will also prevent feedback and cuts out surrounding noise when making a phone call. A telephone whose earpiece emits a magnetic field that can be easily picked up by a hearing aid telephone coil is said to be hearing aid compatible.

211

The telephone coil can also be used to easily and conveniently enable a hearing aid to work with various other types of ALDs.

Can I do anything to make my existing phone louder?

There is a portable snap-on telephone amplifier which can be used with virtually any telephone; however, it may have to be attached and then removed each time the phone is used so that the phone can hang up properly. Also available are in-line telephone amplifiers which can be used with modular phones (where the handset can be unplugged and separated from the desk set) as long as they do not have the dialing keypad in the handset. These can be attached to just about any phone and can be left in place.

What about cordless phones?

There are cordless phones with built-in extra amplification that are available. In addition, some of them have jacks that can be used with a hands-free accessory. Some models also have a special jack into which special accessories such as a neck loop can be plugged.

I travel a lot and sometimes have trouble using local telephones—any suggestions?

Many travelers find the portable snap-on telephone amplifiers very useful. In addition, this device can also be used to turn a non-hearing-aid-compatible telephone into one that is hearing aid compatible.

What is a TTY?

A TTY (teletypewriter; or TDD [telecommunication device for the deaf]) is a device by means of which an individual can type to someone at the other end of the phone line who also has a TTY and can then read the response that has been typed back.

What if I want to communicate with a TTY user but don't have a TTY?

You can go through the national relay system by means of which you speak to a special relay operator (called a communication assistant or CA) who would then type (or relay) the information to the TTY user. The TTY user's typed response is then read back to the hearing caller. This service is available throughout the United States and is accessed by dialing a special toll-free telephone number or by dialing 711.

No matter how loud I turn up my amplified phone, I still have a lot of trouble understanding what is being said— what can I do? I might consider using a TTY but can't type.

Many hard of hearing people who can no longer use a conventional telephone are using a TTY with the relay system in a manner known as voice carry over or VCO. When used in this way, the TTY user is able to read the response of the person at the other end of the line which is typed by the relay operator. When it comes time for the TTY user to respond, he or she can just speak the way he or she normally would and his or her voice is then heard directly by the party at the other end. There are VCO/TTY telephones available that are specially designed to do this.

What about using a cell phone with my hearing aid?

There can be problems of interference when using a hearing aid with a telephone coil with a digital cell phone; however, there are certain digital cell phones that do seem to work well with hearing aids with t-switches. For those cell phones that do cause interference, there are accessories available such as hearing-aid-compatible, hands-free attachments or special neck loop or silhouette coils that permit the cell phone to be used at some distance away from the hearing aid, thus reducing or eliminating this interference.

My TV is not clear and my neighbors complain that I have it on too loud. What can I do?

A very simple solution would be the use of a remote loudspeaker that serves to bring the sound closer to the listener, which would permit lower volume to be used and result in a clearer sound. Another option would be the use of a TV radio which does the same thing but will work only for transmitted channels numbers two through thirteen and not for special cable channels. There are also special radio frequency and infrared systems described below.

I wear a hearing aid and have a particularly difficult time in noise—what can I do?

Anything that will bring the speaker closer to your hearing aid will significantly improve this situation and to this end, an external microphone used with direct audio input (DAI) is highly recommended. DAI allows you to plug external devices into your hearing aid but only if your hearing aid has this feature.

What if I am twenty-five feet away from the speaker?

Because a twenty-five-foot cord would be cumbersome, you could use a personal FM system that consists of a microphone and small body-worn radio transmitter worn by the speaker and a small radio receiver that you wear that can be used either with headphones or with your hearing aid if your hearing aid has a telephone switch and/ or direct audio input. A personal FM system and external microphone do essentially the same thing, with the difference being that the FM system gives you a wireless capability and is a lot more expensive.

I have an especially hard time understanding what is being said at the theater or at a movie. What can I do?

Wireless headsets (either infrared or FM) should be available at theaters. You can also buy your own system to use at home with TV and then take the receiver with you to the theater or movies but keep in mind that these systems are not standardized and the headset you bring with you may not be compatible with the system in the theater. In addition to various listening systems, some movie theaters and some live theater as well are presenting special performances or showings that are captioned. Also keep in mind that at the movies, even though you may be using very good quality equipment, spoken dialogue may be difficult to understand because of background music and sound effects.

I know that some TV programs are captioned so that I can read what is being said but my TV set does not have this feature. What can I do?

If you own a TV that does not have a built-in decoder chip (a set purchased prior to 1994), you can get an external decoder which will let you see the captions. Please keep in mind that although external decoders are still available, the easiest and most convenient thing to do might be to just purchase a new TV set.

I know that some people who wear hearing aids can use DAI and/or T coils to connect to external devices but I use a cochlear implant—what can I do?

There are special cords known as patch cords that are available which will allow you to connect a telephone or other device directly to your cochlear implant processor if it has an external audio input jack.

Where can I see and try different ALDs?

There are many centers available. You can check with your local Hearing Loss Association of America chapter for local resources.

Where can I purchase ALDs?

ALDs can be purchased from a number of sources, including hearing aid dealers. There are a number of companies that specialize in this type of equipment, most of whom have excellent catalogues. They may also have very informative Internet websites through which devices may be ordered on line.

Section 15.3

Captions for Deaf and Hard of Hearing Viewers

Reprinted from "Captions for Deaf and Hard-of-Hearing Viewers," National Institute on Deafness and Other Communication Disorders, National Institutes of Health, NIH Publication No. 00-4834, July 2002.

On August 5, 1972, Julia Child, "The French Chef," in a program televised from WGBH studios in Boston, taught viewers how to make one of her prized chicken recipes. The significance of that day stretched far beyond the details of the entrée to have a profound and lasting impact on human communication. It was the first time Americans who are deaf and hard of hearing could enjoy the audio portion of a national television program through the use of captions.

Since then, captions have opened the world of television to people who are deaf and hard of hearing. At first, special broadcasts of some of the more popular programs were made accessible through the Public Broadcasting Service. Now, more than two thousand hours of entertainment, news, public affairs, and sports programming are captioned each week on network, public, and cable television. Captions are no longer a novelty; they have become a necessity.

What Are Captions?

Captions are words displayed on a television screen that describe the audio or sound portion of a program. Captions allow viewers who are deaf or hard of hearing to follow the dialogue and the action of a program simultaneously. They can also provide information about who is speaking or about sound effects that may be important to understanding a news story, a political event, or the plot of a program.

Captions are created from the transcript of a program. A captioner separates the dialogue into captions and makes sure the words appear in sync with the audio they describe. A specially designed computer software program encodes the captioning information and combines it with the audio and video to create a new master tape or digital file of the program.

Types of Captions

Open and Closed Captions

Captions may be "open" or "closed." To view closed captions, viewers need a set-top decoder or a television with built-in decoder circuitry. Open captions appear on all television sets and can be viewed without a decoder. In the past, some news bulletins, presidential addresses, or programming created by or for deaf and hard-of-hearing audiences were open captioned. With the widespread availability of closed-caption technology, open captions are rarely used.

Digital Closed Captioning

Closed captioning has become available for digital television sets, such as high-definition television (HDTV) sets, manufactured after July 1, 2002.[1] Digital captioning provides greater flexibility by enabling the viewer to control the caption display, including font style, text size and color, and background color.

Real-Time Captioning

Real-time captions are created as an event takes place. A captioner (often trained as a court reporter or stenographer) uses a stenotype machine with a phonetic keyboard and special software. A computer translates the phonetic symbols into English captions almost instantaneously. The slight delay is based on the captioner's need to hear the word and on the computer processing time. Real-time captioning can be used for programs that have no script; live events, including congressional proceedings; news programs; and nonbroadcast meetings, such as the national meetings of professional associations.

Although most real-time captioning is more than 98 percent accurate, the audience will see occasional errors. The captioner may mishear a word, hear an unfamiliar word, or have an error in the software dictionary. Often, real-time captions are produced at a different location from the programming and are transmitted by phone lines. In addition to live, real-time captioning, captions are being put on prerecorded video, rental movies on tape and DVD, and educational and training tapes using a similar process but enabling error correction.

Electronic Newsroom Captions

Electronic newsroom captions (ENR) are created from a news script computer or TelePrompTer and are commonly used for live newscasts. Only material that is scripted can be captioned using this technique. Therefore, spontaneous commentary, live field reports, breaking news, and sports and weather updates may not be captioned using ENR, and real-time captioning is needed.

Edited and Verbatim Captions

Captions can be produced as either edited or verbatim captions. Edited captions summarize ideas and shorten phrases. Verbatim captions include all of what is said. Although there are situations in which edited captions have been preferred for ease in reading (such as for children's programs), most people who are deaf or hard of hearing prefer the full access provided by verbatim texts.

Rear Window Captioning

More and more movie theaters across the country are offering this type of captioning system. An adjustable Lucite panel attaches to the viewer's seat and reflects the captions from a light-emitting diode (LED) panel on the back of the theater.

Current Research

Researchers are studying caption features, speeds, and the effects of visual impairments on reading captions. This research will help the broadcast television industry understand which caption features should be retained and which new features should be adopted to better serve consumers. Other research is examining the potential for captions as a learning tool for acquiring English-language and reading skills. These studies are looking at how captions can reinforce vocabulary, improve literacy, and help people learn the expressions and speech patterns of spoken English.

The Law

The Americans with Disabilities Act (ADA) of 1990 requires that businesses and public accommodations ensure that disabled individuals are not excluded from or denied services because of the absence of auxiliary aids. Captions are considered one type of auxiliary aid. Since the passage of the ADA, the use of captioning has expanded. Entertainment, educational, informational, and training materials are captioned for deaf and hard-of-hearing audiences at the time they are produced and distributed.

The Television Decoder Circuitry Act of 1990 requires that all televisions larger than thirteen inches sold in the United States after July 1993 have a special built-in decoder that enables viewers to watch closed-captioned programming. The Telecommunications Act of 1996 directs the Federal Communications Commission (FCC) to adopt rules requiring closed captioning of most television programming.

Captions and the FCC

The FCC rules on closed captioning became effective January 1, 1998. They require people or companies that distribute television programs directly to home viewers to make sure those programs are captioned. Under the rules, 100 percent of nonexempt programs shown on or after January 1, 1998, must be closed captioned by January 1, 2006. Also, 75 percent of nonexempt programs shown before January 1, 1998, must be closed captioned by January 1, 2008. The rules do not apply to videotapes, laser disks, digital video disks, or video game cartridges.

Who Is Required to Provide Closed Captions?

The rules apply to people or companies that distribute television programs directly to home viewers (video program distributors). Some examples are local broadcast television stations, satellite television services, and local cable television operators. In some situations, video program providers are responsible for captioning programs. A video program provider can be a television program network (for example, ABC, NBC, UPN, Lifetime, A&E) or other company that makes a particular television program. However, since networks do not distribute television programs directly to home viewers, they are not responsible for complying with the captioning rules and are not required to respond to complaints from viewers. However, broadcast and cable networks and program producers pay close attention to captioning issues and, along with the U.S. Department of Education, are the primary source for funding of captioning.

When Will I See More Closed-Captioned Programming?

The FCC rules can create transition periods during which the amount of closed-captioned programming will gradually increase. During 2000 and 2001, video program distributors were required to provide captioning for 450 hours per channel per calendar quarter of new programs (programs shown on or after January 1, 1998). In 2002 and 2003, distributors were required to increase the hours per channel of captioned programming to 900 per calendar quarter for new programs. In 2004 and 2005, 1,350 hours per channel per calendar quarter of new programs were required to be captioned.

If a video program distributor is already providing more than the required number of hours per channel during a specific calendar quarter, that distributor must continue to provide captioned programming at substantially the same level as the average level it provided during the first six months of 1997.

For programming shown before January 1, 1998, at least 30 percent of a channel's programming during each calendar quarter was required to be captioned as of January 1, 2003.

What Programs Are Exempt?

Some advertisements, public service announcements, non-English-language programs (with the exception of Spanish programs), locally produced and distributed non-news programming, textual programs, early-morning programs, and nonvocal musical programs are exempt from captioning. The FCC plans to review the program exemptions later to determine whether any changes are necessary.

Notes

1. Zenith Electronics Corporation, July 1, 2002.

Section 15.4

Better Communication with People Who Are Hard of Hearing

In the United States more than thirty-one million people have some
level of hearing loss. Hearing loss is usually due to genetics or being
exposed to too much loud noise.

If you have a friend, family member or coworker who has a hearing loss, how can you help?

General Tips

Always face the person when you are talking to him or her. Keep
you hands away from your face.

You do not need to talk loud, or to shout. Do talk clearly, without
mumbling, and try not to talk so fast.

If you think the person you know has a hearing loss, encourage him
or her to get a hearing screening. Studies show that most people who
decide to get their hearing checked do so because a friend or family
member suggested it.

Tips for Social Gatherings in Your Home

Turn up the lights. Most people who are hard of hearing rely on
seeing the person talking to help them communicate. So while low
lights might seem cozy and relaxing, it might be a communication
hindrance for your guest(s).

Turn down the music. Perhaps the biggest hindrance to effective
communication for people who are hard of hearing is background
noise. Loud stereos or televisions can be a real source of frustration.

Tips for Visiting a Restaurant

Consider the acoustics. Hardwood floors and high ceilings make it difficult to communicate. Look for places that are carpeted and that have seating areas off to the side, or in more private areas.

When are you going? Friday nights at the Mexican restaurant with the Mariachi band may sound like fun, but your guest(s) who are hard of hearing may not hear a thing you say. Plan on going out to eat at times when there are fewer people, or when there will not be live entertainment.

Tips for a Meeting at Work

Visual information helps. Typed agendas, PowerPoint presentations, and so on are great helps for people with hearing loss.

One at a time. If two people are having their own private conversation, or more than one person is talking at a time, everyone is distracted, especially a person who is hard of hearing. It can also be helpful if the person leading the meeting calls on a person preparing to talk, or at least gestures towards him or her. It often takes a few seconds for a hard of hearing person to figure out where the voice is coming from, so a cue from the leader can really help.

Is this the best place? Environmental noise such as phones ringing, copying machines running, and the like really make it harder for a person who has a hearing loss. Try to find a room where the door can be closed and people can sit as close together as possible.

While all of us sometimes struggle to communicate effectively, people who have a hearing loss face an even greater challenge. By following a few simple strategies those of us who are friends, families, and coworkers can make this challenge less difficult and probably find ourselves communicating more effectively with everyone around us.

Many people who begin to lose their hearing may deny the problem and begin to withdraw and isolate themselves. Hearing aids and other technologies can really make a difference in someone's life. Encourage your family and friends to do something about their hearing loss.

Part Three

Vestibular Disorders

Chapter 16

Vestibular Disorders: An Overview

Chapter Contents

Section 16.1

Vestibular (Balance) Disorders

Reprinted from "Balance Disorders," National Institute on Deafness
and Other Communication Disorders, National Institutes of Health,
NIH Publication No. 00-4374, April 22, 2005.

What is a balance disorder?

A balance disorder is a disturbance that causes an individual to feel
unsteady, giddy, woozy, or have a sensation of movement, spinning, or
floating. An organ in our inner ear, the labyrinth, is an important part
of our vestibular (balance) system. The labyrinth interacts with other
systems in the body, such as the visual (eyes) and skeletal (bones and
joints) systems, to maintain the body's position. These systems, along
with the brain and the nervous system, can be the source of balance
problems.

Three structures of the labyrinth, the semicircular canals, let us know
when we are in a rotary (circular) motion. The semicircular canals, the
superior, posterior, and horizontal, are fluid-filled. Motion of the fluid
tells us if we are moving. The semicircular canals and the visual and
skeletal systems have specific functions that determine an individual's
orientation. The vestibule is the region of the inner ear where the semicircular canals converge, close to the cochlea (the hearing organ). The
vestibular system works with the visual system to keep objects in focus
when the head is moving. Joint and muscle receptors also are important in maintaining balance. The brain receives, interprets, and processes the information from these systems that control our balance.

How does the balance system work?

Movement of fluid in the semicircular canals signals the brain
about the direction and speed of rotation of the head—for example,
whether we are nodding our head up and down or looking from right
to left. Each semicircular canal has a bulbed end, or enlarged portion,
that contains hair cells. Rotation of the head causes a flow of fluid,
which in turn causes displacement of the top portion of the hair cells
that are embedded in the jelly-like cupula. Two other organs that are

part of the vestibular system are the utricle and saccule. These are called the otolithic organs and are responsible for detecting linear acceleration, or movement in a straight line. The hair cells of the otolithic organs are blanketed with a jelly-like layer studded with tiny calcium stones called otoconia. When the head is tilted or the body position is changed with respect to gravity, the displacement of the stones causes the hair cells to bend.

The balance system works with the visual and skeletal systems (the muscles and joints and their sensors) to maintain orientation or balance. For example, visual signals are sent to the brain about the body's position in relation to its surroundings. These signals are processed by the brain and compared to information from the vestibular and the skeletal systems. An example of interaction between the visual and vestibular systems is called the vestibular-ocular reflex. The nystagmus (an involuntary rhythmic eye movement) that occurs when a person is spun around and then suddenly stops is an example of a vestibular-ocular reflex.

What are the symptoms of a balance disorder?

When balance is impaired, an individual has difficulty maintaining orientation. For example, an individual may experience the "room spinning" and may not be able to walk without staggering, or may not even be able to arise. Some of the symptoms a person with a balance disorder may experience are:

- A sensation of dizziness or vertigo (spinning);
- Falling or a feeling of falling;
- Lightheadedness or feeling woozy;
- Visual blurring;
- Disorientation.

Some individuals may also experience nausea and vomiting, diarrhea, faintness, changes in heart rate and blood pressure, fear, anxiety, or panic. Some reactions to the symptoms are fatigue, depression, and decreased concentration. The symptoms may appear and disappear over short time periods or may last for a longer period of time.

What causes a balance disorder?

Infections (viral or bacterial), head injury, disorders of blood circulation affecting the inner ear or brain, certain medications, and aging may change our balance system and result in a balance problem. Individuals who have illnesses, brain disorders, or injuries of the visual or skeletal systems, such as eye muscle imbalance and arthritis, may also experience balance difficulties. A conflict of signals to the brain about the sensation of movement can cause motion sickness (for instance, when an individual tries to read while riding in a car). Some symptoms of motion sickness are dizziness, sweating, nausea, vomiting, and generalized discomfort. Balance disorders can be due to problems in any of four areas:

- **Peripheral vestibular disorder,** a disturbance in the labyrinth.

- **Central vestibular disorder,** a problem in the brain or its connecting nerves.

- **Systemic disorder,** a problem of the body other than the head and brain.

- **Vascular disorder,** or blood flow problems.

What are some types of balance disorders?

Some of the more common balance disorders are:

- **Benign Paroxysmal Positional Vertigo (BPPV):** a brief, intense sensation of vertigo that occurs because of a specific positional change of the head. An individual may experience BPPV when rolling over to the left or right upon getting out of bed in the morning, or when looking up for an object on a high shelf. The cause of BPPV is not known, although it may be caused by an inner ear infection, head injury, or aging.

- **Labyrinthitis:** an infection or inflammation of the inner ear causing dizziness and loss of balance.

- **Ménière disease:** an inner ear fluid balance disorder that causes episodes of vertigo, fluctuating hearing loss, tinnitus (a ringing or roaring in the ears), and the sensation of fullness in the ear. The cause of Ménière disease is unknown.

- **Vestibular neuronitis:** an infection of the vestibular nerve, generally viral.

- **Perilymph fistula:** a leakage of inner ear fluid to the middle ear. It can occur after head injury, physical exertion or, rarely, without a known cause.

How are balance disorders diagnosed?

Diagnosis of a balance disorder is complicated because there are many kinds of balance disorders and because other medical conditions—including ear infections, blood pressure changes, and some vision problems—and some medications may contribute to a balance disorder. A person experiencing dizziness should see a physician for an evaluation.

The primary physician may request the opinion of an otolaryngologist to help evaluate a balance problem. An otolaryngologist is a physician/surgeon who specializes in diseases and disorders of the ear, nose, throat, head, and neck, with expertise in balance disorders. He or she will usually obtain a detailed medical history and perform a physical examination to start to sort out possible causes of the balance disorder. The physician may require tests to assess the cause and extent of the disruption of balance. The kinds of tests needed will vary based on the patient's symptoms and health status. Because there are so many variables, not all patients will require every test.

Some examples of diagnostic tests the otolaryngologist may request are a hearing examination, blood tests, an electronystagmogram (ENG—a test of the vestibular system), or imaging studies of the head and brain.

The caloric test may be performed as part of the ENG. In this test, each ear is flushed with warm and then cool water, usually one ear at a time; the amount of nystagmus resulting is measured. Weak nystagmus or the absence of nystagmus may indicate an inner ear disorder.

Another test of the vestibular system, posturography, requires the individual to stand on a special platform capable of movement within a controlled visual environment; body sway is recorded in response to movement of the platform and/or the visual environment.

How are balance disorders treated?

There are various options for treating balance disorders. One option includes treatment for a disease or disorder that may be contributing to the balance problem, such as ear infection, stroke, or multiple sclerosis. Individual treatment will vary and will be based upon symptoms, medical history, general health, examination by a physician, and the results of medical tests.

Another treatment option includes balance retraining exercises (vestibular rehabilitation). The exercises include movements of the head and body specifically developed for the patient. This form of therapy is thought to promote compensation for the disorder. Vestibular retraining programs are administered by professionals with knowledge and understanding of the vestibular system and its relationship with other systems in the body.

For people diagnosed with Ménière disease, dietary changes such as reducing intake of sodium may help. For some people, reducing alcohol and caffeine and avoiding nicotine may be helpful. Some aminoglycoside antibiotics, such as gentamicin and streptomycin, are used to treat Ménière disease. Systemic streptomycin (given by injection) and topical gentamicin (given directly to the inner ear) are useful for their ability to affect the hair cells of the balance system. Gentamicin also can affect the hair cells of the cochlea, though, and cause hearing loss. In cases that do not respond to medical management, surgery may be indicated.

A program of talk therapy or physical rehabilitation may be recommended for people with anxiety.

How can I help my doctor make a diagnosis?

You can take the following steps that may be helpful to your physician in determining a diagnosis and treatment plan.

- Bring a written list of symptoms to your doctor.

- Bring a list of medications currently being used for balance disorders to your doctor.

- Be specific when you describe the nature of your symptoms to your doctor. For example, describe how, when, and where you experience dizziness.

Lastly, remember to write down any instructions or tips your doctor gives you.

What research is being done for balance disorders?

Scientists are working to understand the various balance disorders and the complex interactions between the labyrinth, other balance-sensing organs, and the brain. Scientists are studying eye movement to understand the changes that occur in aging, disease, and injury. Scientists are collecting data about eye movement and posture to improve diagnosis and treatment of balance disorders. Scientists are also studying the effectiveness of certain exercises as a treatment option.

Recent findings from studies supported by the National Institute on Deafness and Other Communication Disorders (NIDCD) suggest that the vestibular system plays an important role in modulating blood pressure. The information from these studies has potential clinical relevance in understanding and managing orthostatic hypotension (lowered blood pressure related to a change in body posture). Other studies of the otolithic organs, the detectors of linear movement, are exploring how these organs differentiate between downward (gravitational) motion and linear (forward-to-aft, side-to-side) motion.

Other projects supported by NIDCD include studies of the genes essential to normal development and function in the vestibular system. Scientists are also studying inherited syndromes of the brain that affect balance and coordination.

The institute supports research to develop new tests and refine current tests of balance and vestibular function. For example, scientists have developed computer-controlled systems to measure eye movement and body position by stimulating specific parts of the vestibular and nervous systems. Other tests to determine disability, as well as new physical rehabilitation strategies, are under investigation in clinical and research settings.

NIDCD, along with other institutes at the National Institutes of Health, joined the National Aeronautics and Space Administration (NASA) for Neurolab, a research mission dedicated to the study of life sciences. Neurolab focused on the most complex and least understood part of the human body, the nervous system (including the balance system).

Exposure to the weightlessness of space is known to temporarily disrupt balance on return to Earth and to gravity. A team of NIDCD and NASA investigators had previously studied the effects of microgravity exposure on balance control in astronauts who had returned from short-duration space flight missions, but these studies did not include an aged individual. During the October 29–November 7, 1998, Space Shuttle *Discovery* mission, NIDCD and NASA collaborated in another study of postflight balance control. For the first time, a previously experienced, but now elderly astronaut, Senator John Glenn, participated. Data collected during this mission, which are still being analyzed, may help to explain the mechanisms of recovery from balance disorders experienced on Earth as well as in the space environment. Scientists also hope that this data will help to develop strategies to prevent injury from falls, a common occurrence among people with balance disorders, particularly as they grow older.

Section 16.2

Pediatric Vestibular Disorders

Vestibular disorders in children are generally considered uncommon. They are not as easily recognized as vestibular disorders in adults, in part because children cannot describe their symptoms as well.

Symptoms and signs that may indicate vestibular dysfunction in children include developmental and reflex delays, visual-spatial problems, hearing loss, tinnitus, motion sensitivity, abnormal movement patterns, clumsiness, decreased eye-hand and eye-foot coordination, ataxia, falls, nystagmus, seizures, dizziness, nausea, ear pressure, difficulty moving in the dark, behavioral changes, and/or delays in performance of developmental activities such as riding a bicycle, hopping, and stair climbing involving alternating left-right leg movements.

Possible causes include head-neck trauma, chronic ear infections, maternal drug or alcohol abuse during pregnancy, cytomegalovirus, immune-deficiency disorders, migraine with or without headache, meningitis, metabolic disorders (e.g., diabetes), ototoxic medications, neurological disorders (e.g., cerebral palsy, hydrocephalus), genetic syndromes (e.g., branchiootorenal syndrome, Mondini dysplasia, Wallenberg syndrome), posterior brain tumors (e.g., malignant medulloblastomas or the less frequently seen benign acoustic neuromas), and a family history of vertigo, motion sensitivity, hearing loss, or vestibular disorders. Dizziness can be the first symptom of depression in a teenager. Alcohol intoxication can produce dizziness, imbalance, staggering, and abnormal eye movements.

Children may also develop a vestibular disorder for no known reason. The underlying reasons often cannot be determined even with the most aggressive testing. This does not preclude successful treatment or recovery.

Children can experience the same vestibular disorders as adults. Benign paroxysmal positional vertigo (BPPV) in children is typically associated with physical trauma and can result from accidents, falls, or sports injuries. Infrequently, BPPV has also been observed following cochlear implantation. Vestibular neuritis or labyrinthitis occurs in children, as well as ototoxicity. Children that experience ototoxicity can have severe imbalance, falls, and visual-motor problems, including oscillopsia (bouncing vision).

Less common in children is Ménière's disease, enlarged vestibular aqueduct, perilymph fistula, autoimmune disease, and vascular insufficiencies.

In addition to all the vestibular disorders that adults are subject to, children have two of their own. Childhood paroxysmal vertigo, often referred to as migraine equivalent, is typically seen in children two to twelve years old and is characterized by true spinning vertigo, nystagmus, nausea, and vomiting. Children tend to "grow out of" this condition, but it may progress into benign positional vertigo or migraine-associated vertigo in adulthood. Paroxysmal torticollis of infancy consists of head-tilt spells that may be associated with nausea, vomiting, pallor, agitation, and ataxia.

Evaluation and Treatment

Age-specific techniques are used for assessment and treatment of vestibular dysfunction in children. A diagnostic work-up might include a history and physical exam, a hearing test, and possibly brain scans to rule out other pathologies. In addition, a vestibular therapist can help evaluate the child's ability to use the vestibular system for balance and visual-motor control, as well as test the child's developmental reflexes that have control mechanisms in the vestibular system.

Using these results, the therapist develops vestibular-therapy exercises, which are tailored to the individual child. Children with vestibular disorders can respond well to such intervention. In fact, children typically respond more quickly than adults, because of their greater plasticity—the ability of their neurological systems to more quickly compensate for and adapt to vestibular deficits. In addition, children tend to be less fearful of movement than adults, so they participate well in the balance and movement aspects of therapy. Vestibular therapy can be effective for reducing or eliminating vertigo, improving visual-motor control, improving balance and coordination, and promoting normal development in children with vestibular disorders.

Section 16.3

Presbyastasis

As we get older, both the hearing and balance parts of the inner
ear tend to lose sensitivity, causing an age-related hearing loss and
a gradual loss of balance function. For many people this loss is felt
as dizziness or a loss of balance and an increase in falling. This age-
related balance disruption is called presbyastasis (presby = elder,
stasis = balance), and age-related hearing loss is called presbycusis
(cusis = hearing). The degree of loss varies widely. Some people have
no trouble with balance and others are severely impaired. It is not
possible to predict whether this will happen or how bad it might become.

Our balance system involves a complicated interaction of information coming in from many senses (inner ears, vision, joints, and
muscles) to our brain. Our brain processes this information and tells
our muscles what to do to maintain balance. If any part of this system is not working, our balance may be affected. If more than one part
is affected, we have even more difficulty. For people with no inner ear
balance function, walking can be very difficult without a cane, and
walking in the dark (which removes visual clues) may be impossible.

Just as hearing loss can be made worse by toxic chemicals, certain
medications, and hazardous noise exposure, so too can balance function be made worse by certain agents.

In addition, because many older people have brittle bones, falls can
result in fractures, a potentially very serious problem. With this section we hope to lower the risk of falls as a result of the balance problem, and to help you stay as mobile as possible.

Background

The balance part of the inner ear is known as the vestibular system, the main components of which are the semicircular canals. Each

of the three canals is oriented in a specific directional plane, each responding to different stimuli, and designed to help us keep our balance and steady our vision. When we turn our head while looking at an object, the inner ear helps our eyes turn in the opposite direction so that the object does not appear to "move." One way to understand this is to look at a video made by someone carrying the camera on his or her shoulder: The horizon seems to move up and down with the footsteps. When we walk we do not see this type of movement because our vestibular system stabilizes our gaze, so that the horizon appears steady.

The vestibular system consists of five sensory structures within each inner ear. Three of these sensory structures are located in curved canals that detect rotation of our head or body. One of these semicircular canals is in the horizontal plane, while the other two are in the vertical plane. The most common rotation we do is looking to the left or to the right. This stimulates the horizontal canal to keep our gaze fixed straight ahead. Sensors in the other two canals detect body and head motion in other planes, such as bending over, or turning from side to side.

The two remaining sensors, the utricle and saccule, detect the pull of gravity on our body as well as motion in a straight line, such as moving on a sled or bouncing on a trampoline. The signals from the five sensors work together. For example, turning the head to the right makes the right sensor increase its signals and the left side decrease. Thus the brain gets a balanced set of signals that it interprets as motion. A common problem occurs when the two sides are not balanced, as happens after a viral infection of the inner ear (labyrinthitis), and we feel like we are spinning in a circle. This spinning sensation is known as vertigo.

Symptoms

The most common symptom of presbyastasis is dizziness when the head is moved or when there is a change in body position. This is because the inner ear no longer stabilizes our gaze: the world around us appears to move. After a fraction of a second we adjust our vision and the dizziness stops. However, if this happens every time we move our head, after awhile it accumulates and we become uncomfortable, even progressing to the sensation of being sick to our stomach. Walking, especially down the aisle of a supermarket (where we turn our heads and eyes looking for items) can be very difficult. For people with no inner ear function, walking becomes extremely difficult, not only because of difficulty in keeping balance but because of the apparent movement of the world around us.

The second problem with presbyastasis is keeping our balance, particularly in the dark. People with a visual loss will be especially prone to these problems. Because many people develop cataracts and other visual problems with age, presbyastasis, in conjunction with other difficulties, may make it very difficult to get around.

Most people who get seasick stop having symptoms after two to three days because their brain compensates and adapts for this changed environment. As you get older your ability to adapt decreases, thus you may be more prone to these difficulties. Moreover, the sensitivity of the system decreases with age and you may have difficulty with walking, getting up from a chair, rolling over in bed, or other every day movements.

Diagnosis

The diagnosis of presbyastasis is made by the physician's examination, by measurement of posture and balance on the posturography platform and vestibular tests such as the ENG or the rotating chair. These tests can help determine the diagnosis and judge its severity. The ENG and rotating chair tests indicate how much impairment of the inner ear function exists, whereas the platform test helps determine if other parts of the balance system are involved. It is important to remember that balance is maintained by a combination of vestibular, eye, and muscle sensations. People can balance fairly well on two of these systems, but cannot balance on just one.

Electronystagmography

Electronystagmography (ENG) is a method for measuring the sensitivity of one of the vestibular sensors. It consists of an eye movement test (to assure that one's eyes move normally) and an ear function test in which cold and then warm air is directed into the ear canal. This changes the temperature in the horizontal canal. This change stimulates the sensor, resulting in a jerky movement of the eyes, called nystagmus. When the eyes are moving like this, the world seems to turn and this gives the sensation of motion known as vertigo. The ENG electrodes detect how fast the eyes are moving, and the speed indicates the sensitivity of the inner ear. You may feel a little vertigo with the test but this should stop promptly as soon as the ear temperature returns to normal. Some people feel nausea after this test. It is advisable to have someone accompany you home in case of such an event.

Computerized Dynamic Posturography

Computerized dynamic posturography (CDP) is used to test your balance. It provides diagnostic information on your ability to maintain balance under different sensory environments. The CDP test assesses your ability to use visual, vestibular, and somatosensory (muscles and joint) information together to maintain balance. When one or more of these sensory systems becomes interrupted due to aging, trauma, or disease, your ability to maintain your balance can become severely affected.

Most often, trouble maintaining your balance results from dysfunction of the inner ear(s), the eye(s), or the muscles and joints. The combination of CDP with traditional tests of vestibular function can help your doctor localize which information system(s), if any, is causing you to lose your balance.

During the CDP test, you will stand on a mobile platform and will be surrounded by a mobile visual wall. At different times during the test, the wall, the platform, or both will gently move as you move. Your job during this test is to maintain your balance in each of these sensory situations. The CDP test takes about fifteen minutes to complete and will provide your doctor with important information regarding your balance problem.

Depending on the results of your test(s), you might be referred to a physical therapist specially trained in vestibular rehabilitation or to a specialty clinic for further assessment.

Rotating Chair

In this test, you will sit in a motorized chair in a dark room. As the chair rocks gently back and forth, the eyes move back and forth in the opposite direction. The eye movements (nystagmus) are the same as with the ENG except that both ears are stimulated at once. The chair is much more sensitive than the ENG and is used when the ENG is normal or ambiguous.

These examinations can help the physician determine whether balance rehabilitation therapy will be a benefit and help a therapist in planning a strategic program.

Treatment

Medical Therapy

Medications are generally of little help, and surgery is not recommended in the treatment of presbyastasis. Most patients are referred for balance therapy. In addition, your doctor will review the medication you are taking for other disorders to be sure they are not contributing to your balance problem.

Balance Therapy

The goals of balance therapy are to decrease dizziness, improve balance, and increase activity level to help maintain those gains. Balance therapy is given by a physical therapist with special training in this area. An individualized exercise program is set up to help stabilize your vision and improve your balance. Sometimes, specific strengthening and flexibility exercises are also helpful, especially for the legs and ankles. In addition, walking safety is evaluated. The overall goal of physical therapy is to help you remain independent, safe, and active.

Follow-Up

It is important to keep in touch with your doctor and monitor your progress. Sometimes, repeat CDP testing will show improvement. Being as active as possible and taking part in an exercise program is essential for keeping fit and keeping balanced. Exercise and activity are the keys to staying fit. Even if you can't walk, there are many exercise machines and even water exercises that can help.

Section 16.4

Allergies and Vestibular Disorders

Generally speaking, can people who have inner ear disorders or ear damage and allergies have increased symptoms during allergy season?

Yes, this is true. The allergy will cause congestion of the eustachian tube with perhaps even some middle ear effusion, and perilymph fistula and/or endolymphatic hydrops can be aggravated from this, and other vestibular problems also can be adversely affected.

Does treating with antihistamines during allergy season help both the allergy and vertigo?

The antihistamines certainly help the allergy, assuming that the antihistamines are selectively chosen. Whether the dizziness would be helped would depend to a large degree on the cause of the dizziness (vertigo) and whether the vertigo is the only problem or is part of a broader inner ear disorder.

If allergies are severe and a person is having increased vestibular symptoms, would an allergy treatment program help?

I would certainly recommend allergy treatment for anyone having severe allergy problems. Again, the vestibular difficulty would respond in varying degrees depending on the complexity of the inner ear disorder.

Can allergies and sinus problems set off the vestibular system and cause vertigo?

The answer is a qualified yes. The flu virus is often the cause of what is known as toxic labyrinthitis. Patients with the flu sometimes also

239

have allergy and often are described as having "sinus trouble." A more precise definition of sinus trouble is always a help. And by vertigo, do we mean a true whirling sensation or a light- headedness/syncope?

Would an allergist be knowledgeable of the vestibular system or have had some emphasis of study in this area in school?

If the allergist is also trained as an otolaryngologist, yes. Otherwise, probably not.

Is there anything in an allergy desensitizing therapy program that might make a person worse?

If the diluent for allergy injections is normal saline with 0.45 percent phenol in solution (Coca's solution), probably not so long as the therapeutic dosage is at a reasonable level. If the dosage level is raised too quickly or to an extraordinary amount, then a patient could develop real problems. Again, it would depend upon the knowledge and skill of the treating physician.

If an allergist knew a patient had a vestibular disorder (for example, Ménière's disease or hydrops), would that change his or her method of treatment?

Well, such a situation would call for some caution and a more extended progression of dosage in reaching the optimum level of treatment—that is, smaller increments. And, of course, the hydrops or Ménière's disease should also be treated on its own merits.

Do people react to antihistamines? How?

There are various ways of reacting to antihistamines. Some of the common undesired reactions are drowsiness, dryness, bladder retention of urine in men with prostrate problems, the bad taste of milk in nursing mothers, a feeling of heaviness in the head or outright headache, gastric irritation—to give some examples. Fortunately, most people have minimal problems with antihistamines. The desired effects are relief of the allergy and control of sneezing, drainage, and itchy eyes, and so on.

Would it ever be suggested that a vestibular patient undergo an antihistamine therapy treatment program to

control a vestibular problem even if he or she didn't have allergies?

In some patients, a trial on antihistamine therapy might be advantageous in helping control the congestion of the middle ear/eustachian tube complex. A vestibular dysfunction without other accompanying signs or symptoms of congestion—such as BPPN or benign paroxysmal positional nystagmus—probably would not be likely to respond.

Would treatment of a patient be different if it was suspected that the patient had an open fistula?

Well, again, an open fistula means a leak of perilymph from the inner ear into the middle ear, and treatment would more likely involve bed rest for an extended time and/or surgery. Now, if such a patient also had significant allergy problems, then an antihistamine could be efficacious.

Are there certain antihistamines that a doctor always tries first?

No. All antihistamines are derived from about half a dozen chemical roots. Patients vary in their tolerance for and response to antihistamines. Generally, I ask patients to try perhaps a dozen different antihistamines, with or without an ephedrine class of decongestant to try to find at least two compounds that are well tolerated and that provide adequate coverage for the allergy symptoms. The problem of tolerance is then handled by moving from choice number one to number two and back as needed.

Additional precautionary note: Combinations of drugs such as Seldane and erythromycin (and other combinations) can be lethal. Always inform your doctor about any drugs you may be taking in addition to your allergy drug(s).

Additional note on Claritin D: Some people have difficulty swallowing the twenty-four-hour dose of Claritin D. Taking the dose with water may help.

Section 16.5

Vestibular Testing

Reprinted from "Vestibular Testing," by Timothy C. Hain, M.D.
Copyright © 2004 American Hearing Research Foundation.
Reprinted with permission.

Vestibular testing consists of a number of tests that help determine if there is something wrong with the vestibular (balance) portion of the inner ear. These tests can help isolate dizziness symptoms to a specific cause that can often be treated.

Getting Vestibular Tests

If dizziness is not caused by the inner ear, it might be caused by the brain, by medical disorders such as low blood pressure, or by psychological problems such as anxiety. Recent studies have documented that vestibular tests are more accurate than clinical examination in identifying inner ear disorders (Gordon et al, 1996). Hearing pathway tests (audiometry, auditory brainstem response, electrocorticography) can also be used for the same purpose, and are frequently combined with vestibular tests.

Vestibular tests can help determine if more expensive tests, such as magnetic resonance imaging (MRI), are needed. Recent studies (Levy and Arts, 1996) have shown that vestibular testing is much more accurate than clinical symptoms in predicting whether neuroimaging tests will be abnormal. Vestibular tests can also document objectively vestibular conditions such as benign paroxysmal positional vertigo (BPPV) and perilymph fistula, which commonly occur after head injury; and bilateral vestibular ototoxicity, which commonly is a side effect of medication.

The following vestibular tests are described:

- electronystagmography (ENG)
- electrocochleography (ECOG)
- rotational chair test
- posturography

- fistula test
- new and emerging tests

References

Gordon CR, Shupak A, Spitzer O, Doweck I, Melamed Y. Nonspecific vertigo with normal otoneurological examination. The role of vestibular laboratory tests. *Laryngol Otol* 1996 Dec; 110(12):1133–37.

Levy RA, Arts HA. Predicting neuroradiologic outcome in patients referred for audiovestibular dysfunction. *AJNR Am J Neuroradiol* 1996 Oct; 17(9):1717–24.

Stewart MG and others. Cost-effectiveness of the diagnostic evaluation of vertigo. *Laryngoscope,* 109:600–605, 1999.

Electronystagmography (ENG) Test

The ENG test is used to determine whether or not dizziness may be due to inner ear disease. It consists of carefully measuring involuntary eye movement (nystagmus) while the subject's balance system is stimulated in different ways. There are four main parts to the ENG: the calibration test, the tracking test, the positional test, and the caloric test.

The calibration test evaluates rapid eye movements. The tracking test evaluates movement of the eyes as they follow a visual target. The positional test measures dizziness associated with positions of the head. The caloric test measures responses to warm and cold water circulated through a small, soft tube in the ear canal.

The present best method to measure eye movements is an infrared/video system. Other methods include electrooculography (EOG) and infrared reflectance. Video systems are usually more accurate than the older EOG method because they are less sensitive to lid artifact and are not affected by electrical noise generated by muscle. Infrared reflectance is little used in recent times because of nonlinearity.

The ENG test is the "gold standard" for diagnosis of ear disorders affecting one ear at a time. For example, the ENG is excellent for diagnosis of acoustic neuroma as well as vestibular neuritis. The ENG is also useful in diagnosis of BPPV and bilateral vestibular loss, although the rotational chair test is better at the diagnosis of bilateral vestibular disorders than is the ENG. The calibration and tracking tests are intended to diagnose central nervous system disorders. These tests are generally insensitive compared to an examination by a neurologist or a magnetic resonance imaging (MRI) scan. ENG, however, is much less expensive than an MRI in most institutions.

Electrocochleography (ECOG)

ECOG is a variant of brainstem audio evoked response (BAER). It is not a vestibular test at all but rather a test of hearing. It is intended to diagnose Ménière disease, and, in particular, hydrops. In this test, a recording electrode (gold sponge) is inserted into the subject's ear canal, a wire or spring is placed on the ear canal, or a needle that transfixes the eardrum is inserted into the ear. The subject receives a series of audible clicks.

The objective is to record wave one (there are five waves) with greater accuracy and to detect the summating potential, which is a shoulder on wave one. Needle type ECOGs have fallen out of favor because they are generally judged to be unreasonably invasive.

Noise can be a major problem with ECOG. Because of this, it is not an easy test to perform. Generally, the results are reported as a ratio of the summating potential to the action potential (the SP/AP ratio), for which generally a ratio of 0.5 or greater is considered abnormal. It is important when interpreting ECOG to consider the noise level, which is generally assessed by obtaining multiple trials. If they are all similar, then the standard error is small and the result is likely to be correct. If they vary widely, the reliability of the average SP/AP ratio may be questionable. Subjects with poor high-frequency hearing are likely to have higher noise levels, and therefore the limit of normal for their ECOG should be set higher.

Recently, Gamble and others (1999) reported that salt-loaded ECOG may be useful in subjects who have normal ECOGs but a history suggestive of Ménière disease. Similarly it has been suggested that ECOG may be useful in detecting allergic Ménière disease. ECOG is performed before and after challenge with an allergen (Noell et al, 2001).

References for ECOG Testing

Gamble BA, and others. Salt-load electrocochleography. *Am J. Otol* 20:325–30, 1999.

Noell CA, Roland PS, Mabry RL, Shoup AG. Inhalant allergy and Ménière disease: Use of electrocochleography and intranasal allergen challenge as investigational tools. *Otolaryngol Head Neck Surg* 2001; 125:346–50.

Rotational Chair Test

The purpose of rotational chair testing is to determine whether or not dizziness may be due to a disorder of inner ear or brain. There are three parts to the test: the chair test, the optokinetic test, and the fixation test. The rotational chair tests actually test for dizziness by recording eye movement (nystagmus) while the chair is moved in various ways and the subject looks at different lights.

The chair test measures dizziness while the subject is being turned slowly in a motorized chair. Subjects with inner ear disease become less dizzy than do normal persons. The optokinetic test measures dizziness caused by viewing of moving stripes. Optokinetic testing is sometimes useful in diagnosis of bilateral vestibular loss and central conditions. The fixation test measures dizziness while the subject is being rotated, and while the subject is looking at a dot of light that is rotating with him or her. Fixation suppression is impaired by central nervous system conditions and improved by bilateral vestibular loss.

Rotatory chair tests are the "gold standard" for diagnosis of bilateral vestibular loss. ENG tests by themselves may be falsely positive (they are rarely falsely negative) as, for example, when wax blocks one ear canal. Rotatory chair testing is not affected by mechanical obstructions of the ear. Rotatory chair testing is thus a valuable adjunct to ENG testing by confirming an abnormality.

There are several other alternative procedures involving rotation that provide a subset of rotational chair testing. Two tests use active head movement—brand names for these devices are VAT and VORTEQ. Both of these tests provide a part of the rotational chair test information (the high frequencies), and measure something a little different: the contribution of both the inner ear and neck inputs to nystagmus rather than the contribution of the inner ear alone. If you have a rotational chair test, there is no need to get a VAT or VORTEQ test since the information supplied is largely redundant. However, if a rotational chair test is not available, these tests may have some value.

Posturography

Moving platform posturography (MVP), or posturography for short, is a method of quantifying balance (although the definition of balance

245

can be tricky). It is most applicable in situations where balance needs to be followed quantitatively, to determine whether a disorder is getting better or worse, or the response to treatment.

Posturography is insensitive to vestibular disorders, and normal posturography should not be considered indicative of normal vestibular function (Di Fabio, 1995). It may add sensitivity to a vestibular battery, when combined with other tests of vestibular function. Stewart et al. (1999) suggested that audiometry combined with posturography was a cost-effective method of documenting a vestibular disorder.

Posturography is also very useful in medical legal situations where malingering is a possibility. The main vendor of posturography equipment used in clinical context is Neurocom Incorporated. Other vendors include Micromedical Technology and several makers of research balance equipment (e.g., AMTI).

References for Posturography Testing

Di Fabio, RP. Sensitivity and specificity of platform posturography for identifying patients with vestibular dysfunction. *Phys Ther* 1995: 75:290–305.

Gordon CR, Shupak A, Spitzer O, Melamed Y. Nonspecific vertigo with normal otoneurological examination. The role of vestibular laboratory tests. *J. Laryngology and Otology* 110(12):1133–37, 1996.

Stewart MG and others. Cost-effectiveness of the diagnostic evaluation of vertigo. *Laryngoscope*, 109:600–605, 1999.

Fistula Test

The purpose of this test is to detect perilymph fistula. Pressure is applied to each ear in turn, and eye movements are recorded with a sensitive infrared recording device. For this reason, fistula testing is about ten times more sensitive than conventional electrooculography (EOG) based recordings.

Fistula testing can also be done at the bedside. Pressure is applied to the ear, while eye movement is either directly observed or measured with an EOG, infrared (IR) examining microscope, or posturography.

Dizziness Questionnaires

Most practices that evaluate substantial numbers of dizzy patients use questionnaires to quantify symptoms. Table 16.1 provides a list of some questionnaires.

Table 16.1. Dizziness Questionnaires

Questionnaire used to quantify balance dysfunction	Source
Activities specific Balance Confidence Scale (ABC)	Powell and Meyers, 1995; Whitney et al, 1999
Modified falls efficacy scale (MFES)	Hill, Schwartz, and others, 1996
Medical outcomes study short form 36 (SF-36)	Enloe and Sheilds, 1997
Dizziness Handicap Inventory	Jacobson and Newman, 1990
Vestibular Activities of Daily Living	Cohen et al, 2000

The Dizziness Handicap Inventory (DHI) is the most commonly used questionnaire at this writing (2002).

References for Questionnaire Section

Cohen, H. S., et al. (2000). "Development of the vestibular disorders activities of daily living scale." *Arch Otolaryngol Head Neck Surg* 126(7): 881–87.

Cohen, H. S., et al. (2000). "Application of the vestibular disorders activities of daily living scale." *Laryngoscope* 110(7): 1204–9.

Enloe, L. J. and R. K. Shields (1997). "Evaluation of health-related quality of life in individuals with vestibular disease using disease-specific and general outcome measures." *Phys Ther* 77(9): 890–903.

Hill, K. D., J. A. Schwarz, et al. (1996). "Fear of falling revisited." *Arch Phys Med Rehabil* 77(10): 1025–29.

Jacobson, G. P. and J. H. Calder (1998). "A screening version of the Dizziness Handicap Inventory (DHI-S)." *Am J Otol* 19(6): 804–8.

Jacobson, G. P. and C. W. Newman (1990). "The development of the Dizziness Handicap Inventory." *Arch Otolaryngol Head Neck Surg* 116(4): 424–7.

Jacobson, G. P., C. W. Newman, et al. (1991). "Balance function test correlates of the Dizziness Handicap Inventory." *J Am Acad Audiol* 2(4): 253–60.

Powell, L. E. and A. M. Myers (1995). "The Activities-specific Balance Confidence (ABC) Scale." *J Gerontol A Biol Sci Med Sci* 50A(1): M28–34.

Whitney, S. L., M. T. Hudak, et al. (1999). "The activities-specific balance confidence scale and the dizziness handicap inventory: a comparison." *J Vestib Res* 9(4): 253–59.

New and Emerging Tests

As there are five individual motion sensors in each ear, and most of the testing described above is relevant to only one of them (the lateral semicircular canal), there clearly is plenty of room for new tests. In theory, four-fifths of your inner ear could be destroyed yet conventional vestibular testing might not even detect it. Table 16.2 provides an outline of the present status of vestibular testing.

Table 16.2. New and Emerging Tests

Part of the labyrinth	Test
Lateral (horizontal) semicircular canal	Caloric test, rotatory chair test
Superior semicircular canal	No test exists that isolates one canal. New approaches are needed.
Anterior semicircular canal	No test exists that isolates one canal. New approaches are needed.
Utricle	Ocular counter roll, subjective vertical. Neither test isolates a single utricle.
Saccule	Vestibular evoked myogenic potential. This test does assess a single saccule.

Considering first tests of the vertical semicircular canals, very little progress has been made over the last twenty years. In essence, this is because no one has developed a practical way of stimulating individual vertical semicircular canals (the caloric test does this for the lateral semicircular canal). Rotatory chair tests come the closest, but at best they stimulate two vertical canals on opposite sides of the head together.

Considering next the otoliths, the situation is slightly better. With respect to measuring the utricle, there are several methods of detecting ocular counter roll as well as subjective tilting of the visual world (or absence of it). None of these tests have become popular yet, but at least the technology exists. For example, SMI as well as Synapsys sell devices that can measure ocular counter roll (twisting of the eye with head tilt vs. gravity). Micromedical Technology supplies a commercial device that will measure subjective tilting of the vertical.

For the saccule, recently, sound evoked vestibulocollic evoked potentials have been described as useful in diagnosing Tullio phenomenon from superior canal dehiscence (Brantberg et al, 1999; Watson et al, 2000). This test is called vestibular evoked myogenic potential (VEMP). It is still considered investigational and it may be difficult to locate a laboratory that does it. It requires use of loud sounds to stimulate the inner ear.

Finally, it is possible to test the entire vestibular nerve using galvanic stimulation. This is an old technique in which an electrical current is passed into the ear, and eye movements or postural sway are recorded. This technology is presently not commercial and limited because it is difficult to pass enough current into the ear without causing pain. Nevertheless, it may increase in use once vestibular prostheses become available to substitute for the vestibular system of persons who have had severe bilateral vestibular loss.

Section 16.6

Vestibular Rehabilitation Therapy (VRT)

The information in this section is reprinted with permission from the
Vestibular Disorders Association (VEDA), http://www.vestibular.org.
© 2005 VEDA. All rights reserved.

Why is therapy needed?

If the brain cannot rely on the information it receives from the vestibular system, a person's ability to maintain posture and coordinate balance can become overly dependent on vision or on the information received from the muscles and joints (proprioception).

This can lead to developing new patterns of movement to compensate for the change and to avoid head movements that are apt to create symptoms of dizziness and nausea. For example, a person might adopt an exaggerated hip sway as a method of balancing, might swivel the entire body rather than just the head in turning to look at something, or might always look down at the floor to avoid what appears as a confusing swirl of activity.

Unfortunately, these types of adaptation can result in headache, neck ache, muscle stiffness, general fatigue, and a decrease in the ability to retrain the brain to adjust to the vestibular problem, hence making the symptoms much worse.

The goal of VRT is to retrain the brain to recognize and process signals from the vestibular system in coordination with information from vision and proprioception. This often involves desensitizing the balance system to movements that provoke symptoms.

What happens during vestibular therapy?

A qualified therapist will first perform a thorough evaluation. This includes observing posture, balance, movement, and compensatory strategies.

Using the result of this evaluation, the therapist will develop an individualized treatment plan that will include exercises to be performed both in the therapy department and at home and that combine specific head and body movements with eye exercises. Many times, treatment may also include increasing activities and exercise in order to strengthen muscles and increase tolerance for certain stimuli.

Some of the exercise and activities may at first cause an increase in symptoms, as the body and brain attempt to sort out the new pattern of movements. But with time and consistent work, the coordination of signals from the eyes, proprioception, and vestibular system will occur.

How does therapy help?

In most cases, balance improves if the exercises are correctly and faithfully performed. Muscle tension, headaches, and fatigue will diminish, and symptoms of dizziness, vertigo, and nausea will decrease or disappear. Many times, vestibular VRT is so successful that no other treatment is required.

If surgery is required to correct an inner ear problem, therapy will also be an important part of treatment. A therapist may perform a vestibular evaluation before surgery, make daily visits during the hospital stay to help with the temporary increase in balance problems that often accompanies surgery, and provide a series of simple exercises to do for home care after discharge from the hospital. Often, therapists provide further therapy after a person has recovered from the surgery.

Chapter 17

Vestibular Schwannoma

What is a vestibular schwannoma (acoustic neuroma)?

A vestibular schwannoma (also known as acoustic neuroma, acoustic neurinoma, or acoustic neurilemoma) is a benign, usually slow-growing tumor that develops from the balance and hearing nerves supplying the inner ear. The tumor comes from an overproduction of Schwann cells—the cells that normally wrap around nerve fibers like onion skin to help support and insulate nerves. As the vestibular schwannoma grows, it presses against the hearing and balance nerves, usually causing unilateral (one-sided) or asymmetric hearing loss, tinnitus (ringing in the ear), and dizziness/loss of balance. As the tumor grows, it can interfere with the face sensation nerve (the trigeminal nerve), causing facial numbness. Vestibular schwannomas can also press on the facial nerve (for the muscles of the face), causing facial weakness or paralysis on the side of the tumor. If the tumor becomes large, it will eventually press against nearby brain structures (such as the brainstem and the cerebellum), becoming life threatening.

How is a vestibular schwannoma diagnosed?

Unilateral or asymmetric hearing loss, tinnitus, and loss of balance or dizziness are early signs of a vestibular schwannoma. Unfortunately,

Reprinted from "Vestibular Schwannoma (Acoustic Neuroma) and Neurofibromatosis," National Institute on Deafness and Other Communication Disorders, National Institutes of Health, NIH Publication No. 99-580, February 2004.

early detection of the tumor is sometimes difficult because the symptoms may be subtle and may not appear in the beginning stages of growth. Also, hearing loss, dizziness, and tinnitus are common symptoms of many middle and inner ear problems (the important point here is that unilateral or asymmetric symptoms are the worrisome ones). Once the symptoms appear, a thorough ear examination and hearing test (audiogram) are essential for proper diagnosis. Computerized tomography (CT) scans, enhanced with intravenous dye (contrast), and magnetic resonance imaging (MRI) are critical in the early detection of a vestibular schwannoma and are helpful in determining the location and size of a tumor and in planning its microsurgical removal.

How is a vestibular schwannoma treated?

Early diagnosis of a vestibular schwannoma is key to preventing its serious consequences. There are three options for managing a vestibular schwannoma: (1) surgical removal; (2) radiation; and (3) monitoring. Typically, the tumor is surgically removed (excised). The exact type of operation done depends on the size of the tumor and the level of hearing in the affected ear. If the tumor is very small, hearing may be saved and accompanying symptoms may improve. As the tumor grows larger, surgical removal is more complicated because the tumor may have damaged the nerves that control facial movement, hearing, and balance and may also have affected other nerves and structures of the brain.

The removal of tumors affecting the hearing, balance, or facial nerves can make the patient's symptoms worse because sections of these nerves may also need to be removed with the tumor.

As an alternative to conventional surgical techniques, radiosurgery (that is, radiation therapy—the "gamma knife" or LINAC) may be used to reduce the size or limit the growth of the tumor. Radiation therapy is sometimes the preferred option for elderly patients, patients in poor medical health, patients with bilateral vestibular schwannoma (tumor affecting both ears), or patients whose tumor is affecting their only hearing ear. In some cases, usually elderly or medically infirm patients, it may be reasonable to "watch" the tumor for growth. Repeat MRI over time is used to carefully monitor the tumor for any growth.

What is the difference between unilateral and bilateral vestibular schwannomas?

Unilateral vestibular schwannomas affect only one ear. They account for approximately 8 percent of all tumors inside the skull; one out of every 100,000 individuals per year develops a vestibular schwannoma.

Symptoms may develop at any age but usually occur between the ages of thirty and sixty years. Unilateral vestibular schwannomas are not hereditary.

Bilateral vestibular schwannomas affect both hearing nerves and are usually associated with a genetic disorder called neurofibromatosis type 2 (NF-2). Half of affected individuals have inherited the disorder from an affected parent and half seem to have a mutation for the first time in their family. Each child of an affected parent has a 50 percent chance of inheriting the disorder. Unlike those with a unilateral vestibular schwannoma, individuals with NF-2 usually develop symptoms in their teens or early adulthood. In addition, patients with NF-2 usually develop multiple brain and spinal cord related tumors. They also can develop tumors of the nerves important for swallowing, speech, eye and facial movement, and facial sensation. Determining the best management of the vestibular schwannomas as well as the additional nerve, brain, and spinal cord tumors is more complicated than deciding how to treat a unilateral vestibular schwannoma. Further research is needed to determine the best treatment for individuals with NF-2.

Scientists believe that both unilateral and bilateral vestibular schwannomas form following the loss of the function of a gene on chromosome 22. (A gene is a small section of DNA responsible for a particular characteristic like hair color or skin tone). Scientists believe that this particular gene on chromosome 22 produces a protein that controls the growth of Schwann cells. When this gene malfunctions, Schwann cell growth is uncontrolled, resulting in a tumor. Scientists also think that this gene may help control the growth of other types of tumors. In NF-2 patients, the faulty gene on chromosome 22 is inherited. For individuals with unilateral vestibular schwannoma, however, some scientists hypothesize that this gene somehow loses its ability to function properly.

What is being done about vestibular schwannoma?

Scientists are working to better understand how the gene works so they can begin to develop gene therapy to control the overproduction of Schwann cells in individuals with vestibular schwannoma. Also, learning more about the way genes help control Schwann cell growth may help prevent other brain tumors.

Chapter 18

Bilateral Vestibulopathy

What is bilateral vestibulopathy?

Bilateral vestibulopathy occurs when the balance portions of both inner ears are damaged. The symptoms typically include imbalance and visual problems. The imbalance is worse in the dark, or in situations where footing is uncertain. Spinning vertigo is unusual. The visual symptoms, called oscillopsia, only occur when the head is moving (J.C., 1952). Oscillopsia is often common during walking (Freyss et al., 1988). Quick movements of the head are associated with transient visual blurring.

What causes bilateral vestibulopathy?

About 5 percent of all dizziness is due to bilateral vestibulopathy. In about 50 percent of cases, bilateral vestibulopathy is due to exposure to an ototoxic medication. Gentamicin is an antibiotic medication and gentamicin toxicity is the most common single known cause of bilateral vestibulopathy, accounting for 15 to 50 percent of all cases. Ototoxicity can also be due to infection (meningitis, about 10 percent); Ménière disease; sarcoidosis; bilateral ear surgery, such as for certain forms of acoustic neuroma or bilateral vestibular neuritis; congenital disorders with deafness, such as the Mondini malformation; and,

Reprinted from "Bilateral Vestibulopathy," by Timothy C. Hain, M.D., last revision January 2002. © 2002 American Hearing Research Foundation. Reprinted with permission.

very rarely, from disorders of the immune system. One rare familial form, migraine-associated vertigo (MAV), is associated with migraine. Advanced age is another risk factor, since normally vestibular ganglion cell counts decrease with age so that by the age of eighty years, about 50 percent of vestibular neurons remain. In about one-third of all cases, no cause can be identified for bilateral vestibulopathy (Syms and House, 1997).

There is also accumulating evidence that free radical generation plays an important role in ototoxicity. This information is the basis of experimental treatments to prevent ototoxicity.

How is bilateral vestibulopathy diagnosed?

Your physician can make the diagnosis based on your history, findings on physical examination, and the results of vestibular tests (rotatory chair). On physical examination, the tandem Romberg test, the dynamic visual acuity test, and the ophthalmoscope tests are the three most helpful confirmatory tests. The rotatory chair test is essential to document the characteristic reduced responses to motion of both ears. Based on rotatory chair testing in our laboratory, patients are divided into three groups: mild, moderate, and severe (see Table 18.1). These categories have prognostic significance. Other diagnostic studies may be helpful. Hearing testing (audiogram) is necessary. A test for syphilis (FTA [fluorescent treponemal antibody]) and an antibody test (ANA [antinuclear antibody test]) for autoimmune inner ear disease may be performed. A chest x-ray and ACE test may be done if sarcoid is thought likely, and a Lyme titer may be obtained if there has been exposure (a tick bite in an endemic area).

Table 18.1. Classifications of Bilateral Vestibulopathy

Classification	Rotatory Chair	ENG caloric responses
Mild	Increased phase, steeper than normal slope to gain vs. frequency plot	Normal and symmetric. Total response greater than or equal to 20.
Moderate	Increased phase, steep slope, gain greater than 0.2 at highest frequencies	Total response between 0 and 10
Severe	No response at all frequencies except (possibly) highest (0.64 Hz)	No response to usual temperatures as well as ice water

The categories shown in Table 18.1 are based on testing done at the author's institution, and might not be applicable to other protocols at other institutions. Pathologic correlation is minimal for these categories; however, recent data suggests that "severe" losses are associated with roughly an 80 percent or more loss of hair cells.

How is bilateral vestibulopathy treated?

Treatment involves finding out the cause and treating it, if possible. If the damage has already been done, then the focus of treatment is upon avoidance of vestibular suppressants and ototoxins. Vestibular rehabilitation is important to speed recovery and prevent setbacks. We recommend that you tell health care workers that you cannot take drugs that end in mycin (like Azithromycin and Erythromycin), because of possible reaction. This will keep you from contact with the most common ototoxins. Aspirin and nonsteroidal anti-inflammatory drugs can also affect hearing. It may be prudent to avoid these drugs, or at least large doses of them. Antihistamines, like Antivert (meclizine) or Dramamine, and benzodiazepines (Valium-like drugs like Klonopin, Xanax, and Ativan) are temporary vestibular suppressants. While they won't permanently harm you, typically they make imbalance temporarily worse. A list of the most common problem medication follows.

What medications are associated with potential problems?

Medications that can cause a temporary worsening of dizziness or hearing symptoms are generally vestibular suppressants, including the following:

- Antihistamines, such as meclizine and Phenergan
- Antidepressants, such as amitriptyline and other tricyclic type antidepressants
- Aspirin or NSAIDs (drugs like ibuprofen and naproxen) in large doses
- Diazepam (Valium), alprazolam (Xanax), lorazepam (Ativan), clonazepam (Klonopin), and related drugs
- Verapamil and other calcium channel blockers

Medications that can cause permanent or temporary worsening of dizziness or hearing include the following:

- Cisplatinum (a chemotherapy drug) and other platinum based drugs

- Gentamicin and other mycin antibiotics, including large doses of erythromycin (although this is actually in a different group than Gentamicin)

- Furosemide (Lasix) and ethacrynic acid (Edecrin) loop diuretics

- Quinine and related drugs (they usually have a quin in their name)

These medications need not be avoided at all costs but reasonable judgment should be exercised. Medications that cause only temporary unsteadiness (for example, meclizine), may still be useful in some situations. Medications that are ototoxic (such as gentamicin) may still be useful in cases of bilateral vestibulopathy when there is no reasonable alternative, or when the damage done is already so extensive that there is nothing more to lose.

How might bilateral vestibulopathy affect my life?

This is a condition that realistically often causes some permanent disability. In patients with gentamicin-induced ototoxicity, the symptoms generally peak at three months from the last dose of gentamicin. In the long run, however, (five years) most patients are substantially better. There are multiple reasons why people get better. First, there is evidence that the damaged vestibular hair cells in the inner ear can regenerate, although the extent to which this occurs and the degree to which they are functional is not presently clear (Forge et al. 1993; Warchol et al. 1993). Some recovery presumably occurs because marginal hair cells recover, because the brain rewires itself to adapt to the new situation (plasticity), and because people change they way they do things to adjust to their situation.

One can predict prognosis based on the amount of damage done initially, modified by other factors such as age, and other medical problems. Gillespie and Minor (1993) reported that recovery is related to various factors, including severity of lesion. In our experience, rotatory chair testing done at six months following onset (or later) helps to establish prognosis by dividing individuals into three categories. Individuals with mild abnormalities on rotatory testing are nearly always subjectively normal at one year. Individuals with moderate vestibular loss are usually able to continue to work productively, with some modifications in their behavior. For example, most people with moderate or severe loss never return to driving at night. In situations where there is complete or near-complete loss of vestibular function, vision and balance usually remain impaired permanently; however, most individuals do return to work, especially if their job does not require good head-eye coordination or balance. Frequently, job modification or accommodation occurs.

While balance is poorer than normal, given that normal vision and sensation in the feet and ankles is present, most patients with bilateral loss appear, at least on casual inspection, to have a normal gait. Falls are more frequent in persons with bilateral vestibulopathy (Herdman et al. 2000). Reading is generally more difficult than for persons with normal vestibular systems, but quite feasible, as the head can be steadied during reading. Many people with bilateral vestibulopathy complain of a mild confusion or "brain fog," which is attributed to the increased attention needed to maintain balance and vision. This reduces the amount of attention that is available for other thinking tasks.

While crutches, canes, walkers, and wheelchairs may be necessary in the first three months, these appliances are rarely needed by one year. After twenty years, most patients have returned to near-normal for their age. To some extent this return to "normal" is related to the aging of the patient's peers, since vestibular function normally declines with age. Other aspects of recovery involve use of other senses such as neck position sensors (the COR or cervico-ocular reflex), vision, and compensation through prediction.

You will want to change your lifestyle to adjust to your reduced balance and inability to see when your head is in motion. You will want to take precautions to avoid falls. You may need to change your occupation if your present one requires good balance and an ability to see while the head is in motion. For example, it would not be safe to continue as a truck driver, construction worker, or a roofer if you developed a significant bilateral vestibulopathy. A job where you work at a desk is usually a good choice.

What research studies are underway regarding bilateral vestibulopathy?

Considerable research is ongoing regarding bilateral vestibulopathy. Presently, efforts are ongoing to develop a vestibular prosthesis (ARO abstracts 743-747, 2001) as well as mechanisms to stimulate regeneration of hair cells within the inner ear. Both of these projects seem likely to be successful within ten years. Methods of preventing loss through protective agents and predicting susceptibility to gentamicin through genetic testing are also currently hot topics.

Help with research efforts is much needed to speed progress in this disorder. You may wish to volunteer to be a research subject, to contribute funds for research efforts aimed at treating or preventing ototoxicity, or to contribute your inner ear in the event of your death. At this writing, donations of the inner ear of individuals with gentamicin toxicity are sorely needed by the National Temporal Bone Bank, as no usable specimens presently exist in the collection (Tsuji et al., 1999).

At the American Hearing Research Foundation (AHRF), we have funded basic research on bilateral vestibulopathy in the past, and are very interested in funding additional research on bilateral vestibulopathy in the future. We are particularly interested in projects that might lead to prevention of ototoxicity in those who are exposed to aminoglycosides.

References

ARO abstracts—Association for Research in Otolaryngology. 2001 Annual meeting.

Baloh RW. Idiopathic bilateral vestibulopathy. *Neurology*, 39:272–75, 1989.

Baloh RW and others. Clinical-pathologic correlation in a patient with selective loss of hair cells in the vestibular endorgans. *Neurology* 49(5): 1377–82, 1997.

Begg EJ, Barclay ML. Aminoglycosides—50 years on. *Br. J. of Clinical Pharm*, 39:597–603, 1995.

Borradori C, Fawer CL, Buclin T, Calame A. Risk factors of sensorineural hearing loss in preterm infants. *Biology of the Neonate* 71(1):1–10, 1997.

Fife TD, Baloh RW. Disequilibrium of unknown causes in older people. *Ann Neurol* 34:594–702, 1993.

Forge et al.., *Science* 259:1616–19, 1993.

Forge A, Li Li, and Nevil, GJ. *Comp. Neurol*. 397:69–88, 1998

Kuntz AL, Oesterle EC, *J. Comp. Neurol*. 399: 413–23, 1998.

Freyss G, Vitte E, Semont A, Tran-Ba-Huy P, Gaillard P. Computation of eye-head movements in oscilloptic patients: modifications: modifications induced by reeducation. *Adv ORL* 42:294–300, 1988.

Gillespie MB, Minor LB. Prognosis in bilateral vestibular hypofunction. *Laryngoscope*, 109:35–41, 1999.

Herdman SJ, Blatt P, Schubert MC, Tusa RJ. Falls in patients with vestibular deficits. *Am J. Otol* 21:847–51, 2000.

Hodgson et al. Encephalopathy and Vestibulopathy following short-term hydrocarbon exposure. *J. Occup Med*, 1989, 51–54.

J.C. Living without a balancing mechanism. *New England Journal of Medicine* 246:458, 1952.

Moffat DA. *Ototoxicity in Scott-Brown's Otolaryngology*, vol. 3, 5th ed., London: Butterworths.

Rennie J. Healing Hearing. *Scientific American*, July 1993, 26–27.

Syms CA 3rd, House JW. Idiopathic Dandy's syndrome. *Otol HNS* 116(1):75–78, 1997.

Tsuji K, Merchant SN, Rauch S, Wall C. Vestibular otopathology in aminoglycoside toxicity. *ARO abstracts*, 1999, #460.

Warchol et al., *Science* 259:1619–22, 1993.

Chapter 19

Vestibular Neuritis and Labyrinthitis

What are vestibular neuritis and labyrinthitis?

Vestibular neuritis causes dizziness due to a viral infection of the vestibular nerve. The vestibular nerve carries information from the inner ear about head movement. When one of the two vestibular nerves is infected, there is an imbalance between the two sides, and vertigo appears. Vestibular neuronitis is another term that is used for the same clinical syndrome. The various terms for the same clinical syndrome probably reflect our lack of ability to localize the site of lesion.

While there are several different definitions for vestibular neuritis in the literature, with variable amounts of vertigo and hearing symptoms, we will use the definition of Silvoniemi (1988), who stated that the syndrome is confined to the vestibular system. Hearing is unaffected.

Labyrinthitis is a similar syndrome to vestibular neuritis, but with the addition of hearing symptoms (sensory type hearing loss or tinnitus).

The symptoms of both vestibular neuritis and labyrinthitis typically include dizziness or vertigo, disequilibrium or imbalance, and nausea. Acutely, the dizziness is constant. After a few days, symptoms are often precipitated only by sudden movements. A sudden turn of the head is the most common "problem" motion. While patients with these disorders can be sensitive to head position, it is generally not related to the side of the head that is down (as in BPPV [benign paroxysmal positional vertigo]), but rather just whether the patient is lying down or sitting up.

About 5 percent of all dizziness (and perhaps 15 percent of all vertigo) is due to vestibular neuritis or labyrinthitis. It occurs in all age groups, but cases are rare in children.

What is recurrent vestibular neuritis (benign recurrent vertigo)?

Fortunately, in the great majority of cases (at least 95 percent) vestibular neuritis is a one-time experience. Rarely the syndrome is recurrent, coming back year after year. When it is recurrent, the symptom complex often goes under other names. These include benign paroxysmal vertigo in children (Basser, 1964), benign recurrent vertigo (Slater 1979, Moretti et al., 1980), or Ménière disease (Rassekh and Harker, 1992). Many authors attribute this syndrome to migraine-associated vertigo. There is often a familial pattern (Oh et al., 2001).

What causes vestibular neuritis and labyrinthitis?

In vestibular neuritis, the virus that causes the infection is thought to be usually a member of the herpes family, the same group that causes cold sores in the mouth as well as a variety of other disorders (Arbusow et al., 2000). This is not the same herpes virus involved in genital herpes. It is also thought that a similar syndrome, indistinguishable from vestibular neuritis, can be caused by loss of blood flow to the inner ear (Fischer, 1967). However, present thought is that inflammation, presumably viral, is much more common than loss of blood flow.

In labyrinthitis, it is also thought that generally viruses cause the infection, but rarely labyrinthitis can be the result of a bacterial middle ear infection. In labyrinthitis, hearing may be reduced or distorted in tandem with vertigo. Both vestibular neuritis and labyrinthitis are rarely painful—when there is pain it is particularly important to get treatment rapidly, as there may be a treatable bacterial infection or herpes infection.

There are several possible locations for the damage to the vestibular system that manifests as vestibular neuritis. There is good evidence for occasional lesions in the nerve itself, as this can be seen lighting up on MRI scan. There is also reasonable evidence that vestibular neuritis often spares part of the vestibular nerve, the inferior division (Fetter and Dichgans, 1996; Goebel et al., 2001). Because the inferior division supplies the posterior semicircular canal and saccule, even a "complete" loss on vestibular testing may be associated with some retained canal function. Furthermore, it is common to have another dizziness syndrome, BPPV, follow vestibular neuritis. Presumably this happens because the utricle is damaged (supplied by the superior vestibular nerve) and deposits loose otoconia into the preserved posterior canal.

There is also neuropathological evidence for loss of vestibular ganglion lesions. For example, pathologic study of a single patient documented findings compatible with an isolated viral infection of Scarpa ganglion (the vestibular ganglion). There was loss of hair cells, epithelialization of the utricular maculae and semicircular canal cristae on the deafferented side, and reduced synaptic density in the ipsilateral vestibular nucleus (Baloh et al., 1996).

Finally, there is also some evidence for viral damage to the brainstem vestibular nucleus (Arbusow et al., 2000). Since the vestibular neurons are distinct from cochlear neurons in the brainstem, a brainstem localization as well as the vestibular ganglion makes more sense than the nerve lesions in persons with no hearing symptoms. Nevertheless, if the nerve were involved after it separates from the cochlear nerve, neuritis would still be a reasonable mechanism. Prior to death and autopsy there is no way to make a clear distinction.

How are vestibular neuritis and labyrinthitis diagnosed?

Acutely, in uncomplicated cases, while a thorough examination is necessary, no additional testing is usually required. Certain types of specialists, namely otologists, neurotologists, and otoneurologists, are especially good at making these diagnoses, and seeing one of these doctors early on may make it possible to avoid unnecessary testing. In large part, the process involves ascertaining that the entire situation can be explained by a lesion in one or the other vestibular nerve. It is not possible on clinical examination to be absolutely certain that the picture of vestibular neuritis is not actually caused by a brainstem or cerebellar stroke, so mistakes are possible. Nevertheless, this happens so rarely that it is not necessary to perform magnetic resonance imaging (MRI) scans or the like very often.

Signs of vestibular neuritis include spontaneous nystagmus and unsteadiness. Occasionally other ocular disturbances will occur such as skew deviation (Safran et al., 1994) and asymmetric gaze evoked nystagmus.

However, if symptoms persist beyond one month, reoccur periodically, or evolve with time, testing may be proposed. In this situation, nearly all patients will be asked to undergo an audiogram and an electronystagmography (ENG). An audiogram is a hearing test needed to distinguish between vestibular neuritis and other possible diagnoses such as Ménière disease and migraine. The ENG test is essential to document the characteristic reduced responses to motion of one ear. An MRI scan will be performed if there is any reasonable possibility of a stroke or brain tumor. Occasionally one can visualize the inflammation of the vestibular nerve. In most instances, it is most cost effective to see a neurologist prior to obtaining an MRI. Blood tests for diabetes, thyroid disorders, Lyme disease, collagen vascular disease, and syphilis are sometimes performed, looking for these treatable illnesses. However, it is rare that these are ever positive.

How are vestibular neuritis and labyrinthitis treated?

Acutely, vestibular neuritis is treated symptomatically, meaning that medications are given for nausea (anti-emetics) and to reduce dizziness (vestibular suppressants). Typical medications used are Antivert (meclizine), Ativan (lorazepam), Phenergan, Compazine, and Valium (diazepam). When a herpes virus infection is strongly suspected, a medication called acyclovir or a relative may be used. Steroids (prednisone, methylprednisolone, or Decadron) are also used for some cases. Acute labyrinthitis is treated with the same medications as vestibular neuritis, plus an antibiotic such as amoxicillin if there is evidence for a middle ear infection (otitis media), such as ear pain and an abnormal ear examination suggesting fluid, redness, or pus behind the eardrum. Occasionally, especially for persons whose nausea and vomiting cannot be controlled, an admission to the hospital is made to treat dehydration with intravenous fluids. Generally, admission is brief, just long enough to rehydrate the patient and start him or her on an effective medication to prevent vomiting.

It usually takes three weeks to recover from vestibular neuritis or labyrinthitis. Recovery happens due to a combination of the body fighting off the infection and the brain getting used to the vestibular imbalance (compensation). Some persons experience persistent vertigo or discomfort on head motion even after three weeks have gone by. After two to three months, testing (that is, an ENG, audiogram, and others) is indicated to be certain that this is indeed the correct diagnosis. A vestibular rehabilitation program may help speed full recovery via compensation.

How might vestibular neuritis and labyrinthitis affect my life?

You will probably be unable to work for one or two weeks. You may be left with some minor sensitivity to head motion, which will persist for several years and may reduce your ability to perform athletic activities such as racquetball or volleyball. After the acute phase is over, for a moderate deficit, falls are no more likely than in persons of your age without vestibular deficit (Herdman et al., 2000).

Are there any current research studies in vestibular neuritis and labyrinthitis?

Vestibular neuritis and labyrinthitis are well recognized clinical syndromes. In our view, research is needed to quickly sort out the cause of this syndrome. We also hope that eventually better treatment, such as antivirals, may be found. The American Hearing Research Foundation (AHRF) has funded research on similar conditions in the past.

References

Arbusow V and others. Detection of herpes simplex virus type 1 in human vestibular nuclei. *Neurology* 55:880–82, 2000.

Baloh RW, Ishyama A, Wackym PA, Honrubia V. Vestibular neuritis: clinical-pathologic correlation. *Otolaryngology HNS* 114(4):586–92, 1996.

Basser L. Benign paroxysmal vertigo of childhood: a variety of vestibular neuritis. *Brain* 87:141–52.

Coats AC. Vestibular neuronitis. *Acta Otolaryngol (Stockh) (suppl)* 251:1–32, 1969.

Fetter M, Dichgans J. Vestibular neuritis spares the inferior division of the vestibular nerve. *Brain* 119:755–63, 1996.

Fischer CM. Vertigo in cerebrovascular disease. *Arch Otolaryngol* 85:529–34, 1967.

Goebel JA, O'Mara W, Gianoli G. Anatomic considerations in vestibular neuritis. *Otol Neurotol* 22:512–18, 2001.

Hart CW. Vestibular paralysis of sudden onset and probably viral etiology. *Ann ORL* 74:33–47, 1965.

Herdman SJ, Blatt P, Schubert MC, Tusa RJ. Falls in patients with vestibular deficits. *Am J. Otol* 21:847–51, 2000.

Hotson JR, Baloh RW. Acute vestibular syndrome. *NEJM* 9/3/1998, 680–85.

Moretti G, Manzoni G, Caffara P, Parma M. Benign recurrent vertigo and its connection with migraine. *Headache* 20:344–46, 1980.

Oh AK and others. Familial recurrent vertigo. *Am J. Med Gen* 100:287–91, 2001.

Rasekh CH, Harker LA. The prevalence of migraine in Ménière disease. *Laryngoscope* 102:135–38, 1992.

Safran AB, Vibert D, Issoua D, Hausler R. *Am J. Ophthalm.* 118(2): 238–45, 1994.

Silvoniemi P. Vestibular neuronitis: an otoneurological evaluation. *Acta Otolaryngol (Stockh) (Suppl)* 453:1–72, 1988.

Schuknecht HF, Kitamura K. Vestibular Neuritis. *Ann ORL* 79:1–19, 1981.

Slater R. Benign recurrent vertigo. *J. NNNP* 42:363–67, 1979.

Zajtchuk J, Matz G, Lindsay J. Temporal bone pathology in herpes oticus. *Ann ORL* 81:331–38, 1972.

Chapter 20

Vertigo

Chapter Contents

Section 20.1

Benign Paroxysmal Positional Vertigo

Vertigo is described as feeling like you are turning around when you are standing still—the experience is similar to how you feel when spinning on a playground roundabout. Vertigo has also been described as the sensation of standing still within a spinning room.

Benign paroxysmal positional vertigo (BPPV) is a condition characterized by episodes of sudden and severe vertigo when the head is moved around. Common triggers include rolling over in bed, getting out of bed, and lifting the head to look up. BPPV tends to come and go for no apparent reason. An affected person may have attacks of vertigo for a few weeks, then a period of time with no symptoms at all. Usually, BPPV affects only one ear. It is thought that BPPV is caused by particles within the balance organ of the inner ear. Other names for BPPV include benign postural vertigo, positional vertigo, and top shelf vertigo (because you get dizzy looking up).

Symptoms

The symptoms of BPPV can include the following:

- Sudden episodes of violent vertigo
- Nausea
- The vertigo may last half a minute or so
- The eyes may drift and flick uncontrollably (nystagmus)
- Movements of the head trigger the attacks

"Ear Rocks"

Inside the inner ear is a series of canals filled with fluid. These canals are at different angles. When the head is moved, the rolling of the fluid inside these canals tells the brain exactly how far, how fast, and in what direction the head is moving. BPPV is thought to be caused by little calcium carbonate crystals (otoconia) within the canals. Usually, these crystals are held in special reservoirs within other structures of the inner ear (saccule and utricle). It is thought that injury or degeneration of the utricle may allow the "ear rocks" to escape into the balance organ and interfere with the fluid flow.

A Range of Possible Causes

Factors that may allow calcium carbonate crystals to migrate into the balance organ include the following:

- Head injury
- Ear injury
- Ear infection, such as otitis media
- Ear surgery
- Degeneration of the inner ear structures
- Vestibular neuritis (viral infection of the inner ear)
- Ménière disease (disorder of the inner ear)
- Some types of minor strokes
- In around half of BPPV cases, the cause can't be found (idiopathic BPPV).

Diagnosis Methods

Dizziness and vertigo are common to a wide range of medical conditions, so careful diagnosis is important. Diagnosis methods may include the following:

- **Medical history:** illnesses such as cardiac arrhythmia, low blood pressure, and multiple sclerosis can include symptoms of vertigo.
- **Physical examination:** this could include a range of tests. For example, the patient lies on the examination bed while the doctor deliberately moves his or her head into positions that are known to trigger BPPV within a few seconds. The doctor will also check for nystagmus.
- **Electronystagmography (ENG):** a special eye test that checks for the presence of nystagmus.

- **Ear tests:** such as hearing tests.

- **Scans:** such as magnetic resonance imaging, to check for the presence of otoconia in the balance organ.

Treatment Options

Generally, BPPV resolves by itself within six months or so. Treatment options in the meantime could include medications to help control nausea and special maneuvers designed to dislodge otoconia. These maneuvers boast an 80 percent success rate and include the following:

- **The Semont maneuver:** the patient lies down, then is quickly rolled from one side to the other.

- **The Epley maneuver:** also known as canalith repositioning procedure. The patient's head is moved into four different postures. The head is held in each postural position for about half a minute.

- **After-treatment care:** it is important to sit still for at least ten minutes after the Semont or Epley maneuver to allow the otoconia to settle. For the next forty-eight hours, keep the head still and upright and sleep in a semi-sitting position. For the next five days, strictly avoid any postures that have triggered BPPV in the past. After one week, deliberately try to induce BPPV to see if your symptoms have improved. Report to your doctor.

- **Brandt-Daroff exercises:** if the above maneuvers don't work, the next stage of treatment is Brandt-Daroff exercises. This is a more complex series of postures that have to be performed three times every day for two weeks.

Self-Help Suggestions

Certain lifestyle changes could help to manage BPPV and reduce the frequency of attacks. Suggestions include the following:

- Sleep with your head raised higher than usual—for example, use two pillows instead of one.

- In bed, try to avoid lying on the affected side.

- Remember that lying on your back may bring on symptoms too.

- When rising in the morning, move slowly. Rest for a few minutes at each posture.

- Whenever possible, avoid moving your head quickly.

- You may have to avoid sporting activities that rely on quick changes of movement and posture (such as football or tennis).

- Remember that any activity that requires you to tip your head back could bring on vertigo. This could include activities such as getting your hair washed at the hairdresser or having a dental check-up.

Surgery May Be Needed in Severe Cases

If nonsurgical treatments fail and the symptoms continue for more than twelve months, an operation may be needed. Generally, the nerve that services part of the balance organ (posterior semicircular canal) is cut. The risks of this type of operation include hearing loss.

Things to Remember

- Benign paroxysmal positional vertigo (BPPV) is a condition characterized by episodes of sudden and severe vertigo when the head is moved around.

- Common triggers include rolling over in bed, getting out of bed, and lifting the head to look up.

- It is thought that BPPV is caused by particles within the balance organ of the inner ear.

Section 20.2

Epileptic Vertigo

Reprinted from "Epileptic Vertigo," by Timothy C. Hain, M.D., last revised March 2002. © 2004 American Hearing Research Foundation. Reprinted with permission.

What is epileptic vertigo?

While epilepsy is commonly accompanied by dizziness or vertigo, vertigo is only rarely caused by epilepsy. This arises primarily because vertigo is much more commonly caused by ear conditions. Epileptic vertigo is due to brain injury, typically the part of the temporal lobe that processes vestibular signals. Loss of consciousness usually occurs at the time of injury. The typical symptom is "quick spins," although this symptom has other potential causes (for example, BPPV or vestibular neuritis).

What causes epileptic vertigo?

Epileptic vertigo is felt to be caused by abnormal stimulation of parts of the cortex that represent the vestibular system—parietal, temporal, and frontal cortex. Specific areas include the superior lip of the intraparietal sulcus, the posterior superior temporal lobe, and the temporal-parietal border regions (Penfield, 1954).

How is epileptic vertigo diagnosed?

Epileptic vertigo is only a diagnostic problem when the person does not have a full seizure—in other words, he or she does not have convulsions, psychomotor symptoms, or twitching characteristic of classic partial or generalized seizures.

In most instances, it presents as a "quick spin" type symptom. The person notes that the world makes a quick horizontal movement, lasting roughly one to two seconds at most. Quick spins must be differentiated from a variety of other conditions including vestibular neuralgia, Ménière disease, and BPPV, among others.

Diagnostic tests that are particularly helpful include the electro-encephalograph (EEG) and magnetic resonance imaging (MRI) scan of the head.

How is epileptic vertigo treated?

Treatment of epileptic vertigo is generally supervised by a neurologist. Epileptic vertigo generally responds well to traditional anticonvulsants such as carbamazepine and its relatives. There are many anticonvulsant medications that can be used.

Are any research studies in epileptic vertigo ongoing?

As of March 2002, a visit to the National Library of Medicine's search engine, PubMed, revealed 195 research articles concerning epilepsy and vertigo published since 1966. The American Hearing Research Foundation (AHRF) has funded basic research on vertiginous conditions in the past, and is interested in funding sound research on vertigo in the future.

References

Kluge M, and others. Epileptic vertigo: evidence for vestibular representation in human frontal cortex. *Neurology* 2000; 55:1906–8.

Penfield W, Jasper H. *Epilepsy and functional anatomy of the human brain*. Boston: Little, Brown, 1954.

Tusa RJ, Kaplan PW, Hain TC, Naidu S. Ipsiversive eye deviation and epileptic nystagmus. *Neurology*. 1990.

Section 20.3

Vestibular Migraine

Migraine, a disorder usually associated with headache, can cause several vestibular syndromes. Migraine is extremely common. Studies suggest that more than twenty million people in the United States suffer from migraine and that about 25 percent of these experience dizziness during attacks.

The International Headache Society classifies migraine disorders into several types. Migraine without aura consists of periodic headaches that are usually throbbing and one-sided, made worse by activity, and associated with nausea and increased sensitivity to light and noise. Vertigo can occur before, during, or separately from the episodes of migrainous headache. Migraine with aura, or classic migraine, is associated with short-lived symptoms (noises, flashes of light, tingling, numbness, vertigo, and others) known as the aura. These symptoms usually precede the headache and usually last five to twenty minutes. In a variation called migraine with prolonged aura, these symptoms may last a week. Migraine patients may experience migraine with aura on some occasions and migraine without aura on other occasions. Symptoms of basilar migraine include vertigo, tinnitus, decreased hearing, and ataxia (loss of coordination).

Several vestibular syndromes are caused by migraine. Benign recurrent vertigo of adults (not to be confused with BPPV, or benign paroxysmal positional vertigo) consists of spells of vertigo, occasionally with tinnitus but without hearing loss. Doctors must rule out other possible causes before making a diagnosis of migraine-induced vertigo. Benign paroxysmal vertigo of childhood (not to be confused with BPPV) consists of spells of imbalance and vertigo without hearing loss or tinnitus (ringing in the ears). The majority of cases occur between the ages of one and four but may occur up to age ten. Migrainous infarction or complicated migraine is a migraine with aura associated with a stroke (blood-flow problem resulting in cell death); one of the symptoms may be vertigo.

In addition to the syndromes caused by migraine, several vestibular disorders have been associated with migraine. Studies indicate that people with migraine are much more likely than other people to experience severe motion sickness and may be more likely to suffer from Ménière's disease or BPPV.

Stress, anxiety, hypoglycemia, fluctuating estrogen, certain foods, smoking, and other factors can trigger migraine. Vertigo and imbalance secondary to migraine usually respond to the same treatment used for migraine headaches. Treatment of migraine includes eliminating from the diet substances known to trigger migraine attacks, such as chocolate, nuts, cheese, red wine, and other foods. Medications may also be prescribed.

Section 20.4

Post-Traumatic Vertigo

Reprinted from "Post-Traumatic Vertigo," by Timothy C. Hain, M.D., last revised April 2002. © 2002 American Hearing Research Foundation. Reprinted with permission.

What is post-traumatic vertigo?

Head injuries are sustained by 5 percent of the population annually. Post-traumatic vertigo refers to dizziness that follows a neck or head injury. While injuries to other parts of the body might, in theory, be associated with dizziness, in practice this is almost never the case. Because of the high incidence of litigation associated with post-traumatic vertigo, most clinicians are extremely cautious in making this diagnosis.

What causes post-traumatic vertigo?

There are many potential causes of post-traumatic vertigo:

1. **Positional vertigo,** and particularly benign paroxysmal positional vertigo (BPPV). This is the most common type of severe

dizziness, and it is also common after head injury. It is easily recognized by the pattern of dizziness that is brought only when the head is placed in certain positions. There are several good treatments for BPPV and the prognosis for this syndrome, in the proper hands, is excellent. It is also possible to have rarer causes of positional vertigo, including mainly utricular injury, vestibular atelectasis, and various forms of central vertigo caused by cerebellar or brainstem disturbances.

2. **Post-traumatic Ménière disease,** also sometimes called hydrops. Episodes of dizziness accompanied by noises in the ear, fullness, or hearing changes. The mechanism is thought to be bleeding into the inner ear, followed by disturbance of fluid transport. The onset of symptoms may vary from immediately to as long as one year later. There are frequently legal implications to this diagnosis. The probability of Ménière disease being reasonably attributed to post-traumatic mechanisms is a function of the severity of injury (severe makes it more likely), the latency from the injury (longer is less likely), the presence of a pre-existing condition, and the presence of secondary gain. Persons with the large vestibular aqueduct syndrome are felt to be more likely to develop these symptoms (Berettini et al., 2000).

3. **Labyrinthine "concussion."** A nonpersistent hearing or labyrinthine disturbance which follows a head injury, not caused by another mechanism. A hearing loss or a nystagmus must be present to make this diagnosis with a reasonable degree of medical certainty. While the name implicates an inner ear disturbance, this symptom complex may be impossible to differentiate from other entities.

4. **Post-traumatic migraine.** Dizziness combined with migraine headaches. Headaches and vertigo are common after head injuries. The main difficulty in this situation is to determine whether they are related or coincidental.

5. **Cervical vertigo.** Imbalance following a severe neck injury. While nearly all dizziness specialists agree that cervical vertigo does exist, there is controversy regarding the frequency with which it occurs (Brandt T, 1996).

6. **Temporal bone fracture.** Severe dizziness after the injury, with skull or temporal bone CT scan indicating a fracture. Often accompanied by hearing loss or peripheral facial weakness Bell's

palsy. Temporal bone fractures, especially the oblique variety, may impair hearing and cause dizziness. There often is blood seen behind the eardrum (hemotympanum). Either a conductive or a sensorineural hearing loss may be present. Vestibular deficits are also common, especially in the oblique variety. Bilateral vestibular problems are exceedingly rare. Treatment is conservative. Prophylactic antibiotics are given, usually for four weeks. Myringotomy and insertion of a ventilating tube may be indicated, especially for serious otitis that persists after one month (Pulek and Deguine, 2001).

7. **Perilymph fistula.** Usually symptoms of imbalance and dizziness provoked by straining or blowing the nose. People with fistula may also get dizzy with loud noises (called Tullio phenomenon). The frequency with which this syndrome occurs is controversial, but general opinion holds that it is rare.

8. **Factitious vertigo.** Complaints of vertigo related to psychological causes such as depression, anxiety, or an attempt to obtain compensation (also known as "malingering"). Anxiety and depression may result from traumatic brain injury that creates a self-perpetuating psychological reaction (Alexander, 1998).

9. **Epileptic vertigo.** Vertigo due to brain injury, typically the part of the temporal lobe that processes vestibular signals. Loss of consciousness usually occurs at the time of injury. The typical symptom is "quick spins," although this symptom has other potential causes (BPPV, vestibular neuritis). Treatment is with anticonvulsants.

10. **Diffuse axonal injury (DAI).** Pure deceleration forces can produce diffuse axonal injury (Gennarelli et al., 1982). In some individuals who come to autopsy after a twisting type injury of the head or neck, small areas of bleeding (petechial hemorrhage), and interruption of neuronal circuits (axonal damage) can be found. Complaints of dizziness attributed to brainstem injuries which cannot be imaged with a good MRI. This is an autopsy diagnosis—it cannot be made with certainty prior to death. Historically, significant DAI is not felt to occur in awake humans who do not report loss of consciousness. A thirty-minute loss seems likely to be needed for a significant DAI (Alexander, 1998).

11. **Postconcussion syndrome.** A combination of headache, dizziness, and mental disturbance which follows a head injury,

without an identifiable etiology (cause). If an etiology can be determined for symptoms, a more specific diagnosis should be used. Postconcussion syndrome is often attributed to traumatic brain injury (TBI), which is a general term for a head injury affecting the brain. While dizziness and nausea symptoms usually resolve over six weeks, cognitive symptoms and headaches may be persist longer. Occasionally symptoms are permanent. As noted above, in many cases, chronic symptoms are psychological in origin.

12. **Whiplash injury syndrome.** Very similar to postconcussion syndrome, but with the addition of neck complaints. Possibly related to cervical vertigo, dizziness occurs 20 to 60 percent of the time. This syndrome can persist for years; however, about 75 percent of patients are recovered by one year (Radanov et al., 1994).

How is post-traumatic vertigo diagnosed?

First, the doctor will want to know exactly when and how the head or neck was injured, and the character of the dizziness (for example. is there spinning, unsteadiness, confusion?). The doctor will also want to know if you were unconscious and, if so, the duration of time. All available records from the emergency room or hospital where you were seen after the injury should be obtained if possible.

Next, a specialized examination for dizziness will be performed. Balance will be measured. A search for nystagmus will be made, related to head and/or neck position or to vibration of the neck. You will be checked for pressure sensitivity with the fistula test.

Laboratory tests will be ordered. In most instances these will include an audiogram, electronystagmography (ENG), possibly an MRI scan or CT scan of the inner ear. An EEG may be obtained. In patients with hearing disturbance, an electrocochleography (ECOG) may be done. Moving platform posturography and psychological testing is sometimes done in persons who have entirely normal test results. They can document subtle imbalance and cognitive difficulties.

How is post-traumatic vertigo treated?

Treatment is individualized to the diagnosis. Treatment usually includes a combination of medication, changes in lifestyle, and possibly physical therapy. Occasionally, surgery may be recommended.

Is AHRF involved in any research studies in post-traumatic vertigo?

The American Hearing Research Foundation (AHRF) has funded basic research on related conditions in the past.

References

Alexander MP. In the pursuit of proof of brain damage after whiplash injury. *Neurology* 51:336–40, 1998.

Berrettini, S., E. Neri, et al. Large Vestibular Aqueduct in distal renal tubular acidosis. High- resolution MR in three cases. *Acta Radiol* 42(3): 320–22, 2001.

Brandt. Cervical Vertigo—Reality or fiction? *Audiol Neurootol* 1:187–96, 1996.

Feneley, M. R. and P. Murthy. Acute bilateral vestibulo-cochlear dysfunction following occipital fracture. *J Laryngol Otol* 108(1): 54–56, 1994.

Genarelli and others. Diffuse axonal injury and traumatic coma in the primate. *Ann Neurol* 12:564–74, 1982.

Pulec JL, DeGuine C. Hemotympanum from trauma. *ENT journal,* l80:486, 2001.

Radanov BP, Surzenegger M, Schnidrig A. Relation between ... *Br. J. Rheum* 33:442–48, 1994.

Rubin AM. Dizziness associated with head-and-neck trauma. *Audio Digest* 30(22), 1997.

Tusa RJ, Kaplan PW, Hain TC, Naidu S. Ipsiversive eye deviation and epileptic nystagmus. *Neurology*. 1990.

Section 20.5

Mal de Debarquement

Reprinted from "Mal de Debarquement (MDD)," by Timothy C. Hain, M.D., last revised November 2002. © 2002 American Hearing Research Foundation. Reprinted with permission.

What is mal de debarquement?

Mal de debarquement (MDD) is a type of vertigo and imbalance that occurs after getting off of a boat, or sometimes, after a long airplane ride. Most individuals with this diagnosis are women between the ages of forty and fifty who go on a seven-day cruise. After getting off the boat, or "debarking" (debarquement), they develop a rocking sensation, as if they are still on the boat. The rocking sensation may persist for months or even years! Most people seem to have it for a month or less. Nevertheless, a recent study of MDD (Hain et al., 1999) showed that it can last much longer.

What causes mal de debarquement?

Little is known about this rare disorder. It is clear, however, that MDD is not caused by an injury to the ear or brain. Some dizziness experts believe that MDD is caused by a variant of migraine. Because the condition largely occurs in females, it may also have something to do with sex hormones, such as estrogen or progesterone. It could also be genetic, related to two copies of the X chromosome perhaps combined with other susceptibility factors. It seems unlikely to be a psychological disturbance; although it is always difficult to entirely exclude psychological problems, the male to female ratio and other aspects of this disorder would make this unlikely.

How is mal de debarquement diagnosed?

The diagnosis is made by a combination of the history (rocking after prolonged exposure to a boat) and exclusion of reasonable alternatives. Tests to exclude Ménière disease should be done, and if there is a history of plane flight, perilymph fistula should also be considered. A typical person is a woman of appropriate age who has gone on a cruise and who is now rocking.

The following diagnostic tests are generally performed:

- **Rotatory chair and video-ENG** (usually normal; occasionally there may be unusually strong or prolonged optokinetic or vestibular responses, and there is also sometimes positional nystagmus)

- **Audiogram** (expect normal; abnormal suggests other disorders)

- **Blood tests for autoimmune disorders involving the ear** {antinuclear antibody [ANA], antimicrosomal antibodies)

How is mal de debarquement treated?

Medical Treatment: After the MDD has started, most medications that work for other forms of dizziness or motion sickness are ineffective. Specifically, Antivert, Bonine, meclizine, Dramamine, and scopolamine seem to be of little use. Valium and related medications such as Klonopin are helpful in some persons. There is some worry that these medications may prolong the duration of symptoms (although this worry has not yet been tested by a research study). An antidepressant called amitriptyline may also be helpful. Hormonal medications such as estrogen or progesterone might be problematic— it might be worth a trial of stopping them if this is practical. Anecdotally, nonsteroidal anti-inflammatory medications such as Celebrex can help. Also anecdotally, phenytoin, carbamazepine, and related drugs may be useful in reducing symptoms. A controlled trial of these medications may be in order, if more evidence accumulates.

Prevention: It is possible that medications taken prior to and during boat travel might prevent development of MDD. Again, this possibility has not been tested by a research study. Nevertheless, medications that suppress the inner ear or block adaptation to inner ear signals might be useful. Anecdotal evidence suggests that while meclizine and scopolamine are ineffective, some people can prevent MDD by taking diazepam or lorazepam prior to getting on the boat or airplane. Avoidance of motion is clearly helpful. If you get dizzy from riding on boats, don't do it!

Physical Therapy: Physical therapy may be helpful in MDD but the evidence really isn't there. In one study (Hain et al., 1999), ten out of fifteen persons who had vestibular rehabilitation reported improvement. However, as there were no controls in this study, the improvement might have occurred in any case, and it is the trend for MDD to gradually improve over months. Zimbelman has written a review of rehabilitation in MDD.

How might mal de debarquement affect my life?

Persons with MDD often have impaired balance. They often choose to travel less to avoid motion exposures. MDD is not life-threatening.

Are there any current research studies in mal de debarquement?

Little research has been done on MDD, and what has been done largely relates to attempts to quantify how often the condition occurs. We know of no formal research regarding treatment of MDD. The American Hearing Research Foundation (AHRF) has funded basic research on dizziness and balance disorders in the past, and is interested in funding research on MDD in the future.

References

Brown JJ, Baloh RW. Persistent Mal de Debarquement Syndrome: a motion-induced subjective disorder of balance. *Am J Otolaryngol* 1987: 219–22.

Gorden CR, Spitzer O, Shupak A, Doweck I. Survey of mal de debarquement. *British Medical J* 1992:304, 544.

Gorden CR, Spitzer O, Doweck, Melemed Y, Shupak A. Clinical features of Mal De Debarquement: adaptation and habituation to sea conditions. *JVR* 5(5):363–69, 1995.

Hain TC, Hanna PA, Rheinberger MA. Mal de Debarquement. *Arch Otolaryngol Head Neck Surg* 125:615–20, 1999.

Murphy TP. Mal de Debarquement syndrome: a forgotten entity ? *Otol HNS* 109:10–13, 1993.

Mair IWS. The mal de debarquement syndrome. *J. Audiological Med* 5:21–25, 1996.

Zimbelman JL, Walton TM. Vestibular rehabilitation of a patient with persistent Mal de Debarquement. *Physical Therapy Case Reports* 2(4):129–37, 1999.

Chapter 21

Dizziness and Motion Sickness

Each year more than two million people visit a doctor for dizziness, and an untold number suffer with motion sickness, which is the most common medical problem associated with travel.

What is dizziness?

Some people describe a balance problem by saying they feel dizzy, lightheaded, unsteady, or giddy. This feeling of imbalance or disequilibrium, without a sensation of turning or spinning, is sometimes due to an inner ear problem.

What is vertigo?

A few people describe their balance problem by using the word *vertigo*, which comes from the Latin verb "to turn". They often say that they or their surroundings are turning or spinning. Vertigo is frequently due to an inner ear problem.

What is motion sickness and seasickness?

Some people experience nausea and even vomiting when riding in an airplane, automobile, or amusement park ride, and this is called motion sickness. Many people experience motion sickness when riding on a boat or ship, and this is called seasickness even though it is the same disorder.

Motion sickness or seasickness is usually just a minor annoyance and does not signify any serious medical illness, but some travelers are incapacitated by it, and a few even suffer symptoms for a few days after the trip.

How does the body maintain balance?

Dizziness, vertigo, and motion sickness all relate to the sense of balance and equilibrium. Researchers in space and aeronautical medicine call this sense spatial orientation, because it tells the brain where the body is "in space": what direction it is pointing, what direction it is moving, and if it is turning or standing still.

Your sense of balance is maintained by a complex interaction of the following parts of the nervous system:

- The **inner ears** (also called the labyrinth), which monitor the directions of motion, such as turning, or forward-backward, side-to-side, and up-and-down motions

- The **eyes,** which monitor where the body is in space (i.e., upside down, right side up, etc.) and also directions of motion

- The **skin pressure receptors** such as in the joints and spine, which tell what part of the body is down and touching the ground

- The **muscle and joint sensory receptors,** which tell what parts of the body are moving

- The **central nervous system** (the brain and spinal cord), which processes all the bits of information from the four other systems to make some coordinated sense out of it all

The symptoms of motion sickness and dizziness appear when the central nervous system receives conflicting messages from the other four systems.

For example, suppose you are riding through a storm, and your airplane is being tossed about by air turbulence. But your eyes do not detect all this motion because all you see is the inside of the airplane. Then your brain receives messages that do not match with each other. You might become "air sick."

Or suppose you are sitting in the back seat of a moving car, reading a book. Your inner ears and skin receptors will detect the motion of your travel, but your eyes see only the pages of your book. You could become "car sick."

Or, to use a true medical condition as an example, suppose you suffer inner ear damage on only one side from a head injury or an infection. The damaged inner ear does not send the same signals as the healthy ear. This gives conflicting signals to the brain about the sensation of rotation, and you could suffer a sense of spinning, vertigo, and nausea.

What medical conditions cause dizziness?

Circulation: If your brain does not get enough blood flow, you feel lightheaded. Almost everyone has experienced this on occasion when standing up quickly from a lying down position. But some people have lightheadedness from poor circulation on a frequent or chronic basis. This could be caused by arteriosclerosis or hardening of the arteries, and it is commonly seen in patients who have high blood pressure, diabetes, or high levels of blood fats (cholesterol). It is sometimes seen in patients with inadequate cardiac (heart) function or with anemia.

Certain drugs also decrease the blood flow to the brain, especially stimulants such as nicotine and caffeine. Excess salt in the diet also leads to poor circulation. Sometimes circulation is impaired by spasms in the arteries caused by emotional stress, anxiety, and tension.

If the inner ear fails to receive enough blood flow, the more specific type of dizziness that occurs is vertigo. The inner ear is very sensitive to minor alterations of blood flow, and all of the causes mentioned for poor circulation to the brain also apply specifically to the inner ear.

Injury: A skull fracture that damages the inner ear produces a profound and incapacitating vertigo with nausea and hearing loss. The dizziness will last for several weeks, then slowly improve as the normal (other) side takes over.

Infection: Viruses, such as those causing the common cold or flu, can attack the inner ear and its nerve connections to the brain. This can result in severe vertigo, but hearing is usually spared. However, a bacterial infection such as mastoiditis that extends into the inner ear will completely destroy both the hearing and the equilibrium function of that ear. The severity of dizziness and recovery time will be similar to that of skull fracture.

Allergy: Some people experience dizziness or vertigo attacks when they are exposed to foods or airborne particles (such as dust, molds, pollens, danders, etc.) to which they are allergic.

Neurological Diseases: A number of diseases of the nerves can affect balance, such as multiple sclerosis, syphilis, tumors, and so on. These are uncommon causes, but your physician will think about them during the examination.

What will the physician do for my dizziness?

The doctor will ask you to describe your dizziness, whether it is lightheadedness or a sensation of motion, how long and how often the dizziness has troubled you, how long a dizzy episode lasts, and whether it is associated with hearing loss or nausea and vomiting. You might be asked for circumstances that might bring on a dizzy spell. You will need to answer questions about your general health, any medicines you are taking, head injuries, recent infections, and other information about your ears and neurological system.

Your physician will examine your ears, nose, and throat and do tests of nerve and balance function. Because the inner ear controls both balance and hearing, disorders of balance often affect hearing and vice versa. Therefore, your physician will probably recommend hearing tests (audiograms). The physician might order skull x-rays, a CT or MRI scan of your head, or special tests of eye motion after warm or cold water is used to stimulate the inner ear (ENG: electronystagmography). In some cases, blood tests or a cardiology (heart) evaluation might be recommended.

Not every patient will require every test. The physician's judgment will be based on each particular patient. Similarly, the treatments recommended by your physician will depend on the diagnosis.

What can I do to reduce dizziness?

- Avoid rapid changes in position, especially from lying down to standing up or turning around from one side to the other.

- Avoid extremes of head motion (especially looking up) or rapid head motion (especially turning or twisting).

- Eliminate or decrease use of products that impair circulation, such as nicotine, caffeine, and salt.

- Minimize your exposure to circumstances that precipitate your dizziness, such as stress and anxiety or substances to which you are allergic.

- Avoid hazardous activities when you are dizzy, such as driving an automobile or operating dangerous equipment, or climbing a step ladder, and so on.

What can I do for motion sickness?

Always ride where your eyes will see the same motion that your body and inner ears feel (e.g., sit in the front seat of the car and look at the distant scenery; go up on the deck of the ship and watch the horizon; sit by the window of the airplane and look outside. In an airplane choose a seat over the wings where the motion is the least).

- Do not read while traveling if you are subject to motion sickness, and do not sit in a seat facing backward.

- Do not watch or talk to another traveler who is having motion sickness.

- Avoid strong odors and spicy or greasy foods immediately before and during your travel. Medical research has not yet investigated the effectiveness of popular folk remedies such as soda crackers and Seven Up® or cola syrup over ice.

- Take one of the varieties of motion sickness medicines before your travel begins, as recommended by your physician.

Some of these medications can be purchased without a prescription (i.e., Dramamine®, Bonine®, Marezine®, etc.) Stronger medicines such as tranquilizers and nervous system depressants will require a prescription from your physician. Some are used in pill or suppository form.

Remember: Most cases of dizziness and motion sickness are mild and self-treatable disorders. But severe cases and those that become progressively worse deserve the attention of a physician with specialized skills in diseases of the ear, nose, throat, equilibrium, and neurological systems.

Chapter 22

Ménière Disease

Ménière disease is an abnormality of the inner ear causing a host of symptoms, including vertigo or severe dizziness, tinnitus or a roaring sound in the ears, fluctuating hearing loss, and the sensation of pressure or pain in the affected ear. The disorder usually affects only one ear and is a common cause of hearing loss. Named after French physician Prosper Ménière, who first described the syndrome in 1861.

What causes Ménière disease?

The symptoms of Ménière disease are associated with a change in fluid volume within a portion of the inner ear known as the labyrinth. The labyrinth has two parts: the bony labyrinth and the membranous labyrinth. The membranous labyrinth, which is encased by bone, is necessary for hearing and balance and is filled with a fluid called endolymph. When your head moves, endolymph moves, causing nerve receptors in the membranous labyrinth to send signals to the brain about the body's motion. An increase in endolymph, however, can cause the membranous labyrinth to balloon or dilate, a condition known as endolymphatic hydrops.

Many experts on Ménière disease think that a rupture of the membranous labyrinth allows the endolymph to mix with perilymph, another inner ear fluid that occupies the space between the membranous

Reprinted from " Ménière's Disease," National Institute on Deafness and Other Communication Disorders, National Institutes of Health, NIH Publication No. 98-3404, November 2001.

labyrinth and the bony inner ear. This mixing, scientists believe, can cause the symptoms of Ménière disease. Scientists are investigating several possible causes of the disease, including environmental factors, such as noise pollution and viral infections, as well as biological factors.

What are the symptoms of Ménière disease?

The symptoms of Ménière disease occur suddenly and can arise daily or as infrequently as once a year. Vertigo, often the most debilitating symptom of Ménière disease, typically involves a whirling dizziness that forces the sufferer to lie down. Vertigo attacks can lead to severe nausea, vomiting, and sweating and often come with little or no warning.

Some individuals with Ménière disease have attacks that start with tinnitus (ear noises), a loss of hearing, or a full feeling or pressure in the affected ear. It is important to remember that all of these symptoms are unpredictable. Typically, the attack is characterized by a combination of vertigo, tinnitus, and hearing loss lasting several hours. People experience these discomforts at varying frequencies, durations, and intensities. Some may feel slight vertigo a few times a year. Others may be occasionally disturbed by intense, uncontrollable tinnitus while sleeping. Ménière disease sufferers may also notice a hearing loss and feel unsteady all day long for prolonged periods. Other occasional symptoms of Ménière disease include headaches, abdominal discomfort, and diarrhea. A person's hearing tends to recover between attacks but over time becomes worse.

How is Ménière disease diagnosed?

Based on a recent study, the National Institute on Deafness and Other Communication Disorders (NIDCD) estimates that there are currently approximately 615,000 individuals with diagnosed Ménière disease in the United States and 45,500 newly diagnosed cases each year. Proper diagnosis of Ménière disease entails several procedures, including a medical history interview and a physical examination by a physician, hearing and balance tests, and medical imaging with magnetic resonance imaging (MRI). Accurate measurement and characterization of hearing loss are of critical importance in the diagnosis of Ménière disease.

Through the use of several types of hearing tests, physicians can characterize hearing loss as being sensory, arising from the inner ear,

or neural, arising from the hearing nerve. Recording the aud
brain stem response, which measures electrical activity in the hearing nerve and brain stem, is useful in differentiating between these
two types of hearing loss. Electrocochleography, recording the electrical activity of the inner ear in response to sound, helps confirm the
diagnosis.

To test the vestibular or balance system, physicians irrigate the
ears with warm and cool water or air. This procedure, known as caloric testing, results in nystagmus, rapid eye movements that can help
a physician analyze a balance disorder. Since tumor growth can produce symptoms similar to Ménière disease, an MRI is a useful test to
determine whether a tumor is causing the patient's vertigo and hearing loss.

How is Ménière disease treated?

There is no cure for Ménière disease. However, the symptoms of
the disease are often controlled successfully by reducing the body's
retention of fluids through dietary changes (such as a low-salt or salt-
free diet and no caffeine or alcohol) or medication. Changes in medications that either control allergies or improve blood circulation in
the inner ear may help. Eliminating tobacco use and reducing stress
levels are more ways some people can lessen the severity of their
symptoms.

Different surgical procedures have been advocated for patients
with persistent, debilitating vertigo from Ménière disease. Labyrinth-
ectomy (removal of the inner ear sense organ) can effectively control
vertigo, but sacrifices hearing and is reserved for patients with nonfunctional hearing in the affected ear. Vestibular neurectomy, selectively severing a nerve from the affected inner ear organ, usually
controls the vertigo while preserving hearing, but carries surgical
risks. Recently, the administration of the ototoxic antibiotic gentamicin directly into the middle ear space has gained popularity worldwide for the control of the vertigo of Ménière disease.

What research is being done?

Scientists are investigating environmental and biological factors
that may cause Ménière disease or induce an attack. They are also
studying how fluid composition and movement in the labyrinth affect
hearing and balance. By studying hair cells in the inner ear, which are
responsible for proper hearing and balance, scientists are learning how

the ear converts the mechanical energy of sound waves and motion into nerve impulses. Insights into the mechanisms of Ménière disease will enable scientists to develop preventive strategies and more effective treatment.

Chapter 23

Perilymph Fistula

A perilymph fistula, or PLF, is an abnormal opening in the fluid-filled inner ear. There are several possible places that there can be an opening—between the air-filled middle ear/mastoid sinus, into the intracranial cavity, or into other spaces in the temporal bone. In most instances it is a tear or defect in one or both of the small, thin membranes between the middle and inner ears. These membranes are called the oval window and the round window.

A dehiscence is similar to a fistula, but not as severe. Bone is missing, usually over the top (superior) semicircular canal, uncovering a membrane. This dehiscence makes the ear more sensitive to pressure and noise.

PLF is a very rare condition compared to most other causes of dizziness and hearing loss.

Symptoms of a Fistula

The changes in air pressure that occur in the middle ear (for example, when your ears "pop" in an airplane) normally do not affect your inner ear. When a fistula is present, changes in middle ear pressure will directly affect the inner ear, stimulating the balance and/or hearing structures within and causing typical symptoms. There are a number of other conditions that can also cause pressure sensitivity, such as Ménière disease and vestibular fibrosis.

The symptoms of perilymph fistula may include dizziness, vertigo, imbalance, nausea, and vomiting. Usually, however, patients report an unsteadiness that increases with activity and that is relieved by rest. Some people experience ringing or fullness in the ears, and many notice a hearing loss. Some people with fistulas find that their symptoms get worse with coughing, sneezing, or blowing their noses, as well as with exertion and activity. This sort of symptom goes under the general rubric of "Valsalva-induced dizziness," and it can also be associated with other medical conditions in entirely different categories—for example, the Chiari malformation, and a heart condition called "IHSS." Returning to fistula, it is not unusual to notice that use of one's own voice or a musical instrument will cause dizziness (this is called the Tullio phenomenon).

A closely related condition is alternobaric vertigo (Wicks, 1989). Here dizziness is associated with a difference in pressure between the ears. This condition remains difficult to document. Some patients with sleep apnea on CPAP may have vertigo due to this mechanism.

Fistula Types and Usual Causes

Window Fistulae

- Oval window type
  - Stapedectomy surgery (for otosclerosis)
  - Head trauma or barotrauma (pressure injury)
  - Acoustic trauma
- Round window type
  - Barotrauma—Scuba diving, airplane pressurization
  - Congenital malformations (such as Mondini)

Canal Type

There is usually no opening in the inner ear membranes with this type of fistula.

- Cholesteatoma (chronic infection [Magliulo et al., 1997])
- Fenestration surgery (obsolete surgery for otosclerosis)
- Superior canal dehiscence (congenital weakness in bone combined with head trauma [Minor, 2000])
- Head trauma

Other Otic Capsule Type (Not in Canal)

- Congenital weakness in bone, located in neither the canal nor window areas
- Cochlear implant

Head trauma is the most common cause of fistulas, usually involving a direct blow to the ear. Fistulas may also develop following rapid or profound changes in intracranial or atmospheric pressure, such as may occur with Scuba diving, or even just dives into a swimming pool (Rozsasi et al., 2003). The damage of pressure fluctuations probably arises via coupling through the middle ear, as tympanic membrane perforations protect animals from barotrauma (Meller et al., 2003). Forceful coughing, sneezing, or straining as in lifting a heavy object may rarely cause a fistula. In pregnancy, collagen changes throughout the body, and fistulae may arise spontaneously or in association with delivery.

Children are likely more prone to develop fistulae because of more widely open pathways between the inner ear and the spinal fluid.

Ear surgery, particularly "stapes" surgery for otosclerosis (stapedectomy or stapedotomy), often creates a fistula. These are thought to generally heal spontaneously. If vertigo persists for a week following stapes surgery, exploration for fistula may be recommended. Vertigo may also occur in a delayed fashion—months to years after stapes surgery. In these cases, exploration and patching of fistula has also been reported to be effective (Albera, Canale et al., 2004). In some of these cases, the stapes prosthesis has become displaced into the oval window.

Some patients develop symptoms attributed to fistula following airplane descent.

Fistulas may be present from birth (usually in association with deafness) or may result from chronic ear infections called cholesteatomas.

Fistulae are also created by a surgical procedure usually done for otosclerosis ("stapedectomy"). A dehiscence was the intended result of another surgical procedure for otosclerosis called a "fenestration"). The purpose of fenestration is to improve hearing. In animals, fenestrations create pressure sensitivity (Hirvonen et al., 2001), and this is nearly always the case in people who have had this obsolete surgery.

Fistulae are usually associated with some event, most commonly barotrauma or head injury (Lehrer et al., 1984), but rarely, fistulae occur spontaneously (Kohut, 1996).

297

Fistulas may occur in one or both ears, but bilateral fistulas are thought to be exceedingly rare (Sismanis et al., 1990).

How Does the Doctor Know If I Have a Fistula?

There is considerable controversy about how to make the diagnosis of fistula. Ménière disease, which is much more common than fistula, can have identical symptoms, including pressure sensitivity. For this reason, fistula diagnoses made in patients without barotrauma are easily questioned. A second problem is that at the time of surgery, diagnosis is entirely based on the surgeon's judgment, and these judgments have been variable. In non-emergency cases, especially where there has been no barotrauma, we think it is prudent to get two opinions prior to proceeding with surgical remedies. Situations where the diagnosis of fistula is likely to be incorrect are those where fistula is diagnosed without a reasonable cause, or in a diagnosis of bilateral fistula.

Tests recommended when fistula is strongly suspected:

- Fistula test
- Valsalva test (mainly looking for SCD [superior canal dehiscence])
- Audiometry
- Electrocochleography (ECOG)
- ENG
- Temporal bone CT scan, high resolution (looking for SCD)
- MRI scan (looking for cholesteatoma or tumor)
- VEMP (Vestibular evoked myogenic potentials)

A fistula test, which entails making a sensitive recording of eye movements while pressurizing each ear canal with a rubber bulb, will almost always be needed. A positive test is good grounds for surgical exploration. In window fistulae, very little nystagmus is produced, and a positive test may consist of only a slight nystagmus after pressurization. In superior canal dehiscence (SCD), a strong nystagmus may be produced. Simple observation of the patient's eyes with appropriate equipment (such as VNG [videonystagmography]) may also provide the diagnosis of PLF, as in some cases there is a pulse-synchronous oscillation (Rambold, 2001).

Audiometry and an ENG is nearly always necessary in order to establish the side, and to exclude other potential causes of symptoms. Audiometry may show sensorineural hearing reduction. In patients with SCD, audiometry may show bone conduction scores better than air (conductive hyperacusis). If there is a simultaneous sensorineural hearing loss in SCD, the overall picture may mimic the conductive hearing loss pattern of otosclerosis (Mikulec et al., 2004).

An ECOG, or electrocochleography, may be of help also, although only in rare instances. The main role of ECOG is to diagnose Ménière disease, which is a common alternative source of pressure sensitivity. ECOG is technically challenging and it may be difficult to locate a laboratory that does it well.

A CT scan should generally be obtained. CT of the temporal bone is very accurate in identifying canal fistulae (Fuse et al., 1996), although as there is really no other good way to identify canal fistulae, it is hard to be sure that it is picking them all up.

MRI is not the best test for fistulae because it doesn't show the bone and resolution is not as good as with a CT scan. However, MRI is the best way of showing other possibly confounding problems such as acoustic tumors, cholesteatoma, or multiple sclerosis plaques.

A cerebrospinal fluid (CSF) leak can occur from the ear as well as from other places in the head. CSF leaks mainly are a consequence of head injury or surgery (for example, they are fairly common after acoustic neuroma surgery). CSF leaks in the ear can be documented by CT cisternography with a spinal injection of a contrast material. In this test the head is tilted down for three minutes with the patient prone, and a CT scan is done with high-resolution cuts (spiral), in the coronal plane immediately after the prone positioning, to cover the frontal sinus through the mastoid sinus region.

Air in the labyrinth (pneumolabyrinth) is the most convincing finding of fistula. Middle ear effusions may also be suggestive of fistula. Variants in the stapes structure are sometimes a clue that there is a congenital fistula at the level of the oval window. Round window fistulae are generally unaccompanied by CT abnormalities, although an effusion would seem to be possible in this situation. Other congenital abnormalities of the cochlea, vestibule, and vestibular aqueduct may also be documented by CT of the temporal bone (Swartz and Harnsberger, 1998). Unfortunately, these procedures are not 100 percent accurate for all types of fistulae, and in some cases, only direct inspection of the inner ear will confirm or rule out a possible fistula.

Vestibular Evoked Myogenic Potentials (VEMPS)

Recently sound-evoked vestibulocollic evoked potentials have been described as useful in diagnosing Tullio phenomenon (sound-induced dizziness) from superior canal dehiscence (Brantberg et al., 1999; Watson et al., 2000). These are also called "VEMP," for vestibular evoked myogenic potential. The side with the larger VEMP or lower threshold is the abnormal side. This test is not generally available, however.

Click-Evoked Vestibulo-Ocular Reflex (VOR)

This test was described very recently by Halmagyi and others (2003). Event-triggered averaging is used to detect electro-oculographic responses to loud clicks—intensities ranging from 80 to 110 Db. One hundred twenty-eight clicks were delivered at a rate of five per second from 60 to 110 db, in 10 db steps. Normal subjects have no or a very low amplitude response of < 0.25 deg at 110. The latency was 8 msec. This test is not generally available, but appears promising.

Fluorescence Endoscopy

A method of documenting a fistula without operation is to inject a fluorescent material that gets into perilymph and observe it with an endoscope (Kleeman et al., 2001). There are several difficulties. First, getting the dye into the perilymph may be problematic. While perilymph is connected to some extent to CSF, the connection is not as open in some people as in others. Injection of dye into other fluids, such as intravenously, leaves open the question as to whether the fluid seen that fluoresces is serum or perilymph. This procedure is not widely available.

Questionable Tests

There are several tests for fistula which we do not think are necessary or reliable.

The pressure posturography test is one. This test involves measuring postural sway after pressurization of the ear. This test appears to us to be prone to false positives.

The glycerin test has also been advocated for fistula (Leherer, 1980). We are concerned that this test is diagnosing Ménière (hydrops) rather than fistula.

How Are Fistulas Treated?

Conservative Approach

In many cases, perhaps 90 percent, a window fistula will heal itself if your activity is restricted. In such cases, strict bed rest is recommended for one week or more to give the fistula a chance to close. It is usual to wait six months before embarking on surgical repair, given that hearing function is reasonable and is stable or improving. With respect to air travel, while it is certainly safest to avoid air travel altogether, in some instances it may be unavoidable. In this case, we suggest using a nasal decongestant at least one half hour prior to landing. Some of our patients have indicated that earplugs are helpful in this situation also. The "ear plane" earplugs are designed to reduce pressure fluctuation, and may be useful.

Surgery: Ventilation Tubes

It is our opinion that frequently a ventilation tube will help. The rationale for this is that the ill effects of barotrauma appear to require an intact tympanic membrane (Meller et al., 2003). We conjecture that this positive effect is due to reduced movement of the tympanic membrane, ossicular chain, and stapes footplate.

Case example: a woman in her thirties began to complain of dizziness during the second trimester of pregnancy. She complained of spinning, fainting, and nausea. Fistula testing induced nausea. A VEMP test revealed a much larger response on the right side. The Tullio test elicited upbeating nystagmus on the right side only. A ventilation tube was recommended on the right. After the tube was placed, symptoms were "75 percent better." However, it plugged up and symptoms returned after that. A bigger tube was placed a few months later, and symptoms again resolved. Nevertheless, surgery was recommended. On surgery there was an active round window fistula. This was patched, and the patient remained much better at last follow-up (two months later).

Surgery: Exploratory Tympanotomy

If you have a canal fistula, if your symptoms are significant and have not responded to the conservative approach outlined above, or if you have a progressive hearing loss, surgical repair of the fistula may be required.

For a window fistula surgery involves placing a soft-tissue graft over the fistula defect in the oval or round window. Otic capsule fistulae do not, in general, heal by themselves. Unfortunately, in our opinion anyway, surgical procedures are not well worked out. Cure rates (with respect to vertigo) are reported to be about 60 percent, but in our experience, we think that failures occur at least two-thirds of the time, if one looks at patients one year out. Patients are often re-operated when it is decided that the graft has failed. Some otologic surgeons operate on the same patient many times (e.g., fourteen times in one publicized case). In our opinion, one or two retries should be the limit.

Surgery: Unusual Procedures

In most instances, shunt of the endolymphatic sac or spinal fluid pathways (e.g. lumbar shunts) are not appropriate treatments for fistulae. When done, the rationale is to reduce CSF and thereby peri-lymph pressure, possibly allowing the ear to heal. A recent paper by Weber and others suggests that fistula surgery does not worsen things in children (Weber et al., 2003).

There have been sporadic reports of endoscope-guided fistula repair (Karhuketo and Puhakka, 2001). While one must admire the skill of the surgeons in these cases, in our opinion, this approach seems ill suited to general use, as fistula diagnosis and repair is difficult even when using a wider exposure.

There is considerable variability among otologic surgeons regarding their diagnosis and surgical management of fistulae (Hughes, 1990). We recommend getting a second opinion when fistula surgery is suggested.

Medications

For persons with plugged up eustachian tubes (such as due to a cold or allergy), decongestants, allergy medication, and ventilating tubes may be of use. Medications in the minor tranquilizer family such as diazepam (Valium), clonazepam, and lorazepam help some individuals. Antivert and Phenergan are also medications that some find helpful.

Activities to Avoid

Patients with fistula should avoid the following:

- Lifting
- Straining
- Bending over
- Popping the ears

- Forceful nose blowing

- Air pressure changes such as due to air travel

- High-speed elevators

- Scuba diving

- Loud noises (such as your own singing or a musical instrument)

A trial of bed rest for one to two weeks may be recommended. In this situation, one attempts to minimize pressure changes in the ear, hoping that scar tissue will seal the leak. For persons with superior canal dehiscence, no treatment will close the bone, so the only reasonable options are avoidance and surgery.

Earplugs are sometimes helpful for those who develop dizziness related to loud noise or rapid fluctuation in air pressure. Custom earplugs, such as the ER/15, which seal the affected ear, seem to work the best. A baffled earplug called the "Ear Plane" may be helpful.

Surgery may be recommended to close the leak. If hearing is good or the diagnosis not that clear, most persons are advised to wait for six months before proceeding with a surgical exploration. The hope is that the body will repair the leak on its own. This is a reasonable hope, as most fistulas do indeed appear to close spontaneously. On the other hand, if in the judgment of your doctor hearing appears to be at risk, then surgery may be advised more quickly.

How Might This Condition Affect My Life?

You may find that modifications in your daily activities will be necessary so that you can cope with your dizziness. For example, you may need to have someone shop for you for a while if going up and down supermarket aisles tends to increase your symptoms.

You should take special precautions in situations where clear, normal vision is not available to you. For example, avoid trying to walk through dark rooms and hallways; keep lights or nightlights on at all times. Don't drive your car at night or during stormy weather when visibility is poor.

Make sure your hallways at home are uncluttered and free of obstructions. Most important, do not place yourself in a situation where you might lose your balance and be at risk for a fall and serious injury; stay off of chairs, stools, ladders, roofs, and so on. If your balance continues to be a serious problem, you may need to consider using a cane or walker for added safety.

References

Albera, R, Canale, A, et al. Delayed vertigo after stapes surgery. *Laryngoscope* 114(5): 860–62, 2004.

Hain TC, Ostrowski, VB. Limits of Normal for Pressure Sensitivity in the Fistula Test. *Audiology and Neuro-otology* 2:384–90, 1997.

Hakuba N, Hato N, Shinomori Y, Sato H, Gyo K. Labyrinthine fistula as a late complication of middle ear surgery using the canal wall down technique. *Otol Neurotol* 23:832–35, 2002.

Hempel JM and others. Labyrinth dysfunction 8 months after cochlear implantation: a Case report. *Otol Neurotol* 25:727–29, 2004.

Hirvonen TP, Carey JP, Liang CJ, Minor LB. Superior canal dehiscence: mechanisms of pressure sensitivity in a chinchilla model. *Arch Otolaryngol Head Neck Surg* 127(11): 1331–36, 2001.

Hughes GB, Sismanis A, House JW. Is there consensus in perilymph fistula management? *Otolaryngol Head Neck Surg* 102(2): 111–17, 1990.

Karhuketo TS, Puhakka HJ. Endoscope-guided round window fistula repair. *Otol Neurotol* 22:869–73, 2001.

Kleeman D, Nofz S, Plank I, Schlottmann A. Rupture of the round window—detection with fluorescence endoscopy. *HNO* 49:89–92, 2001.

Kohut RI, Hinojosa R, Ryu JH. Update on idiopathic perilymphatic fistulas. *Oto Clin NA* 29(2): 343–52, 1996.

Kusuma S, Liou S, Haynes DS. Disequilibrium after cochlear implantation caused by a perilymph fistula. *Laryngoscope* 115:25–26, 2005.

Lehrer JF, Poole DC, Sigil B. Use of the glycerin test in the diagnosis of post-traumatic perilymphatic fistulas. *Am. J. Otolaryngol* 1, 3, 1980.

Lehrer JF, Rubin RC and others. Perilymphatic fistula—a definitive and curable cause of vertigo following head trauma. *Western J. Med* 141:57–60, 1984.

Magliulo G, Terranova G, Varacalli S, Sepe C. Labyrinthine fistula as a complication of cholesteatoma. *Am J. Otol* 18(6): 697–701, 1997.

Meller R, Rostain JC, Luciano M, Chays A, Bruzzo M, Cazals Y, Magnan J. Does repeated hyperbaric exposure to 4 atmosphere absolute cause hearing impairment? Study in Guinea pigs and clinical incidences. *Otol Neurotol* 24(5): 723–27, 2003.

Ostrowski VB, Hain TC, Wiet R. Pressure Induced Ocular Torsion. *Archives in Otolaryngology-Head and Neck Surgery* 123:646–49, 1997.

Rambold H and others. Perilymph fistula associated with pulse synchronous eye oscillations. *Neurology* 56:1769–71, 2001.

Rozsasi A, Sigg O, Keck T. Persistent inner ear injury after diving. *Otol Neurotol* 24(2): 195–200, 2003.

Sismanis A, Hughes GB, Butts F. Bilateral spontaneous perilymph fistulae: a diagnostic and management dilemma. *Otolaryngol Head Neck Surg* 103(3): 436–38, 1990.

Watson SRD, Halmagyi M, Colebatch JG. Vestibular hypersensitivity to sound (Tullio phenomenon). *Neurology* 54:722–28, 2000.

Weber PC, Bluestone CD, Perez B. Outcome of hearing and vertigo after surgery for congenital perilymphatic fistula in children. *Am J Otolaryngol* 24(3):138–42, May–June 2003.

Wicks RE. Alternobaric Vertigo: an aeromedical review. *Aviat Space and Env Med* 1989, 67–72.

Part Four

Disorders of the
Nose and Sinuses

Chapter 24

Introduction to the Nose and Sinuses

Chapter Contents

Section 24.1

Anatomy of the Nose

"What's That Smell? The Nose Knows." This information was provided by KidsHealth, one of the largest resources online for medically reviewed health information written for parents, kids, and teens. For more articles like this one, visit www.KidsHealth.org, or www.TeensHealth.org. © 2004 The Nemours Center for Children's Health Media, a division of The Nemours Foundation.

A big batch of cookies coming out of the oven. Your gym bag full of dirty clothes. How do you smell these smells and thousands more? It's your nose, of course.

Your nose lets you smell and it's a big part of why you are able to taste things. The nose is also the main gate to the respiratory system, your body's system for breathing. Let's be nosey and find out some more about the nose.

Nose Parts

The nose has two holes called nostrils. The nostrils and the nasal passages are separated by a wall called the septum. Deep inside your nose, close to your skull, your septum is made of very thin pieces of bone.

Closer to the tip of your nose, the septum is made of cartilage, which is flexible material that's firmer than skin or muscle. It's not as hard as bone, and if you push on the tip of your nose, you can feel how wiggly it is.

Behind your nose, in the middle of your face, is a space called the nasal cavity. It connects with the back of the throat. The nasal cavity is separated from the inside of your mouth by the palate (roof of your mouth).

Getting the Air in There

When you inhale air through your nostrils, the air enters the nasal passages and travels into your nasal cavity. The air then passes down the back of your throat into the trachea (or windpipe) on its way to the lungs.

Your nose is also a two-way street. When you exhale the old air from your lungs, the nose is the main way for the air to leave your body. But your nose is more than a passageway for air. The nose also warms, moistens, and filters the air before it goes to the lungs.

The inside of your nose is lined with a moist, thin layer of tissue called a mucous membrane. This membrane warms up the air and moistens it. The mucous membrane makes mucus, that sticky stuff in your nose you might call snot. Mucus captures dust, germs, and other small particles that could irritate your lungs. If you look inside your nose, you will also see hairs that can trap large particles, like dirt or pollen.

If something does get trapped in there, you can probably guess what happens next. You sneeze. Sneezes can send those unwelcome particles speeding out of your nose at 100 mph!

Further back in your nose are even smaller hairs called cilia that you can see only with a microscope. The cilia move back and forth to move the mucus out of the sinuses and back of the nose. Cilia can also be found lining the air passages, where they help move mucus out of the lungs.

Sniff, Sniff, Take a Whiff

The nose allows you to make scents of what's going on in the world around you. Just as your eyes give you information by seeing and your ears help you out by hearing, the nose lets you figure out what's happening by smelling. It does this with help from many parts hidden deep inside your nasal cavity and head.

Up on the roof of the nasal cavity (the space behind your nose) is the olfactory epithelium. Olfactory is a fancy word that has to do with smelling. The olfactory epithelium contains special receptors that are sensitive to odor molecules that travel through the air.

These receptors are very small—there are at least ten million of them in your nose! There are hundreds of different odor receptors, each with the ability to sense certain odor molecules. Research has shown that an odor can stimulate several different kinds of receptors. The brain interprets the combination of receptors to recognize any one of about ten thousand different smells.

When the smell receptors are stimulated, signals travel along the olfactory nerve to the olfactory bulb. The olfactory bulb is underneath the front of your brain just above the nasal cavity. Signals are sent from the olfactory bulb to other parts of the brain to be interpreted as a smell you may recognize, like apple pie fresh from the oven. Yum!

Identifying smells is your brain's way of telling you about your environment. Have you ever smelled your toast burning? In an instant, your brain interpreted the smell and a problem and you knew to check on your toast.

You learned to associate a certain smell with burning and now your brain remembers that smell so you recognize it. Your sense of smell also can help you keep safe. For example, it can be warn you not to eat something that smells rotten or help you detect smoke before you see a fire.

Tastes Great!

Most people just think of the tongue when they think about taste. But you couldn't taste anything without some help from the nose! The ability to smell and taste go together because odors from foods allow us to taste more fully.

Take a bite of food and think about how it tastes. Then, pinch your nose and take another bite. Notice the difference? It's just another reason to appreciate your knockout of a nose!

Section 24.2

How the Sinuses Work

What the Sinuses Are

The sinuses are cavities in the face and skull, located above, beside, and behind the nose. These cavities are filled with air.

There are four distinct sinus cavities:

- **Ethmoid Sinuses:** On each side of the nose between the eyes.

- **Frontal Sinuses:** In the forehead.

- **Maxillary Sinuses:** In the cheek above the teeth and below the eyes.

- **Sphenoid Sinuses:** Behind the eyes.

What the Sinuses Do

The sinuses are part of the system that helps you breathe. You can breathe with either your nose or your mouth, but your nose is better equipped for the job because it can humidify and warm the air before the air enters the lungs. Warming the air protects the sensitive tissues of the lungs and bronchial tubes.

Scientists and physicians believe that the sinuses also serve as resonating chambers for speaking and singing. Sinuses also reduce the weight of the skull by replacing dense bone with lighter, air-filled chambers.

How the Sinuses Work

The sinuses connect to the nose by tiny passages that carry sinus mucous into the nose. The sinuses themselves are lined by membranes, similar to but more delicate than the membranes that line the nose.

The membranes lining the sinuses move the mucous through the system. The mucous is important to sinus health because it includes particles that fight infection.

When areas of the sinuses become obstructed, you become susceptible to sinus infections. Not only can the infection-fighting mucous not move through, but the obstruction itself can cause an infection.

What Causes Sinus Problems

A number of different things can cause the sinuses to become obstructed:

- Swelling from a cold
- Swelling from an allergy
- Irritants like cigarette smoke or fumes
- Growths in the nose or sinuses, such as polyps
- Deviated septum or other abnormalities

Many of the factors leading to sinus obstruction, such as growths and anatomic abnormalities, are persistent. The best way to treat these chronic problems is to visit a sinus specialist.

Section 24.3

Diagnostic Tests of the Nose and Sinuses

"Cranial CT Scan" is © 2006 A.D.A.M., Inc. Reprinted with permission. "Nasal Mucosal Biopsy" is © 2006 A.D.A.M., Inc. Reprinted with permission. "Nasal Endoscopy" is reprinted from "Diagnosing Sinus Problems: Nasal Endoscopy," copyright © 2005 Northwestern Nasal and Sinus (http://www.nwnasalsinus.com). All rights reserved. Reprinted with permission.

Cranial CT Scan

Alternative Names

Head CT; CT scan—skull; CT scan—head; CT scan—orbits; CT scan—sinuses

Definition

A cranial CT scan is computed tomography of the head, including the skull, brain, orbits (eye sockets), and sinuses.

How the Test Is Performed

A head CT will produce an image from the upper neck to the top of the head. If the patient cannot keep still, immobilization may be necessary. All jewelry, glasses, dentures, and other metal should be removed from the head and neck to prevent obstruction of the images.

A contrast dye may be injected into a vein to further evaluate a mass (the mass becomes brighter with contrast dye if it has a lot of blood vessels). Contrast dye is also used to produce an image of the blood vessels of the head and brain.

The total amount of time in the CT scanner is usually a few minutes.

How to Prepare for the Test

Generally, there is no preparation necessary.

Infants and children: The preparation you can provide for this test depends on your child's age, previous experiences, and level of trust.

How the Test Will Feel

As with any intravenous iodinated contrast injection, there may be a slight temporary burning sensation in the arm, metallic taste in the mouth, or whole body warmth. This is a normal occurrence and will subside in a few seconds.

Otherwise, the CT scan is painless.

Why the Test Is Performed

A CT scan is recommended to help:

- evaluate acute cranial-facial trauma;
- determine acute stroke;
- evaluate suspected subarachnoid or intracranial hemorrhage;
- evaluate headache;
- evaluate loss of sensory or motor function;
- determine if there is abnormal development of the head and neck.

CT scans are also used to view the facial bones, jaw, and sinus cavities.

What Abnormal Results Mean

There may be signs of:

- trauma;
- bleeding (for example, chronic subdural hematoma or intracranial hemorrhage);
- stroke;
- masses or tumors;
- abnormal sinus drainage;
- sensorineural hearing loss;
- malformed bone or other tissues;
- brain abscess;

- cerebral atrophy (loss of brain tissue);
- brain tissue swelling;
- hydrocephalus (fluid collecting in the skull).

Additional conditions under which the test may be performed:

- acoustic neuroma;
- acoustic trauma;
- acromegaly;
- acute (subacute) subdural hematoma;
- amyotrophic lateral sclerosis;
- arteriovenous malformation (cerebral);
- benign positional vertigo;
- throat cancer;
- central pontine myelinolysis;
- cerebral aneurysm;
- Cushing syndrome;
- deep intracerebral hemorrhage;
- delirium;
- dementia;
- dementia due to metabolic causes;
- drug-induced tremor;
- encephalitis;
- epilepsy;
- essential tremor;
- extradural hemorrhage;
- familial tremor;
- general paresis;
- generalized tonic-clonic seizure;
- hemorrhagic stroke;
- hepatic encephalopathy;
- Huntington disease;
- hypertensive intracerebral hemorrhage;

- hypopituitarism;
- intracerebral hemorrhage;
- juvenile angiofibroma;
- labyrinthitis;
- lobar intracerebral hemorrhage;
- Ludwig angina;
- mastoiditis;
- melanoma of the eye;
- Ménière disease;
- meningitis;
- metastatic brain tumor;
- multi-infarct dementia;
- multiple endocrine neoplasia (MEN) I;
- neurosyphilis;
- normal pressure hydrocephalus (NPH);
- occupational hearing loss;
- optic glioma;
- orbital cellulitis;
- otitis media, chronic;
- otosclerosis;
- partial (focal) seizure;
- partial complex seizure;
- petit mal seizure;
- pituitary tumor;
- primary brain tumor;
- primary lymphoma of the brain;
- prolactinoma;
- retinoblastoma;
- Reye syndrome;
- schizophrenia;

- senile dementia/Alzheimer type;
- acute sinusitis;
- stroke secondary to atherosclerosis;
- stroke secondary to cardiogenic embolism;
- stroke secondary to FMD (fibromuscular dysplasia);
- stroke secondary to syphilis;
- subarachnoid hemorrhage;
- syphilitic aseptic meningitis;
- temporal lobe seizure;
- toxoplasmosis;
- transient ischemic attack (TIA);
- Wilson disease.

What the Risks Are

Iodine is the usual contrast dye. Some patients are allergic to iodine and may experience a reaction that may include hives, itching, nausea, breathing difficulty, or other symptoms.

As with any x-ray examination, radiation is potentially harmful. Consult your health care provider about the risks if multiple CT scans are needed over a period of time.

Special Considerations

A CT scan can decrease or eliminate the need for invasive procedures to diagnose problems in the skull. This is one of the safest means of studying the head and neck.

Nasal Mucosal Biopsy

Alternative Names

Biopsy—nasal mucosa; Nose biopsy

Definition

A nasal mucosal biopsy is surgery in which a small piece of tissue is removed from the lining of the nose and checked for disease.

319

How the Test Is Performed

A pain-killer is sprayed into the nose. In some cases, a numbing shot may be used. A small piece of the tissue that appears abnormal is removed and checked for problems in the laboratory.

How to Prepare for the Test

No special preparation is necessary. You may be asked to fast for a few hours before the biopsy.

How the Test Will Feel

There may be feelings of pressure or tugging during removal of the tissue. After the numbness wears off, the area may be sore for a few days. If there is bleeding, cautery (sealing of blood vessels with electric current or laser) may be needed.

Why the Test Is Performed

Nasal mucosal biopsy is usually done when abnormal tissue is seen during examination of the nose. It may also be done when problems affecting the mucosal tissue of the nose are suspected.

Normal Values

There is normal mucosal tissue, with no abnormal growths or tissues.

What Abnormal Results Mean

- Necrotizing granuloma (granular tumor)
- Wegener disease
- Nasal polyps
- Nasal tumors
- Sarcoid
- Infections (tuberculosis, fungal)

What the Risks Are

- Infection
- Bleeding from the biopsy site

Special Considerations

Avoid blowing your nose after the biopsy.

Nasal Endoscopy

This simple, in-office procedure allows the doctor to get a good look inside your nose and determine the cause and extent of your problems. It enables the doctor to examine the interior of your nasal passages and the openings to your sinuses. As a diagnostic tool, it also confirms whether you will need endoscopic surgery.

Nasal endoscopies work together with CT scans to help the doctor make an accurate diagnosis. While an endoscopy offers the doctor a view of your nasal cavity, a CT scan offers a view inside your sinuses and of the unique structures within your head. When you put the two images together, it provides the complete information necessary to diagnose your individual problem and determine the best steps to take in your care.

What causes sinus problems or blockages?

Your sinuses are chambers within your nose and head that circulate air. They also produce and drain mucus, acting as a drainage system. Colds, infections, allergies, and physical obstructions can all cause blockages that may shut down the sinuses and cause discomfort or pain.

How do I know if I need a nasal endoscopy?

If you have been experiencing sinus problems such as recurrent bacterial sinus infections, difficulty breathing, or severe sinus headaches, you may have a sinus condition. The doctor will discuss these problems with you, along with your complete medical history. The doctor will need to know which medications you have taken to clear your past sinus conditions and how effective they were. And, the doctor will ask you about physical conditions, environmental influences, allergies, or irritants that may be affecting your sinuses. Sometimes the doctor will perform a nasal endoscopy after you've had a CT scan of your sinuses or a sinus x-ray to investigate potential problems identified in the test results.

Does it hurt?

No it doesn't. Actually, nasal endoscopy is a quick and painless procedure. After spraying your nasal passages to anesthetize the lining

321

and shrink the tissue, the doctor inserts a very small, thin tube or endoscope. (A local anesthetic may not be necessary, depending on your nasal anatomy.)

What will the doctor look for?

Through the eyepiece of this instrument, he can see the inside of your nose and nasal passages to check for swelling, polyps, thickened mucus, inflammation, blockages, or other problems.

Will my insurance cover this procedure?

Insurance companies always consider diagnostic endoscopies a surgical procedure. Your insurance company may reimburse surgical services at a different rate than an office visit.

What if I need sinus surgery?

Today, sinus surgery can also be performed endoscopically, usually on an outpatient basis. While you are under general anesthesia, the doctor will use the same basic type of scope as he does during a diagnostic endoscopy. With the help of this scope, he can then insert surgical instruments that will treat or remove sinus obstructions. Because the procedure causes little tissue damage, there is minimal pain and swelling and no visible scarring. You will be back to your normal activities and feeling better in no time.

Chapter 25

Your Stuffy Nose

Chapter Contents

Section 25.1

The Common Cold

Reprinted from "The Common Cold," National Institute of Allergy and Infectious Diseases, National Institute of Health, December 13, 2004.

Overview

Sneezing, scratchy throat, runny nose—everyone knows the first signs of a cold, probably the most common illness known. Although the common cold is usually mild, with symptoms lasting one to two weeks, it is a leading cause of doctor visits and missed days from school and work. According to the Centers for Disease Control and Prevention, twenty-two million school days are lost annually in the United States due to the common cold.

In the course of a year, people in the United States suffer one billion colds, according to some estimates.

Children have about six to ten colds a year. One important reason why colds are so common in children is because they are often in close contact with each other in daycare centers and schools. In families with children in school, the number of colds per child can be as high as twelve a year. Adults average about two to four colds a year, although the range varies widely. Women, especially those aged twenty to thirty years, have more colds than men, possibly because of their closer contact with children. On average, people older than sixty have fewer than one cold a year.

Causes

The Viruses

More than two hundred different viruses are known to cause the symptoms of the common cold. Some, such as the rhinoviruses, seldom produce serious illnesses. Others, such as parainfluenza and respiratory syncytial virus, produce mild infections in adults but can precipitate severe lower respiratory infections in young children.

Rhinoviruses (from the Greek *rhin*, meaning "nose") cause an estimated 30 to 35 percent of all adult colds, and are most active in early fall, spring, and summer. More than 110 distinct rhinovirus types have been identified. These agents grow best at temperatures of about 91 degrees Fahrenheit, the temperature inside the human nose.

Scientists think coronaviruses cause a large percentage of all adult colds. They bring on colds primarily in the winter and early spring. Of the more than thirty kinds, three or four infect humans. The importance of coronaviruses as a cause of colds is hard to assess because, unlike rhinoviruses, they are difficult to grow in the laboratory.

Approximately 10 to 15 percent of adult colds are caused by viruses also responsible for other, more severe illnesses: adenoviruses, coxsackieviruses, echoviruses, orthomyxoviruses (including influenza A and B viruses, which cause flu), paramyxoviruses (including several parainfluenza viruses), respiratory syncytial virus, and enteroviruses.

The causes of 30 to 50 percent of adult colds, presumed to be viral, remain unidentified. The same viruses that produce colds in adults appear to cause colds in children. The relative importance of various viruses in pediatric colds, however, is unclear because it's difficult to isolate the precise cause of symptoms in studies of children with colds.

The Weather

There is no evidence that you can get a cold from exposure to cold weather or from getting chilled or overheated.

Other Factors

There is also no evidence that your chances of getting a cold are related to factors such as exercise, diet, or enlarged tonsils or adenoids. On the other hand, research suggests that psychological stress and allergic diseases affecting your nose or throat may have an impact on your chances of getting infected by cold viruses.

The Cold Season

In the United States, most colds occur during the fall and winter. Beginning in late August or early September, the rate of colds increases slowly for a few weeks and remains high until March or April, when it declines. The seasonal variation may relate to the opening of schools and to cold weather, which prompt people to spend more time indoors and increase the chances that viruses will spread to you from someone else.

Seasonal changes in relative humidity also may affect the prevalence of colds. The most common cold-causing viruses survive better when humidity is low—the colder months of the year. Cold weather also may make the inside lining of your nose drier and more vulnerable to viral infection.

Symptoms

Symptoms of the common cold usually begin two to three days after infection and often include:

- mucus buildup in your nose;
- difficulty breathing through your nose;
- swelling of your sinuses;
- sneezing;
- sore throat;
- cough;
- headache.

Fever is usually slight but can climb to 102 degrees Fahrenheit in infants and young children. Cold symptoms can last from two to fourteen days, but like most people, you'll probably recover in a week. If symptoms occur often or last much longer than two weeks, you might have an allergy rather than a cold.

Colds occasionally can lead to bacterial infections of your middle ear or sinuses, requiring treatment with antibiotics. High fever, significantly swollen glands, severe sinus pain, and a cough that produces mucus may indicate a complication or more serious illness requiring a visit to your healthcare provider.

Transmission

You can get infected by cold viruses by either of these methods:

- Touching your skin or environmental surfaces, such as telephones and stair rails, that have cold germs on them and then touching your eyes or nose
- Inhaling drops of mucus full of cold germs from the air

Treatment

There is no cure for the common cold, but you can get relief from your cold symptoms by:

- resting in bed;

- drinking plenty of fluids;

- gargling with warm salt water or using throat sprays or lozenges for a scratchy or sore throat;

- using petroleum jelly for a raw nose;

- taking aspirin or acetaminophen, Tylenol, for example, for headache or fever.

A word of caution: Several studies have linked aspirin use to the development of Reye syndrome in children recovering from flu or chickenpox. Reye syndrome is a rare but serious illness that usually occurs in children between the ages of three and twelve years. It can affect all organs of the body but most often the brain and liver. While most children who survive an episode of Reye syndrome do not suffer any lasting consequences, the illness can lead to permanent brain damage or death. The American Academy of Pediatrics recommends children and teenagers not be given aspirin or medicine containing aspirin when they have any viral illness such as the common cold.

Over-the-Counter Cold Medicines

Nonprescription cold remedies, including decongestants and cough suppressants, may relieve some of your cold symptoms but will not prevent or even shorten the length of your cold. Moreover, because most of these medicines have some side effects, such as drowsiness, dizziness, insomnia, or upset stomach, you should take them with care.

Over-the-Counter Antihistamines

Nonprescription antihistamines may give you some relief from symptoms such as runny nose and watery eyes which are commonly associated with colds.

Antibiotics

Never take antibiotics to treat a cold because antibiotics do not kill viruses. You should use these prescription medicines only if you have a rare bacterial complication, such as sinusitis or ear infections. In addition, you should not use antibiotics "just in case" because they will not prevent bacterial infections.

327

Steam

Although inhaling steam may temporarily relieve symptoms of congestion, health experts have found that this approach is not an effective treatment.

Prevention

There are several ways you can keep yourself from getting a cold or passing one on to others.

- Because cold germs on your hands can easily enter through your eyes and nose, keep your hands away from those areas of your body.
- If possible, avoid being close to people who have colds.
- If you have a cold, avoid being close to people.
- If you sneeze or cough, cover your nose or mouth.

Handwashing

Handwashing with soap and water is the simplest and one of the most effective ways to keep from getting colds or giving them to others. During cold season, you should wash your hands often and teach your children to do the same. When water isn't available, CDC recommends using alcohol-based products made for washing hands.

Disinfecting

Rhinoviruses can live up to three hours on your skin. They also can survive up to three hours on objects such as telephones and stair railings. Cleaning environmental surfaces with a virus-killing disinfectant might help prevent spread of infection.

Vaccine

Because so many different viruses can cause the common cold, the outlook for developing a vaccine that will prevent transmission of all of them is dim. Scientists, however, continue to search for a solution to this problem.

Unproven Prevention Methods

Echinacea: Echinacea is a dietary herbal supplement that some people use to treat their colds. Researchers, however, have found that while the herb may help treat your colds if taken in the early stages, it will not help prevent them. One research study funded by the National Center for Complementary and Alternative Medicine, a part of the National Institutes of Health, found that echinacea is not affective at all in treating children aged two to eleven.

Vitamin C: Many people are convinced that taking large quantities of vitamin C will prevent colds or relieve symptoms. To test this

Table 25.1. Is It a Cold or an Allergy?

Symptoms	Cold	Airborne Allergy
Cough	Common	Sometimes
General Aches, Pains	Slight	Never
Fatigue, Weakness	Sometimes	Sometimes
Itchy Eyes	Rare or Never	Common
Sneezing	Usual	Usual
Sore Throat	Common	Sometimes
Runny Nose	Common	Common
Stuffy Nose	Common	Common
Fever	Rare	Never
Duration	3 to 14 days	Weeks (for example, 6 weeks for ragweed or grass pollen seasons)
Treatment	Antihistamines Decongestants Nonsteroidal anti-inflammatory medicines	Antihistamines Nasal steroids Decongestants
Prevention	Wash your hands often Avoid close contact with anyone with a cold	Avoid those things that you are allergic to such as pollen, house dust mites, mold, pet dander, cockroaches
Complications	Sinus infection Middle ear infection Asthma	Sinus infection Asthma

Source: National Institute of Allergy and Infectious Diseases, National Institutes of Health, September 2005.

theory, several large-scale, controlled studies involving children and adults have been conducted. To date, no conclusive data has shown that large doses of vitamin C prevent colds. The vitamin may reduce the severity or duration of symptoms, but there is no clear evidence.

Taking vitamin C over long periods of time in large amounts may be harmful. Too much vitamin C can cause severe diarrhea, a particular danger for elderly people and small children.

Research

Thanks to basic research, scientists know more about the rhinovirus than almost any other virus, and have powerful new tools for developing antiviral drugs. Although the common cold may never be uncommon, further investigations offer the hope of reducing the huge burden of this universal problem.

Research on Rhinovirus Transmission

Much of the research on the transmission of the common cold has been done with rhinoviruses, which are shed in the highest concentration in nasal secretions. Studies suggest a person is most likely to transmit rhinoviruses in the second to fourth day of infection, when the amount of virus in nasal secretions is highest.

Researchers also have shown that using aspirin to treat colds increases the amount of virus in nasal secretions, possibly making the cold sufferer more of a hazard to others.

Section 25.2

Sneezing

"What Makes Me Sneeze?" This information was provided by KidsHealth, one of the largest resources online for medically reviewed health information written for parents, kids, and teens. For more articles like this one, visit www.KidsHealth.org, or www.TeensHealth.org. © 2003 The Nemours Center for Children's Health Media, a division of The Nemours Foundation.

Ahhh-Choo!

If you just sneezed, something was probably irritating or tickling the inside of your nose. Sneezing, also called sternutation, is your body's way of removing an irritation from your nose.

When the inside of your nose gets a tickle, a message is sent to a special part of your brain called the sneeze center. The sneeze center then sends a message to all the muscles that have to work together to create the amazingly complicated process that we call the sneeze.

Some of the muscles involved are the abdominal (belly) muscles, the chest muscles, the diaphragm (the large muscle beneath your lungs that makes you breathe), the muscles that control your vocal cords, and muscles in the back of your throat. Don't forget the eyelid muscles! Did you know that you always close your eyes when you sneeze?

It is the job of the sneeze center to make all these muscles work together, in just the right order, to send that irritation flying out of your nose. And fly it does—sneezing can send tiny particles speeding out of your nose at up to one hundred miles per hour!

Most anything that can irritate the inside of your nose can start a sneeze. Some common things include dust, cold air, or pepper. When you catch a cold in your nose, a virus has made a temporary home there and is causing lots of swelling and irritation. Some people have allergies, and they sneeze when they are exposed to certain things, such as animal dander (which comes from the skin of many common pets) or pollen (which comes from some plants).

Do you know anyone who sneezes when they step outside into the sunshine? About one out of every three people sneezes when exposed

331

to bright light. They are called photic sneezers (photic means light). If you are a photic sneezer, you got it from one of your parents because it is an inherited trait. You could say that it runs in your family. Most people have some sensitivity to light that can trigger a sneeze.

Have you ever had the feeling that you are about to sneeze, but it just gets stuck? Next time that happens, try looking toward a bright light briefly (but don't look right into the sun)—see if that doesn't unstick a stuck sneeze!

Section 25.3

Rhinitis

Do you suffer from a runny or stuffy nose much of the time? In the United States, about forty million people do. This problem is known as rhinitis. Approximately forty million people in the United States have rhinitis. There are several types of rhinitis.

What are the types of rhinitis?

Allergic Rhinitis: If you sneeze and have a runny or stuffy nose during the spring, summer, or fall allergy seasons, you may have seasonal allergic rhinitis or hay fever. Hay fever is the most common type of allergy problem. It mainly affects the eyes and nose. Hay fever symptoms include sneezing, itching, runny or stuffy nose, and red, watery eyes.

Rhinitis can be a problem all year or only some of the year. It can be a problem when inside or when outside. Allergy symptoms are caused when someone has a problem when around a certain substance. These substances are called allergens. They can be inside, such as cats or dust. They can be outside, such as tree and grass pollen in the spring and weed pollen and molds in the summer and fall. Hay fever is mainly an allergy caused by outdoor allergens.

Non-Allergic Rhinitis: This type of rhinitis is not as well understood. Although not triggered by allergy, the symptoms are often the same as seen with allergic rhinitis. Although the symptoms are similar, allergy skin test results are negative. Nasal polyps may also be seen with this type of rhinitis.

Vasomotor Rhinitis: Common symptoms of vasomotor rhinitis are nasal congestion and postnasal drip. A person with this type of rhinitis may have symptoms when exposed to temperature and humidity changes. Symptoms may also occur with exposure to smoke, odors, and emotional upsets. Allergy skin test results are negative.

Infectious Rhinitis: This can occur as a cold, which may clear rapidly or continue with symptoms longer than a week. Some people may also develop an acute or chronic bacterial sinus infection. Symptoms include an increased amount of colored (yellow-green) and thickened nasal discharge and nasal congestion.

Rhinitis Medicamentosa: This type of rhinitis is seen with long-term use of decongestant nasal sprays or recreational use of cocaine. Symptoms may include nasal congestion and postnasal drip. Decongestant nasal sprays are intended for short-term use only. Overuse can cause rebound nasal congestion. It is very important for a person with rebound congestion to work closely with a doctor to gradually decrease the nasal spray.

Mechanical Obstruction: This is most often seen with a deviated septum or enlarged adenoids. Symptoms often include nasal obstruction that may be one-sided.

Hormonal: This type of rhinitis is often seen with changes in the hormones. This often occurs during pregnancy, puberty, menses, or hypothyroidism.

How is rhinitis diagnosed?

Often a person may have more than one type of rhinitis. In making the diagnosis, an evaluation by your doctor may include the following:

- **History:** The doctor will ask questions about your health and your symptoms.

- **Physical exam**

- **Nasal smears**

- **Nasal secretions are examined under a microscope**

- **Allergy testing:** Skin testing by a board-certified allergist is often recommended for someone with recurrent symptoms. A positive skin test often is seen with allergies. In most cases, an allergic person will react to more than one substance. Your doctor will compare your prick skin test results with your history of symptoms.

- **Sinus x-ray or CT scan:** Changes in the sinus x-ray or CT scan may indicate sinusitis (inflammation of the sinuses) with or without infection or nasal polyps.

How can you manage symptoms?

The goal of treatment is to reduce symptoms. This often includes:

- identifying, controlling and/or treating things that make your symptoms worse;

- using and understanding medications.

What makes your symptoms worse?

The best way to prevent allergic rhinitis is to avoid the things to which you are allergic. Because allergic rhinitis is caused by outdoor allergies, this can be hard to do. If you have outdoor allergies there are some things you can do to help:

- Keep your doors and windows shut during pollen season.

- Use an air conditioner to cool your home instead of coolers or fans that bring in outside air.

- Consider pollen counts when planning outdoor activities. It may help to limit your outdoor activities when pollen and mold counts are at their highest.

Pollen and mold counts can vary throughout the day. Peak times are:

- **grass:** afternoon and early evening;

- **ragweed:** early midday;

- **mold:** some types peak during warm, dry, windy afternoons; other types occur at high levels during periods of dampness and rain.

House Dust Mites: If you are allergic to house dust mites and live in a humid area:

- cover your mattress and box spring in zippered, dustproof encasings;
- wash your pillows, sheets, and blankets weekly in hot water. Dust mites will survive in lukewarm water.

Animals: Dander, urine, and saliva from feathered or furry animals is a major year-round allergen. Cats, dogs, birds, hamsters, gerbils, and horses are common pets. If you are allergic to an animal:

- do not keep any furry or feathered pets in your home;
- if you must keep the pet, try to keep it outdoors. If the pet comes indoors, make sure it stays out of your bedroom at all times. After exposure to the pet, wash your hands and change your clothes.

Irritants: Many substances can irritate the nose, throat, or airways. Common irritants include tobacco smoke, smoke from wood-burning stoves, kerosene stoves, and fireplaces, aerosol sprays, strong odors, dust, and air pollution. Reducing exposure to irritants can be very helpful.

- It is important that no one smokes in the home or car.
- Always look for nonsmoking sections in public areas.
- Avoid aerosol spray, perfumes, strong cleaning products, and other odor sources in the home.

What medications treat rhinitis?

Anti-inflammatory medicines control inflammation in the body. This inflammation causes redness and swelling (congestion).

Cromolyn and nedocromil are anti-inflammatory medicines that are not steroids. They may help prevent nasal and eye symptoms.

Nasal steroid sprays work well to reduce nasal symptoms of sneezing, itching, runny and stuffy nose. Nasal steroids may also improve eye symptoms. A steroid nasal spray may work after several hours or take several days to work. Nasal steroids work best if you take them daily.

Common nasal steroid sprays:

- Beconase®, Beconase AQ®, Vancenase®, Vancenase AQ® (beclomethasone)
- Rhinocort® (flunisolide)
- Nasarel® (flunisolide)
- Flonase® (fluticasone)
- Nasonex® (mometasone)
- Nasacort®, Nasacort AQ® (triamcinolone)

Nasal Wash: A nasal wash with salt water may help clean out your nose. When done routinely, this can also lessen post-nasal drip. If you do a nasal wash, do this before using other nasal medicine.

Antihistamine Medicine: Antihistamines can help decrease allergy symptoms. They may be used daily during allergy season or when allergy symptoms occur. There are many different antihistamines. If one doesn't work, another can be tried. Some can make you sleepy and some do not.

Common antihistamines that do not make you sleepy:

- Claritin® (loratadine)
- Clarinex® (desloratadine)
- Allegra® (fexofenadine)
- Zyrtec® (cetirizine) (can cause some people to be sleepy)

Some over-the-counter antihistamines can make you feel sleepy. They may also affect thinking and your reflexes. If you take one of these, use caution when driving or using any kind of machine.

Astelin® (azelastine) is an antihistamine nasal spray. It usually does not make you sleepy.

Decongestant Medicine: Decongestants help when your nose is stuffy (congestion). They are available as pills, liquids, or nasal sprays. Many are available over the counter. A common over-the-counter decongestant is Sudafed (pseudoephedrine). Use caution when taking a decongestant nasal spray. Using one longer than four days can have a rebound effect. This causes you to have more nasal congestion.

Atrovent® (ipratropium bromide) is a nasal spray. Atrovent may be helpful for decreasing symptoms of a runny nose. This nasal spray may be helpful for vasomotor rhinitis.

Immunotherapy (Allergy Shots): Allergy shots may be helpful for specific allergies that aren't controlled with medicine. We recommend that you see a board-certified allergist for allergy testing or allergy shots.

Rhinitis can be managed so you can have an active, fun life. Talk with your doctor if you think you have rhinitis. Your doctor is your partner in your health care.

Section 25.4

Post-Nasal Drip

The glands in your nose and throat continually produce mucus (one to two quarts a day). It moistens and cleans the nasal membranes, humidifies air, traps and clears inhaled foreign matter, and fights infection. Although mucus normally is swallowed unconsciously, the feeling that it is accumulating in the throat or dripping from the back of your nose is called post-nasal drip.

This feeling can be caused by excessive or thick secretions or by throat muscle and swallowing disorders.

What Causes Abnormal Secretions—Thin and Thick

Increased thin clear secretions can be due to colds and flu, allergies, cold temperatures, bright lights, certain foods and spices, pregnancy, and other hormonal changes. Various drugs (including birth control pills and high blood pressure medications) and structural abnormalities can also produce increased secretions. These abnormalities might include a deviated or irregular nasal septum (the cartilage and bony dividing wall that separates the two nostrils).

Increased thick secretions in the winter often result from too little moisture in heated buildings and homes. They can also result from sinus or nose infections and some allergies, especially to certain foods such as dairy products. If thin secretions become thick and green or yellow, it is likely that a bacterial sinus infection is developing. In children, thick secretions from one side of the nose can mean that something is stuck in the nose (such as a bean, wadded paper, or piece of toy, etc.).

Sinuses are air-filled cavities in the skull. They drain into the nose through small openings. Blockages in the openings from swelling due to colds, flu, or allergies may lead to acute sinus infection. A viral "cold" that persists for ten days or more may have become a bacterial sinus infection. With this infection you may notice increased post-nasal drip. If you suspect that you have a sinus infection, you should see your physician for antibiotic treatment.

Chronic sinusitis occurs when sinus blockages persist and the lining of the sinuses swells further. Polyps (growths in the nose) may develop with chronic sinusitis. Patients with polyps tend to have irritating, persistent post-nasal drip. Evaluation by an otolaryngologist may include an exam of the interior of the nose with a fiberoptic scope and CAT scan x-rays. If medication does not relieve the problem, surgery may be recommended.

Vasomotor Rhinitis describes a non-allergic "hyperirritable nose" that feels congested, blocked, or wet.

Swallowing Problems

Swallowing problems may result in accumulation of solids or liquids in the throat that may complicate or feel like post-nasal drip. When the nerve and muscle interaction in the mouth, throat, and food passage (esophagus) aren't working properly, overflow secretions can spill into the voice box (larynx) and breathing passages (trachea and bronchi) causing hoarseness, throat clearing, or cough.

Several factors contribute to swallowing problems:

• With age, swallowing muscles often lose strength and coordination. Thus, even normal secretions may not pass smoothly into the stomach.

• During sleep, swallowing occurs much less frequently, and secretions may gather. Coughing and vigorous throat clearing are often needed when awakening.

- When nervous or under stress, throat muscles can trigger spasms that feel like a lump in the throat. Frequent throat clearing, which usually produces little or no mucus, can make the problem worse by increasing irritation.

- Growths or swelling in the food passage can slow or prevent the movement of liquids and/or solids.

Swallowing problems may be caused also by gastroesophageal reflux disease (GERD). This is a return of stomach contents and acid into the esophagus or throat. Heartburn, indigestion, and sore throat are common symptoms. GERD may be aggravated by lying down, especially following eating. Hiatal hernia, a pouch-like tissue mass where the esophagus meets the stomach, often contributes to the reflux.

Chronic Sore Throat

Post-nasal drip often leads to a sore, irritated throat. Although there is usually no infection, the tonsils and other tissues in the throat may swell. This can cause discomfort or a feeling of a lump in the throat. Successful treatment of the post-nasal drip will usually clear up these throat symptoms.

Treatment for Post-Nasal Drip

A correct diagnosis requires a detailed ear, nose, and throat exam and possible laboratory, endoscopic, and x-ray studies. Each treatment is different.

Bacterial infection, when present, is treated with antibiotics. These drugs may provide only temporary relief. In cases of chronic sinusitis, surgery to open the blocked sinuses may be required.

Allergy is managed by avoiding the cause if possible. Antihistamines and decongestants, cromolyn and steroid (cortisone type) nasal sprays, and other forms of steroids may offer relief. Immunotherapy (allergy shots) also may be helpful. However, some older, sedating antihistamines may dry and thicken post-nasal secretions even more; newer nonsedating antihistamines, available by prescription only, do not have this effect. Decongestants can aggravate high blood pressure, heart, and thyroid disease. Steroid sprays generally may be used safely under medical supervision. Oral and injectable steroids rarely produce serious complications in short-term use. Because significant side effects can occur, steroids must be monitored carefully when used for more than one week.

Gastroesophageal reflux is treated by elevating the head of the bed six to eight inches, avoiding foods and beverages for two to three hours before bedtime, and eliminating alcohol and caffeine from the daily diet. Antacids (e.g., Maalox®, Mylanta®, Gaviscon ®) and drugs that block stomach acid production (e.g., Zantac®, Tagamet®, Pepcid®) or more powerful medications may be prescribed. A trial treatment may be suggested before x-rays and other diagnostic studies are performed.

General measures for thinning secretions so they can pass more easily may be recommended when it is not possible to determine whether an existing structural abnormality is causing the post-nasal drip or if some other condition is to blame.

Many people, especially older persons, need more fluids to thin secretions. Drinking more water, eliminating caffeine, and avoiding diuretics (fluid pills) will help. Mucous-thinning agents such as guaifenesin (Humibid®, Robitussin®) may also thin secretions.

Nasal irrigations may alleviate thickened secretions. These can be performed two to four times a day either with a nasal douche device or a Water Pik® with a nasal irrigation nozzle. Warm water with baking soda or salt (1/2 to 1 tsp. to the pint) or Alkalol®, a nonprescription irrigating solution (full strength or diluted by half warm water), may be helpful. Finally, use of simple saline (salt) nonprescription nasal sprays (e.g., Ocean®, Ayr®, or Nasal®) to moisten the nose is often very beneficial.

Chapter 26

Your Allergic Nose

Introduction

Sneezing is not always the symptom of a cold. Sometimes, it is an allergic reaction to something in the air. Health experts estimate that thirty-five million Americans suffer from upper respiratory tract symptoms that are allergic reactions to airborne allergens. Pollen allergy, commonly called hay fever, is one of the most common chronic diseases in the United States. Worldwide, airborne allergens cause the most problems for people with allergies. The respiratory symptoms of asthma, which affect approximately eleven million Americans, are often provoked by airborne allergens.

Overall, allergic diseases are among the major causes of illness and disability in the United States, affecting as many as forty to fifty million Americans.

This chapter summarizes what health experts know about the causes and symptoms of allergic reactions to airborne allergens, how health care providers diagnose and treat these reactions, and what medical researchers are doing to help people who suffer from these allergies.

What is an allergy?

An allergy is a specific reaction of the body's immune system to a normally harmless substance, one that does not bother most people.

Reprinted from "Airborne Allergens: Something in the Air," National Institute of Allergy and Infectious Diseases, National Institutes of Health, NIH Publication No. 03-7045, April 2003.

People who have allergies often are sensitive to more than one substance. Types of allergens that cause allergic reactions include the following:

- pollens
- house dust mites
- mold spores
- food
- latex rubber
- insect venom
- medicines

Why are some people allergic?

Scientists think that some people inherit a tendency to be allergic from one or both parents. This means they are more likely to have allergies. They probably, however, do not inherit a tendency to be allergic to any specific allergen. Children are more likely to develop allergies if one or both parents have allergies. In addition, exposure to allergens at times when the body's defenses are lowered or weakened, such as after a viral infection or during pregnancy, seems to contribute to developing allergies.

What is an allergic reaction?

Normally, the immune system functions as the body's defense against invading germs such as bacteria and viruses. In most allergic reactions, however, the immune system is responding to a false alarm. When an allergic person first comes into contact with an allergen, the immune system treats the allergen as an invader and gets ready to attack.

The immune system does this by generating large amounts of a type of antibody called immunoglobulin E, or IgE. Each IgE antibody is specific for one particular substance. In the case of pollen allergy, each antibody is specific for one type of pollen. For example, the immune system may produce one type of antibody to react against oak pollen and another against ragweed pollen.

The IgE molecules are special because IgE is the only type of antibody that attaches tightly to the body's mast cells, which are tissue cells, and to basophils, which are blood cells. When the allergen next encounters its specific IgE, it attaches to the antibody like a key fitting into a lock. This action signals the cell to which the IgE is attached to release (and, in some cases, to produce) powerful chemicals like histamine, which cause inflammation. These chemicals act on tissues in various parts of the body, such as the respiratory system, and cause the symptoms of allergy.

Symptoms

The signs and symptoms of airborne allergies are familiar to many:

- sneezing, often with a runny or clogged nose
- coughing and postnasal drip
- itching eyes, nose, and throat
- watering eyes
- conjunctivitis
- "allergic shiners" (dark circles under the eyes caused by increased blood flow near the sinuses)
- "allergic salute" (in a child, persistent upward rubbing of the nose that causes a crease mark on the nose)

In people who are not allergic, the mucus in the nasal passages simply moves foreign particles to the throat, where they are swallowed or coughed out. But something different happens in a person who is sensitive to airborne allergens.

In sensitive people, as soon as the allergen lands on the lining inside the nose, a chain reaction occurs that leads the mast cells in these tissues to release histamine and other chemicals. The powerful chemicals contract certain cells that line some small blood vessels in the nose. This allows fluids to escape, which causes the nasal passages to swell—resulting in nasal congestion. Histamine also can cause sneezing, itching, irritation, and excess mucus production, which can result in allergic rhinitis.

Other chemicals released by mast cells, including cytokines and leukotrienes, also contribute to allergic symptoms.

Some people with allergy develop asthma, which can be a very serious condition. The symptoms of asthma include the following:

- coughing
- wheezing
- shortness of breath

The shortness of breath is due to a narrowing of the airways in the lungs and to excess mucus production and inflammation. Asthma can be disabling and sometimes fatal. If wheezing and shortness of breath accompany allergy symptoms, it is a signal that the airways also have become involved.

Is it an allergy or a cold?

There is no good way to tell the difference between allergy symptoms of runny nose, coughing, and sneezing and cold symptoms. Allergy symptoms, however, may last longer than cold symptoms. Anyone who has any respiratory illness that lasts longer than a week or two should consult a health care provider.

Pollen Allergy

Each spring, summer, and fall, tiny pollen grains are released from trees, weeds, and grasses. These grains hitch rides on currents of air. Although the mission of pollen is to fertilize parts of other plants, many never reach their targets. Instead, pollen enters human noses and throats, triggering a type of seasonal allergic rhinitis called pollen allergy. Many people know this as hay fever.

Of all the things that can cause an allergy, pollen is one of the most common. Many of the foods, medicines, or animals that cause allergies can be avoided to a great extent. Even insects and household dust are escapable. But short of staying indoors, with the windows closed, when the pollen count is high—and even that may not help—there is no easy way to avoid airborne pollen.

What is pollen?

Plants produce tiny—too tiny to see with the naked eye—round or oval pollen grains to reproduce. In some species, the plant uses the pollen from its own flowers to fertilize itself. Other types must be cross-pollinated. Cross-pollination means that for fertilization to take place and seeds to form, pollen must be transferred from the flower of one plant to that of another of the same species. Insects do this job for certain flowering plants, while other plants rely on wind for transport.

The types of pollen that most commonly cause allergic reactions are produced by the plain-looking plants (trees, grasses, and weeds) that do not have showy flowers. These plants make small, light, dry pollen grains that are custom-made for wind transport

Amazingly, scientists have collected samples of ragweed pollen four hundred miles out at sea and two miles high in the air. Because airborne pollen can drift for many miles, it does little good to rid an area of an offending plant. In addition, most allergenic pollen comes from plants that produce it in huge quantities. For example, a single ragweed plant can generate a million grains of pollen a day.

The type of allergens in the pollen is the main factor that determines whether the pollen is likely to cause hay fever. For example, pine tree pollen is produced in large amounts by a common tree, which would make it a good candidate for causing allergy. It is, however, a relatively rare cause of allergy because the type of allergens in pine pollen appear to make it less allergenic.

Among North American plants, weeds are the most prolific producers of allergenic pollen. Ragweed is the major culprit, but other important sources are sagebrush, redroot pigweed, lamb's quarters, Russian thistle (tumbleweed), and English plantain.

Grasses and trees, too, are important sources of allergenic pollens. Although more than one thousand species of grass grow in North America, only a few produce highly allergenic pollen.

It is common to hear people say they are allergic to colorful or scented flowers like roses. In fact, only florists, gardeners, and others who have prolonged, close contact with flowers are likely to be sensitive to pollen from these plants. Most people have little contact with the large, heavy, waxy pollen grains of such flowering plants because this type of pollen is not carried by wind but by insects such as butterflies and bees.

Some grasses that produce pollen include the following:

- Timothy grass
- Kentucky bluegrass
- Johnson grass
- Bermuda grass
- Redtop grass
- Orchard grass
- Sweet vernal grass

Some trees that produce pollen include the following:

- Oak
- Ash
- Elm

345

- Hickory
- Pecan
- Box elder
- Mountain cedar

When do plants make pollen?

One of the most obvious features of pollen allergy is its seasonal nature—people have symptoms only when the pollen grains to which they are allergic are in the air. Each plant has a pollinating period that is more or less the same from year to year. Exactly when a plant starts to pollinate seems to depend on the relative length of night and day—and therefore on geographical location— rather than on the weather. On the other hand, weather conditions during pollination can affect the amount of pollen produced and distributed in a specific year. Thus, in the Northern Hemisphere, the farther north you go, the later the start of the pollinating period and the later the start of the allergy season.

A pollen count, familiar to many people from local weather reports, is a measure of how much pollen is in the air. This count represents the concentration of all the pollen (or of one particular type, like ragweed) in the air in a certain area at a specific time. It is shown in grains of pollen per square meter of air collected over twenty-four hours. Pollen counts tend to be the highest early in the morning on warm, dry, breezy days and lowest during chilly, wet periods. Although the pollen count is an approximate measure that changes, it is useful as a general guide for when it may be wise to stay indoors and avoid contact with the pollen.

Mold Allergy

What is mold?

There are thousands of types of molds and yeasts in the fungus family. Yeasts are single cells that divide to form clusters. Molds are made of many cells that grow as branching threads called hyphae. Although both can probably cause allergic reactions, only a small number of molds are widely recognized offenders.

The seeds or reproductive pieces of fungi are called spores. Spores differ in size, shape, and color among types of mold. Each spore that germinates can give rise to new mold growth, which in turn can produce millions of spores.

What is mold allergy?

When inhaled, tiny fungal spores, or sometimes pieces of fungi, may cause allergic rhinitis. Because they are so small, mold spores also can reach the lungs.

In a small number of people, symptoms of mold allergy may be brought on or worsened by eating certain foods such as cheeses processed with fungi. Occasionally, mushrooms, dried fruits, and foods containing yeast, soy sauce, or vinegar will produce allergy symptoms.

Where do molds grow?

Molds can be found wherever there is moisture, oxygen, and a source of the few other chemicals they need. In the fall, they grow on rotting logs and fallen leaves, especially in moist, shady areas. In gardens they can be found in compost piles and on certain grasses and weeds. Some molds attach to grains such as wheat, oats, barley, and corn, which makes farms, grain bins, and silos likely places to find mold.

Hot spots of mold growth in the home include damp basements and closets, bathrooms (especially shower stalls), places where fresh food is stored, refrigerator drip trays, house plants, air conditioners, humidifiers, garbage pails, mattresses, upholstered furniture, and old foam rubber pillows.

Molds also like bakeries, breweries, barns, dairies, and greenhouses. Loggers, mill workers, carpenters, furniture repairers, and upholsterers often work in moldy environments.

What molds are allergenic?

Like pollens, mold spores are important airborne allergens only if they are abundant, easily carried by air currents, and allergenic in their chemical makeup. Found almost everywhere, mold spores in some areas are so numerous they often outnumber the pollens in the air. Fortunately, however, only a few dozen different types are significant allergens.

In general, *Alternaria* and *Cladosporium* (Hormodendrum) are the molds most commonly found both indoors and outdoors in the United States. *Aspergillus*, *Penicillium*, *Helminthosporium*, *Epicoccum*, *Fusarium*, *Mucor*, *Rhizopus*, and *Aureobasidium* (*Pullularia*) are common as well.

There is no relationship, however, between a respiratory allergy to the mold *Penicillium* and an allergy to the drug penicillin, which is made from mold.

347

Are mold counts helpful?

Similar to pollen counts, mold counts may suggest the types and number of fungi present at a certain time and place. For several reasons, however, these counts probably cannot be used as a constant guide for daily activities.

One reason is that the number and types of spores actually present in the mold count may have changed considerably in twenty-four hours because weather and spore distribution are directly related. Many common allergenic molds are of the dry spore type—they release their spores during dry, windy weather. Other fungi need high humidity, fog, or dew to release their spores. Although rain washes many larger spores out of the air, it also causes some smaller spores to be propelled into the air.

In addition to the effect of weather changes during twenty-four-hour periods on mold counts, spore populations may also differ between day and night. Dry spore types are usually released during daytime, and wet spore types are usually released at night.

Are there other mold-related disorders?

Fungi or organisms related to them may cause other health problems similar to allergic diseases. Some kinds of *Aspergillus* may cause several different illnesses, including both infections and allergies. These fungi may lodge in the airways or a distant part of the lung and grow until they form a compact sphere known as a "fungus ball." In people with lung damage or serious underlying illnesses, *Aspergillus* may grasp the opportunity to invade the lungs or the whole body.

In some people, exposure to these fungi also can lead to asthma or to a lung disease resembling severe inflammatory asthma called allergic bronchopulmonary aspergillosis. This latter condition, which occurs in only a small number of people with asthma, causes wheezing, low-grade fever, and coughing up of brown-flecked masses or mucus plugs. Skin testing, blood tests, x-rays, and examination of the sputum for fungi can help establish the diagnosis. Corticosteroid drugs usually treat this reaction effectively. Immunotherapy (allergy shots) is not helpful.

Dust Mite Allergy

Dust mite allergy is an allergy to a microscopic organism that lives in the dust found in all dwellings and workplaces. House dust, as well as some house furnishings, contains microscopic mites. Dust mites are perhaps the most common cause of perennial allergic rhinitis. House dust mite allergy usually produces symptoms similar to pollen allergy and also can produce symptoms of asthma.

House dust mites, which live in bedding, upholstered furniture, and carpets, thrive in summer and die in winter. In a warm, humid house, however, they continue to thrive even in the coldest months. The particles seen floating in a shaft of sunlight include dead dust mites and their waste products. These waste products, which are proteins, actually provoke the allergic reaction.

What is house dust?

Rather than a single substance, so-called house dust is a varied mixture of potentially allergenic materials. It may contain fibers from different types of fabrics and materials. Here are some examples of house dust components:

- cotton lint, feathers, and other stuffing materials
- dander from cats, dogs, and other animals
- bacteria
- mold and fungus spores (especially in damp areas)
- food particles
- bits of plants and insects
- other allergens peculiar to an individual house or building

Cockroaches are commonly found in crowded cities and in the southern United States. Certain proteins in cockroach feces and saliva also can be found in house dust. These proteins can cause allergic reactions or trigger asthma symptoms in some people, especially children. Cockroach allergens likely play a significant role in causing asthma in many inner-city populations.

Animal Allergy

Household pets are the most common source of allergic reactions to animals. Many people think that pet allergy is provoked by the fur of cats and dogs. Researchers have found, however, that the major allergens are proteins in the saliva. These proteins stick to the fur when the animal licks itself.

Urine is also a source of allergy-causing proteins, as is the skin. When the substance carrying the proteins dries, the proteins can then float into the air. Cats may be more likely than dogs to cause allergic reactions because they lick themselves more, may be held more, and spend more time in the house, close to humans.

Some rodents, such as guinea pigs and gerbils, have become increasingly popular as household pets. They, too, can cause allergic reactions in some people, as can mice and rats. Urine is the major source of allergens from these animals.

Allergies to animals can take two years or more to develop and may not decrease until six months or more after ending contact with the animal. Carpet and furniture are a reservoir for pet allergens, and the allergens can remain in them for four to six weeks. In addition, these allergens can stay in household air for months after the animal has been removed. Therefore, it is wise for people with an animal allergy to check with the landlord or previous owner to find out if furry pets lived on the premises.

Chemical Sensitivity

Some people report that they react to chemicals in their environments and that these allergy-like reactions seem to result from exposure to a wide variety of synthetic and natural substances. Such substances can include those found in substances such as these:

- paints
- carpeting
- plastics
- perfumes
- cigarette smoke
- plants

Although the symptoms may resemble those of allergies, sensitivity to chemicals does not represent a true allergic reaction involving IgE and the release of histamine or other chemicals. Rather than a reaction to an allergen, it is a reaction to a chemical irritant, which may affect people with allergies more than others.

Diagnosis

People with allergy symptoms—such as the runny nose of allergic rhinitis—may at first suspect they have a cold, but the "cold" lingers on. Testing for allergies is the best way to find out if a person is allergic.

Skin Tests

Allergists (doctors who specialize in allergic diseases) use skin tests to determine whether a person has IgE antibodies in the skin that react to a specific allergen. The allergist will use weakened extracts from allergens such as dust mites, pollens, or molds commonly found in the local area. The extract of each kind of allergen is injected under a person's skin or is applied to a tiny scratch or puncture made on the arm or back.

Skin tests are one way of measuring the level of IgE antibody in a person. With a positive reaction, a small, raised, reddened area, called a wheal (hive), with a surrounding flush, called a flare, will appear at the test site. The size of the wheal can give the doctor an important diagnostic clue, but a positive reaction does not prove that a particular allergen is the cause of symptoms. Although such a reaction indicates that IgE antibody to a specific allergen is present, respiratory symptoms do not necessarily result.

Blood Tests

Skin testing is the most sensitive and least costly way to identify allergies. People with widespread skin conditions like eczema, however, should not be tested using this method.

There are other diagnostic tests that use a blood sample to detect levels of IgE antibody to a particular allergen. One such blood test is called the radioallergosorbent test (RAST), which can be performed when eczema is present or if a person has taken medicines that interfere with skin testing.

Some ways to handle airborne allergies include the following:

- avoid the allergen
- take medicine
- get allergy shots

Prevention

Pollen and Molds

Complete avoidance of allergenic pollen or mold means moving to a place where the offending substance does not grow and where it is not present in the air. Even this extreme solution may offer only temporary relief because a person sensitive to a specific pollen or mold may develop allergies to new allergens after repeated exposure to them. For example, people allergic to ragweed may leave their ragweed-ridden communities and relocate to areas where ragweed does not grow, only to develop allergies to other weeds or even to grasses or trees in their new surroundings. Because relocating is not a reliable solution, allergy specialists do not encourage this approach.

There are other ways to reduce exposure to offending pollens:

- Remain indoors with the windows closed in the morning, for example, when the outdoor pollen levels are highest. Sunny, windy days can be especially troublesome.

- Wear a face mask designed to filter pollen out of the air and keep it from reaching nasal passages if you must work outdoors.

- Take your vacation at the height of the expected pollinating period and choose a location where such exposure would be minimal. Vacationing at the seashore or on a cruise, for example, may be effective retreats for avoiding pollen allergies.

House Dust

If you have dust mite allergy, pay careful attention to dust-proofing your bedroom. The worst things to have in the bedroom are items such as these:

- wall-to-wall carpet
- blinds
- down-filled blankets
- feather pillows
- stuffed animals
- heating vents with forced hot air
- dogs and cats
- closets full of clothing

Carpets trap dust and make dust control impossible:

- Shag carpets are the worst type of carpet for people who are sensitive to dust mites.

- Vacuuming doesn't get rid of dust mite proteins in furniture and carpeting, but redistributes them back into the room, unless the vacuum has a special HEPA (high-efficiency particulate air) filter.

- Rugs on concrete floors encourage dust mite growth.

If possible, replace wall-to-wall carpets with washable throw rugs over hardwood, tile, or linoleum floors, and wash the rugs frequently.

Reducing the amount of dust mites in your home may mean new cleaning techniques as well as some changes in furnishings to eliminate dust collectors. Water is often the secret to effective dust removal.

- Clean washable items, including throw rugs, often, using water hotter than 130 degrees Fahrenheit. Lower temperatures will not kill dust mites.

- Clean washable items at a commercial establishment that uses high water temperature, if you cannot or do not want to set water temperature in your home at 130 degrees. (There is a danger of getting scalded if the water is more than 120 degrees.)

- Dust frequently with a damp cloth or oiled mop.

If cockroaches are a problem in your home, the U.S. Environmental Protection Agency suggests some ways to get rid of them:

- Do not leave food or garbage out.

- Store food in airtight containers.

- Clean all food crumbs or spilled liquids right away.

- Try using poison baits, boric acid (for cockroaches), or traps first, before using pesticide sprays.

If you use sprays, remember these guidelines:

- Do not spray in food preparation or storage areas.

- Do not spray in areas where children play or sleep.

- Limit the spray to the infested area.

- Follow instructions on the label carefully.

- Make sure there is plenty of fresh air when you spray.

- Keep the person with allergies or asthma out of the room while spraying.

Pets

If you or your child is allergic to furry pets, especially cats, the best way to avoid allergic reactions is to find them another home. If you are like most people who are attached to their pets, that is usually not a desirable option. There are ways, however, to help lower the levels of animal allergens in the air, which may reduce allergic reactions.

- Bathe your cat weekly and brush it more frequently (ideally, a non-allergic person should do this).
- Keep cats out of your bedroom.
- Remove carpets and soft furnishings, which collect animal allergens.
- Use a vacuum cleaner and room air cleaners with HEPA filters.
- Wear a facemask while house and cat cleaning.

Chemicals

Irritants such as chemicals can worsen airborne allergy symptoms, and you should avoid them as much as possible. For example, if you have pollen allergy, avoid unnecessary exposure to irritants such as insect sprays, tobacco smoke, air pollution, and fresh tar or paint during periods of high pollen levels.

Air Conditioners and Filters

When possible, use air conditioners inside your home or car to help prevent pollen and mold allergens from entering. Various types of air-filtering devices made with fiberglass or electrically charged plates may help reduce allergens produced in the home. You can add these to your present heating and cooling system. In addition, portable devices that can be used in individual rooms are especially helpful in reducing animal allergens.

An allergist can suggest which kind of filter is best for your home. Before buying a filtering device, rent one and use it in a closed room (the bedroom, for instance) for a month or two to see whether your allergy symptoms diminish. The airflow should be sufficient to exchange the air in the room five or six times per hour. Therefore, the size and efficiency of the filtering device should be determined in part by the size of the room.

You should be wary of exaggerated claims for appliances that cannot really clean the air. Very small air cleaners cannot remove dust and pollen. No air purifier can prevent viral or bacterial diseases such as the flu, pneumonia, or tuberculosis.

Before buying an electrostatic precipitator, you should compare the machine's ozone output with federal standards. Ozone can irritate the noses and airways of people with allergies, especially those with asthma, and can increase their allergy symptoms. Other kinds of air filters, such as HEPA filters, do not release ozone into the air. HEPA filters, however, require adequate airflow to force air through them.

Treatment

Medicines

If you cannot adequately avoid airborne allergens, your symptoms often can be controlled by medicines. You can buy medicines without a prescription that can relieve allergy symptoms. If, however, they don't give you relief or they cause unwanted side effects such as sleepiness, your health care provider can prescribe antihistamines and topical nasal steroids. You can use either medicine alone or together.

Antihistamines: As the name indicates, an antihistamine counters the effects of histamine, which is released by the mast cells in your body's tissues and contributes to your allergy symptoms. For many years, antihistamines have proven useful in relieving itching in the nose and eyes; relieving sneezing; and reducing nasal swelling and drainage.

Many people who take antihistamines have some distressing side effects such as drowsiness and loss of alertness and coordination. Adults may interpret such reactions in children as behavior problems.

Antihistamines that cause fewer of these side effects are available over-the-counter or by prescription. These nonsedating antihistamines are as effective as other antihistamines in preventing histamine-induced symptoms, but most do so without causing sleepiness.

Topical Nasal Steroids: You should not confuse topical nasal steroids with anabolic steroids, which athletes sometimes use to enlarge muscle mass and which can have serious side effects. The chemicals in nasal steroids are different from those in anabolic steroids.

Topical nasal steroids are anti-inflammatory medicines that stop the allergic reaction. In addition to other helpful actions, they decrease the number of mast cells in the nose and reduce mucus secretion and nasal swelling. The combination of antihistamines and nasal steroids is a very effective way to treat allergic rhinitis, especially if you have moderate or severe allergic rhinitis.

Although topical nasal steroids can have side effects, they are safe when used at recommended doses.

Cromolyn Sodium: Cromolyn sodium is a nasal spray that in some people helps prevent allergic rhinitis from starting. When used as a nasal spray, it can safely stop the release of chemicals like histamine from mast cells. It has few side effects when used as directed and significantly helps some people manage their allergies.

Decongestants: Sometimes helping the nasal passages to drain away mucus will help relieve symptoms such as congestion, swelling, excess secretions, and discomfort in the sinus areas that can be caused by nasal allergies. Your doctor may recommend using oral or nasal decongestants to reduce congestion along with an antihistamine to control allergic symptoms.

You should not, however, use over-the-counter or prescription decongestant nose drops and sprays for more than a few days. When used for longer periods, these medicines can lead to even more congestion and swelling of the nasal passages. Because of recent concern about the bad effects of decongestant sprays and drops, some have been removed from store shelves.

Immunotherapy

Immunotherapy, or a series of allergy shots, is the only available treatment that has a chance of reducing your allergy symptoms over a longer period of time. You would receive subcutaneous (under the skin) injections of increasing concentrations of the allergen(s) to which you are sensitive. These injections reduce the level of IgE antibodies in the blood and cause the body to make a protective antibody called IgG.

About 85 percent of people with allergic rhinitis will see their hay fever symptoms and need for medicines drop significantly within twelve months of starting immunotherapy. Those who benefit from allergy shots may continue it for three years and then consider stopping. While many are able to stop the injections with good results lasting for several years, others do get worse after the shots are stopped.

One research study shows that children treated for allergic rhinitis with immunotherapy were less likely to develop asthma. Researchers need to study this further, however.

As researchers produce better allergens for immunotherapy, this technique will be become an even more effective treatment.

Allergy Research

Research on allergies is focused on understanding what happens to the human body during the allergic process—the sequence of events leading to the allergic response and the factors responsible for allergic diseases.

Scientists supported by the National Institute of Allergy and Infectious Diseases (NIAID) found that, during the first years of their lives, children raised in a house with two or more dogs or cats may be less likely to develop allergic diseases as compared with children raised without pets. The striking finding here is that high pet exposure early in life appears to protect some children from not only pet allergy but also other types of common allergies, such as allergy to house dust mites, ragweed, and grass. This new finding is changing the way scientists think about pet exposure. Scientists must now figure out how pet exposure causes a general shift of the immune system away from an allergic response.

The results of this and a number of other studies suggest that bacteria carried by pets may be responsible for holding back the immune system's allergic response. These bacteria release molecules called endotoxin. Some researchers think endotoxin is the molecule responsible for shifting the developing immune system away from responding to allergens through a class of lymphocytes called Th-2 cells. (These cells are associated with allergic reactions.) Instead, endotoxin may stimulate the immune system to block allergic reactions.

If scientists can find out exactly what it is about pets or the bacteria they carry that prevents the allergic response, they might be able to develop a new allergy treatment.

Some studies are seeking better ways to diagnose as well as treat people with allergic diseases and to better understand the factors that regulate IgE production to reduce the allergic response. Several research institutions are focusing on ways to influence the cells that participate in the allergic response.

NIAID supports a network of Asthma, Allergic and Immunologic Diseases Cooperative Research Centers throughout the United States. The centers encourage close coordination among scientists studying basic and clinical immunology, genetics, biochemistry, pharmacology, and environmental science. This interdisciplinary approach helps move research knowledge as quickly as possible from the lab into the hands of doctors and their allergy patients.

Educating patients and health care providers is an important tool in controlling allergic diseases. All of these research centers conduct and evaluate education programs focused on methods to control allergic diseases.

Since 1991, researchers participating in NIAID's Inner-City Asthma Study have been examining ways to treat asthma in minority children living in inner-city environments. Asthma, a major cause of illness and hospitalizations among these children, is provoked by a number of possible factors, including allergies to airborne substances.

The success of NIAID's model asthma program led the U.S. Centers for Disease Control and Prevention to award grants to help community-based health organizations throughout the United States implement the program.

Based on the success of the first National Cooperative Inner-City Asthma Study, NIAID and the National Institute of Environmental Health Sciences, also part of NIH, started a second cooperative multi-center study in 1996. This study recruited children with asthma, aged four to eleven, to test the effectiveness of two interventions. One intervention uses a novel communication and doctor education system. Information about the children's asthma severity is provided to their primary care physicians, with the intent that this information will help the doctors give the children the best care possible.

The other intervention involves educating families about reducing exposure to passive cigarette smoke and to indoor allergens, including cockroaches, house dust mites, and mold. Researchers are assessing the effectiveness of both interventions by evaluating their capacity to reduce the severity of asthma in these children.

Early data show that by reducing allergen levels in children's beds by one-third, investigators reduced by nearly one-quarter (22 percent) both the number of days the children wheezed and the number of days the children missed school.

Although several factors provoke allergic responses, scientists know that heredity plays a major role in determining who will develop an allergy. Therefore, scientists are trying to identify and describe the genes that make a person susceptible to allergic diseases.

Because researchers are becoming increasingly aware of the role of environmental factors in allergies, they are evaluating ways to control environmental exposures to allergens and pollutants to prevent allergic disease.

These studies offer the promise of improving the treatment and control of allergic diseases and the hope that one day allergic diseases will be preventable.

Chapter 27

Common Nasal Concerns

Chapter Contents

Section 27.1

Deviated Septum

The shape of your nasal cavity could be the cause of chronic sinusitis. The nasal septum is the wall dividing the nasal cavity into halves; it is composed of a central supporting skeleton covered on each side by mucous membrane. The front portion of this natural partition is a firm but bendable structure made mostly of cartilage and is covered by skin that has a substantial supply of blood vessels. The ideal nasal septum is exactly midline, separating the left and right sides of the nose into passageways of equal size.

Estimates are that 80 percent of all nasal septums are off-center, a condition that is generally not noticed. A "deviated septum" occurs when the septum is severely shifted away from the midline. The most common symptom from a badly deviated or crooked septum is difficulty breathing through the nose. The symptoms are usually worse on one side, and sometimes actually occur on the side opposite the bend. In some cases the crooked septum can interfere with the drainage of the sinuses, resulting in repeated sinus infections.

Septoplasty is the preferred surgical treatment to correct a deviated septum. This procedure is not generally performed on minors, because the cartilaginous septum grows until around age eighteen. Septal deviations commonly occur due to nasal trauma.

A deviated septum may cause one or more of the following:

• Blockage of one or both nostrils

• Nasal congestion, sometimes one-sided

• Frequent nosebleeds

• Frequent sinus infections

• At times, facial pain, headaches, postnasal drip

• Noisy breathing during sleep (in infants and young children)

360

In some cases, a person with a mildly deviated septum has symptoms only when he or she also has a "cold" (an upper respiratory tract infection). In these individuals, the respiratory infection triggers nasal inflammation that temporarily amplifies any mild airflow problems related to the deviated septum. Once the "cold" resolves, and the nasal inflammation subsides, symptoms of a deviated septum often resolve, too.

Diagnosis of a Deviated Septum

Patients with chronic sinusitis often have nasal congestion, and many have nasal septal deviations. However, for those with this debilitating condition, there may be additional reasons for the nasal airway obstruction. The problem may result from a septal deviation, reactive edema (swelling) from the infected areas, allergic problems, mucosal hypertrophy (increase in size), other anatomic abnormalities, or combinations thereof. A trained specialist in diagnosing and treating ear, nose, and throat disorders can determine the cause of your chronic sinusitis and nasal obstruction.

Your First Visit

After discussing your symptoms, the primary care physician or specialist will inquire if you have ever incurred severe trauma to your nose and if you have had previous nasal surgery. Next, an examination of the general appearance of your nose will occur, including the position of your nasal septum. This will entail the use of a bright light and a nasal speculum (an instrument that gently spreads open your nostril) to inspect the inside surface of each nostril.

Surgery may be the recommended treatment if the deviated septum is causing troublesome nosebleeds or recurrent sinus infections. Additional testing may be required in some circumstances.

Septoplasty

Septoplasty is a surgical procedure performed entirely through the nostrils; accordingly, no bruising or external signs occur. The surgery might be combined with a rhinoplasty, in which case the external appearance of the nose is altered and swelling or bruising of the face is evident. Septoplasty may also be combined with sinus surgery.

The time required for the operation averages about one to one and a half hours, depending on the deviation. It can be done with a local

361

or a general anesthetic, and is usually done on an outpatient basis. After the surgery, nasal packing is inserted to prevent excessive postoperative bleeding. During the surgery, badly deviated portions of the septum may be removed entirely, or they may be readjusted and reinserted into the nose.

If a deviated nasal septum is the sole cause for your chronic sinusitis, relief from this severe disorder will be achieved.

Section 27.2

Nasal Polyps

Blocked nose? Food seem less tasty? Thick, discolored nasal drainage? You might be suffering from nasal polyps—a treatable nasal problem.

Nasal polyps are noncancerous growths occurring in the nose or sinuses. Other types of polyps occur in the bowel or urinary bladder, but have no relationship to those in the nose and sinuses. Polyps in the bowel or bladder have a chance of being cancerous; polyps in the nose and sinuses are rarely malignant.

Polyps can cause nasal blockage, making it hard to breathe, but most nasal polyp problems can be helped.

While some polyps are a result of swelling from an infection, most of the time, the cause for the nasal polyps is never known. A few individuals may have a combination of asthma, aspirin sensitivity, and nasal polyps. If aspirin is taken, the asthma and nasal polyps may worsen.

Because polyps block the nose, patients often notice a decrease in the sense of smell. Since much of our sense of taste is related to our sense of smell, patients with nasal polyps may describe a loss of both taste and smell.

Nasal polyps also cause nasal obstruction and may also block the pathways where the sinuses drain into the nose. This blockage by the polyps causes the mucus (which normally forms and drains through the nose) to remain in the sinuses. When this mucous stays in the sinuses too long, it can become infected. It is this infected mucous that the patient experiences as a thick, discolored drainage in the nose and down the throat. This type of nasal obstruction and infection may also cause pressure over the forehead and face.

Many people with nasal polyps have no symptoms and therefore require no treatment. For those patients whose polyps are causing symptoms, medical or surgical management is available.

Medical management to reduce the size of the polyps often requires a series of steroid pills and nasal steroid sprays. Since the nasal steroid sprays have very little absorption into the bloodstream, there are few, if any, side effects. For those patients whose polyps cannot be managed medically or who choose not to manage them medically, surgery is usually effective.

Surgery for nasal polyps is usually done as an outpatient in an ambulatory surgery center where patients go home the same day as the surgery. The polyps are removed from the nose and sinuses using small nasal telescopes, which not only remove the diseased tissue but also preserve the normal structures and reconstruct the normal inflow, outflow, and function of the sinuses.

While most patients with nasal polyps and asthma or nasal polyps, asthma, and aspirin sensitivity have the same 90 percent improvement, eighteen months after surgery 40 percent of patients with asthma and nasal polyps report continued improvement; and 35 percent of patients with the combination of aspirin sensitivity, asthma, and nasal polyps report still feeling well.

The asthmatic patient with nasal polyps is the most difficult to cure, but by using the endoscopic technique, as well as ongoing management with medication after surgery, we are able to help many patients breathe easier, regain their sense of smell, eliminate facial pressure, and have their asthma better controlled.

Section 27.3

Noseobleeds

From "Pediatric Common Questions, Quick Answers," by Donna M. D'Alessandro, M.D., Lindsay Huth, B.A., and Susan Kinzer, M.P.H., revised October 2004. © Donna M. D'Alessandro M.D. All rights reserved. For additional information, visit http://www.virtualpediatrichospital.org.

What causes nosebleeds?

- Nosebleeds can happen if a cold or allergy irritates the inner nose.

- Touching and poking the inner nose can cause nosebleeds.

- Hard nose blowing can cause nosebleeds.

- Nosebleeds can start after the nose is hit or bumped.

- Nosebleeds are common in the winter when the air is dry.

Who can get nosebleeds?

- Nosebleeds are common in children.

- Children who have veins close to the skin in their nose will likely get more nosebleeds than other children.

How are nosebleeds treated?

- Sitting is best. Have the child lean forward with head down. If your child is hurt and needs to lies down, prop her head up on pillows.

- If your child has blood in her mouth, she should spit it out.

- Apply pressure to the nose by squeezing the nostrils together. Hold for ten minutes. Don't peek to see if the bleeding has stopped. You'll need to start over if you do.

- If bleeding doesn't stop, press ice or a towel soaked in cold water on the ridge of the nose.

- Do not stick tissues, gauze, or other things into the nose.
- Have your child avoid rough activities where the nose could be bumped.
- Release a sneeze through the mouth instead of the nose. Blow the nose gently if needed.

How long does a nosebleed last?

- Bleeding should stop within ten to fifteen minutes.

How can nosebleeds be prevented?

Nosebleeds commonly happen for a few days in a row. It takes time for the nose to heal. For a few days after a nosebleed, do as follows:

- Use a cool mist vaporizer or humidifier at night to keep the air moist. Clean daily with bleach and water to kill germs (mix one part bleach to ten parts water).
- Gently put a little petroleum jelly (such as Vaseline) inside the nose with your fingertip to keep it moist.
- Discourage the child from picking her nose.
- Use saline nose drops (such as Ocean Nasal Spray or Ayr) to keep the nose moist. You can buy these at the store without a prescription. Drops will keep blood from crusting.

When should I call the doctor?

- Call the doctor if bleeding lasts for longer than fifteen minutes after pinching the nose without peeking.
- Call the doctor if your child has many nosebleeds.
- Call the doctor if your child has blood in her stool, urine, tears, ears, throat, or gums.
- Call the doctor if your child bruises easily or if blood from injuries is hard to stop.
- Call the doctor if your child has a flat, purplish-red rash on her skin.
- Call the doctor if your child looks sick or pale.
- Call the doctor if she is unusually tired or weak.

- Call the doctor if there is a large amount of blood.
- Call the doctor if your child has an object stuck in her nose.

Quick Answers

- Nosebleeds can start if the inner nose is dry or irritated or if the nose is bumped.
- Nosebleeds are common in children.
- Apply pressure to the nose by squeezing the nostrils together. Hold for ten minutes.
- Bleeding should stop within ten to fifteen minutes.
- For the next few days, keep the inner nose moist. Use nose drops, a humidifier or vaporizer, or petroleum jelly.
- Call the doctor if bleeding lasts for longer than fifteen minutes.

References

Children's Hospital, Boston. *Nosebleeds in Children*. 1993 January (cited 2001 September 5). Available from: URL: http://www.vh.org/Patients/IHB/Emergency/Peds/Nosebleeds.html

Emergency Medicine. *Nosebleeds*. 1992–2001 (cited 2001 September 5). Available from: URL: http://www.vh.org/Patients/IHB/Emergency/Peds/Nosebleeds2.html

Mayo Clinic. *Nosebleeds*. 2001 July 1 (cited 2001 September 5). Available from: URL: http://www.mayoclinic.com/home?id=HQ00105

Section 27.4

Septoplasty and Turbinate Reduction

The nasal septum is the partition that divides one side of the nose from the other. It is rarely perfectly straight—it is slightly crooked in over 80 percent of people. When the septum is so crooked or deviated that it blocks the nasal passage, then a surgical operation called a septoplasty may restore clear breathing.

If your nose is congested on one side during part of the day and later congested on the other side, then it is not just the septum that is causing the nasal obstruction. In this instance, an abnormal turbinate—a structure that projects from the lateral wall of the nose into the nasal cavity—may be the cause. Usually medical treatment (such as a nasal steroid spray) is recommended before considering surgery. If the medical treatments fail to bring relief, then your doctor may also recommend a procedure known as a turbinate reduction. Turbinate reductions can be done in the office or in the operating room.

A septoplasty may be combined with a turbinate reduction so that a normal nasal airway can be restored.

It is important that the turbinate not be removed completely because its removal will result in a very dry, crusty nose that is unable to adequately humidify and warm the air. Occasionally, turbinate tissue will re-grow after turbinate surgery and the procedure may need to be repeated. This is preferable to the situation of totally removing the turbinate.

If your doctor recommends a septoplasty, then this must be done in an operating room. It may be done under general or local anesthesia with sedation. Whether you choose general or local anesthesia, the recuperative period is similar, and patients go home within three to four hours after the operation is completed. A variety of nasal dressings are applied in the nose along the septum. Some surgeons prefer to pack the nose with gauze or special sponge-like material. Other surgeons will use soft plastic splints for the same purpose. In addition, absorbable sutures may also be used.

Because the septal cartilage has "memory"—it has an intrinsic tendency to assume its initial shape—the septal cartilage can sometimes bend after the surgery and cause nasal obstruction. In most cases there is no bruising or black eyes associated with just a septoplasty. If the outside of your nose is crooked, then occasionally this must be fixed along with the septum in order to get a good airway. This procedure is called a septorhinoplasty. In these situations you are much more likely to have bruising and swelling of the nose and possibly black eyes. This bruising usually resolves within two weeks.

Complications of Septoplasty

- It is possible that your airway will not improve.

- Some swelling of the external nose or change in the external appearance is possible.

- A septal perforation (hole in the septum that connects the two sides of the nose) may occur. A septal perforation may be associated with a whistling sound, bleeding, and/or crusting. A severe septal perforation may alter the shape of the external nose. Septal perforations are rare complications of septal surgery.

- Numbness of the tip of the nose or the upper front teeth is not uncommon and usually resolves within several months following the procedure. Rarely, the numbness may persist.

- Bleeding of any significant amount is uncommon. Patients who are undergoing nasal surgery should discontinue aspirin and other non-steroidal anti-inflammatory drugs (NSAIDs, such as Motrin, Advil, ibuprofen, etc.) ten days prior to surgery, since the medications can produce bleeding.

- Septal hematoma occurs when bleeding persists underneath the skin flaps of the septum. This must be recognized within twenty-four hours and drained in order to prevent later saddling of the nose. This is a rare complication.

- Infection is uncommon but can occur. If nasal packing has been used and the patient develops a rash and a high fever, then the patient must immediately contact his or her physician because of the possibility of toxic shock syndrome. This is very rare complication.

- Loss of smell has been reported following septoplasty but is quite rare.

Complications of Turbinate Surgery

- Bleeding usually resolves within several weeks following the procedure.

- Over-resection of the turbinate will result in a dry nose.

- Under-resection may not totally relieve the nasal stuffiness and the procedure may need to be repeated.

- Discomfort following the procedure for more than two weeks is uncommon.

Section 27.5

Rhinoplasty

"Understanding Rhinoplasty Surgery," © 2002.
Reprinted with permission from the American Academy of Facial Plastic and Reconstructive Surgery, www.aafprs.org.

Surgery of the Nose

Every year, half a million people who are interested in improving the appearance of their noses seek consultation with facial plastic surgeons. Some are unhappy with the noses they were born with, and some with the way aging has changed their nose. For others, an injury may have distorted the nose, or the goal may be improved breathing. But one thing is clear: nothing has a greater impact on how a person looks than the size and shape of the nose. Because the nose is the most defining characteristic of the face, a slight alteration can greatly improve one's appearance.

If you have wondered how nose surgery, or rhinoplasty, could improve your looks, self-confidence, or health, you need to know how rhinoplasty is performed and what you can expect. No chapter can answer all your concerns, but this chapter can provide answers to many of the questions you may have.

Successful facial plastic surgery is a result of good rapport between patient and surgeon. Trust, based on realistic expectations and exacting medical expertise, develops in the consulting stages before surgery. Your surgeon can answer specific questions about your specific needs.

Is Rhinoplasty for You?

As with all facial plastic surgery, good health and realistic expectations are prerequisites. Understanding nasal surgery is also critical. Since there is no ideal in rhinoplasty, the goal is to improve the nose aesthetically, making it harmonize better with other facial features.

Skin type, ethnic background, and age are important factors to be considered in discussions with your surgeon prior to surgery. Before the nose is altered, a young patient must reach full growth, usually around age fifteen or sixteen. Exceptions are cases in which breathing is severely impaired.

Before deciding on rhinoplasty, ask your facial plastic surgeon if any additional surgery might be recommended to enhance the appearance of your face. Many patients have chin augmentation in conjunction with rhinoplasty to create a better balance of features.

Making the Decision for Rhinoplasty

Whether the surgery is desired for functional or cosmetic reasons, your choice of a qualified facial plastic surgeon is of paramount importance. Many facial plastic surgeons are trained in both ear, nose, throat, and facial cosmetic surgery, which provides you, the patient, with the highest level of training and expertise. Your surgeon will examine the structure of your nose, both externally and internally, to evaluate what you can expect from rhinoplasty. You are most likely to be pleased with the results of your surgery if you have a realistic idea of what nasal surgery can and cannot do.

You can expect a thorough explanation of the surgeon's expectations and the risks involved in surgery. Following a joint decision by you and your surgeon to proceed with rhinoplasty, the surgeon will take photographs of you and discuss the options available. Your surgeon will explain how the nasal structures, including bone and cartilage, can be sculpted to reshape the nose and indicate how reshaping the chin, for example, could enhance the desired results.

After conducting a thorough medical history, your surgeon will offer information regarding anesthesia, the surgical facility to be used, and the costs for the procedure.

Understanding the Surgery

The definition of rhinoplasty is, literally, shaping the nose. First, incisions are made and the bone and cartilage support system of the nose is accessed. The majority of incisions are made inside the nose, where they are invisible. In some cases, an incision is made in the area of skin separating the nostrils. Next, certain amounts of underlying bone and cartilage are removed, added to, or rearranged to provide a newly shaped structure. For example, when the tip of the nose is too large, the surgeon can sculpt the cartilage in this area to reduce it in size. The angle of the nose in relation to the upper lip can be altered for a more youthful look or to correct a distortion.

The tissues are then redraped over the new frame and the incisions are closed. A splint is applied to the outside of the nose to help retain the new shape while the nose heals. Soft, absorbent material may be used inside the nose to maintain stability along the dividing wall of the air passages called the septum. Alternatively, soft nasal supports that permit nasal breathing post-operatively can be placed.

What to Expect after the Surgery

Immediately after surgery, a small splint will be placed on your nose to protect it and to keep the structure stable for at least five to eight days. If packing is placed inside the nose during surgery, it is removed the morning following the surgery. Your face will feel puffy, especially the first day after surgery. Pain medication may be required. Your surgeon will advise you to avoid blowing your nose for seven days after surgery. In the immediate days following surgery, you may experience bruising and minor swelling in the eye area. Cold compresses often reduce the bruising and discomfort. Absorbable sutures are usually used that do not have to be removed. Nasal dressing and splints are usually removed six or seven days after surgery.

It is crucial that you follow your surgeon's directions, especially instructions to keep your head elevated for a certain period after surgery. Some activities will be prohibited in the weeks after the procedure. Sun exposure, exertion, and risk of injury must be avoided. If you wear glasses, special arrangements must be made to ensure that the glasses do not rest on the bridge of the nose. Tape and other devices are sometimes used to permit wearing glasses without stressing the area where surgery was performed.

Follow-up care is vital for this procedure to monitor healing. Obviously, anything unusual should be reported to your surgeon immediately. It is essential that you keep your follow-up appointments with your surgeon.

Insurance does not generally cover surgery that is purely for cosmetic reasons. Surgery to correct or improve nasal function or surgery for major deformity or injury may be reimbursable in whole or in part. It is the patient's responsibility to check with the insurance carrier for information on the degree of coverage.

Chapter 28

Sinus Problems

Chapter Contents

Section 28.1

Sinusitis

Reprinted from "Sinusitis," National Institute of Allergy and
Infectious Diseases, National Institutes of Health, February 11, 2005.

You're coughing and sneezing and tired and achy. You think that you
might be getting a cold. Later, when the medicines you've been taking
to relieve the symptoms of the common cold are not working and you've
now got a terrible headache, you finally drag yourself to the doctor. After listening to your history of symptoms, examining your face and forehead, and perhaps doing a sinus x-ray, the doctor says you have sinusitis.

Sinusitis simply means your sinuses are infected or inflamed, but
this gives little indication of the misery and pain this condition can
cause. Health care experts usually divide sinusitis cases into these categories:

- Acute, which lasts for three weeks or less

- Chronic, which usually lasts for three to eight weeks but can
  continue for months or even years

- Recurrent, which means several acute attacks within a year

Health care experts estimate that thirty-seven million Americans are
affected by sinusitis every year. Health care providers report nearly
thirty-two million cases of chronic sinusitis to the Centers for Disease
Control and Prevention annually. Americans spend millions of dollars
each year for medications that promise relief from their sinus symptoms.

What Are Sinuses?

Sinuses are hollow air spaces in the human body. When people say,
"I'm having a sinus attack," they usually are referring to symptoms
in one or more of four pairs of cavities, or sinuses, known as paranasal
sinuses. These cavities, located within the skull or bones of the head
surrounding the nose, include these:

- Frontal sinuses over the eyes in the brow area

- Maxillary sinuses inside each cheekbone

- Ethmoid sinuses just behind the bridge of the nose and between the eyes

- Sphenoid sinuses behind the ethmoids in the upper region of the nose and behind the eyes

Each sinus has an opening into the nose for the free exchange of air and mucus, and each is joined with the nasal passages by a continuous mucous membrane lining. Therefore, anything that causes a swelling in the nose—an infection, an allergic reaction, or another type of immune reaction—also can affect the sinuses. Air trapped within a blocked sinus, along with pus or other secretions, may cause pressure on the sinus wall. The result is the sometimes intense pain of a sinus attack. Similarly, when air is prevented from entering a paranasal sinus by a swollen membrane at the opening, a vacuum can be created that also causes pain.

Symptoms

The location of your sinus pain depends on which sinus is affected.

- Headache when you wake up in the morning is typical of a sinus problem.

- Pain when your forehead over the frontal sinuses is touched may indicate that your frontal sinuses are inflamed.

- Infection in the maxillary sinuses can cause your upper jaw and teeth to ache and your cheeks to become tender to the touch.

- Since the ethmoid sinuses are near the tear ducts in the corner of the eyes, inflammation of these cavities often causes swelling of the eyelids and tissues around your eyes, and pain between your eyes. Ethmoid inflammation also can cause tenderness when the sides of your nose are touched, a loss of smell, and a stuffy nose.

- Although the sphenoid sinuses are less frequently affected, infection in this area can cause earaches, neck pain, and deep aching at the top of your head.

Most people with sinusitis, however, have pain or tenderness in several locations, and their symptoms usually do not clearly indicate which sinuses are inflamed.

Other symptoms of sinusitis can include the following:

- Fever
- Weakness
- Tiredness
- A cough that may be more severe at night
- Runny nose (rhinitis) or nasal congestion

In addition, the drainage of mucus from the sphenoid or other sinuses down the back of your throat (postnasal drip) can cause you to have a sore throat. Mucus drainage also can irritate the membranes lining your larynx (upper windpipe). Not everyone with these symptoms, however, has sinusitis.

On rare occasions, acute sinusitis can result in brain infection and other serious complications.

Some Causes of Acute Sinusitis

Most cases of acute sinusitis start with a common cold, which is caused by a virus. These viral colds do not cause symptoms of sinusitis, but they do inflame the sinuses. Both the cold and the sinus inflammation usually go away without treatment in two weeks. The inflammation, however, might explain why having a cold increases your likelihood of developing acute sinusitis. For example, your nose reacts to an invasion by viruses that cause infections such as the common cold or flu by producing mucus and sending white blood cells to the lining of the nose, which congest and swell the nasal passages.

When this swelling involves the adjacent mucous membranes of your sinuses, air and mucus are trapped behind the narrowed openings of the sinuses. When your sinus openings become too narrow, mucus cannot drain properly. This increase in mucus sets up prime conditions for bacteria to multiply.

Most healthy people harbor bacteria, such as *Streptococcus pneumoniae* and *Haemophilus influenzae*, in their upper respiratory tracts with no problems until the body's defenses are weakened or drainage from the sinuses is blocked by a cold or other viral infection. Thus, bacteria that may have been living harmlessly in your nose or throat can multiply and invade your sinuses, causing an acute sinus infection.

Sometimes, fungal infections can cause acute sinusitis. Although fungi are abundant in the environment, they usually are harmless to healthy people, indicating that the human body has a natural resistance to them. Fungi, such as *Aspergillus*, can cause serious illness in people whose immune systems are not functioning properly. Some people with fungal sinusitis have an allergic-type reaction to the fungi.

Chronic inflammation of the nasal passages also can lead to sinusitis. If you have allergic rhinitis or hay fever, you can develop episodes of acute sinusitis. Vasomotor rhinitis, caused by humidity, cold air, alcohol, perfumes, and other environmental conditions, also may be complicated by sinus infections.

Acute sinusitis is much more common in some people than in the general population. For example, sinusitis occurs more often in people who have reduced immune function (such as those with primary immune deficiency diseases or HIV infection) and with abnormality of mucus secretion or mucus movement (such as those with cystic fibrosis).

Causes of Chronic Sinusitis

It can be difficult to determine the cause of chronic sinusitis. Some investigators think it is an infectious disease but others are not certain. It is an inflammatory disease that often occurs in patients with asthma. If you have asthma, an allergic disease, you may have chronic sinusitis with exacerbations. If you are allergic to airborne allergens, such as dust, mold, and pollen, which trigger allergic rhinitis, you may develop chronic sinusitis. An immune response to antigens in fungi may be responsible for at least some cases of chronic sinusitis. In addition, people who are allergic to fungi can develop a condition called "allergic fungal sinusitis." If you are subject to getting chronic sinusitis, damp weather, especially in northern temperate climates, or pollutants in the air and in buildings also can affect you.

If you have an immune deficiency disease or an abnormality in the way mucus moves through and from your respiratory system (e.g., primary immune deficiency, HIV infection, and cystic fibrosis) you might develop chronic sinusitis with frequent flare-ups of acute sinusitis due to infections. In otherwise normal individuals, sinusitis may or may not be infectious. In addition, if you have severe asthma, nasal polyps (small growths in the nose), or severe asthma attacks caused by aspirin and aspirin-like medicines such as ibuprofen, you might have chronic sinusitis.

Diagnosis

Because your nose can get stuffy when you have a condition like the common cold, you may confuse simple nasal congestion with sinusitis.

377

A cold, however, usually lasts about seven to fourteen days and disappears without treatment. Acute sinusitis often lasts longer and typically causes more symptoms than just a cold.

Your doctor can diagnose sinusitis by listening to your symptoms, doing a physical examination, taking x-rays, and if necessary, an MRI or CT scan (magnetic resonance imaging and computed tomography).

Treatment

After diagnosing sinusitis and identifying a possible cause, a doctor can suggest treatments that will reduce your inflammation and relieve your symptoms.

Acute Sinusitis

If you have acute sinusitis, your doctor may recommend the following:

- Decongestants to reduce congestion

- Antibiotics to control a bacterial infection, if present

- Pain relievers to reduce any pain

You should, however, use over-the-counter or prescription decongestant nose drops and sprays for only few days. If you use these medicines for longer periods, they can lead to even more congestion and swelling of your nasal passages.

If bacteria cause your sinusitis, antibiotics used along with a nasal or oral decongestant will usually help. Your doctor can prescribe an antibiotic that fights the type of bacteria most commonly associated with sinusitis.

Many cases of acute sinusitis will end without antibiotics. If you have allergic disease along with sinusitis, however, you may need medicine to relieve your allergy symptoms. If you already have asthma then get sinusitis, you may experience worsening of your asthma and should be in close touch with your doctor.

In addition, your doctor may prescribe a steroid nasal spray, along with other treatments, to reduce your sinus congestion, swelling, and inflammation.

Chronic Sinusitis

Doctors often find it difficult to treat chronic sinusitis successfully, realizing that symptoms persist even after taking antibiotics for a long period. As discussed in the following, many doctors treat with steroids such as steroid nasal sprays. Many doctors do treat chronic sinusitis as though it is an infection, by using antibiotics and decongestants. Other doctors use both antibiotics and steroid nasal sprays. Further research is needed to determine what is the best treatment.

Some people with severe asthma are said to have dramatic improvement of their symptoms when their chronic sinusitis is treated with antibiotics.

Doctors commonly prescribe steroid nasal sprays to reduce inflammation in chronic sinusitis. Although doctors occasionally prescribe these sprays to treat people with chronic sinusitis over a long period, doctors don't fully understand the long-term safety of these medications, especially in children. Therefore, doctors will consider whether the benefits outweigh any risks of using steroid nasal sprays.

If you have severe chronic sinusitis, your doctor may prescribe oral steroids, such as prednisone. Because oral steroids are powerful medicines and can have significant side effects, you should take them only when other medicines have not worked.

Although home remedies cannot cure sinus infection, they might give you some comfort.

- Inhaling steam from a vaporizer or a hot cup of water can soothe inflamed sinus cavities.

- Saline nasal spray, which you can buy in a drug store, can give relief.

- Gentle heat applied over the inflamed area is comforting.

When medical treatment fails, surgery may be the only alternative for treating chronic sinusitis. Research studies suggest that the vast majority of people who undergo surgery have fewer symptoms and better quality of life.

In children, problems often are eliminated by removal of adenoids obstructing nasal-sinus passages.

Adults who have had allergic and infectious conditions over the years sometimes develop nasal polyps that interfere with proper drainage. Removal of these polyps and/or repair of a deviated septum to ensure an open airway often provides considerable relief from sinus symptoms.

The most common surgery done today is functional endoscopic sinus surgery, in which the natural openings from the sinuses are enlarged to allow drainage. This type of surgery is less invasive than conventional sinus surgery, and serious complications are rare.

379

Prevention

Although you cannot prevent all sinus disorders—any more than you can avoid all colds or bacterial infections—you can do certain things to reduce the number and severity of the attacks and possibly prevent acute sinusitis from becoming chronic.

- You may get some relief from your symptoms with a humidifier, particularly if room air in your home is heated by a dry forced-air system.

- Air conditioners help to provide an even temperature.

- Electrostatic filters attached to heating and air conditioning equipment are helpful in removing allergens from the air.

If you are prone to getting sinus disorders, especially if you have allergies, you should avoid cigarette smoke and other air pollutants. If your allergies inflame your nasal passages, you are more likely to have a strong reaction to all irritants.

If you suspect that your sinus inflammation may be related to dust, mold, pollen, or food—or any of the hundreds of allergens that can trigger an upper respiratory reaction—you should consult your doctor. Your doctor can use various tests to determine whether you have an allergy and its cause. This will help you and your doctor take appropriate steps to reduce or limit your allergy symptoms.

Drinking alcohol also causes nasal and sinus membranes to swell.

If you are prone to sinusitis, it may be uncomfortable for you to swim in pools treated with chlorine, since it irritates the lining of the nose and sinuses.

Divers often get sinus congestion and infection when water is forced into the sinuses from the nasal passages.

You may find that air travel poses a problem if you are suffering from acute or chronic sinusitis. As air pressure in a plane is reduced, pressure can build up in your head, blocking your sinuses or eustachian tubes in your ears. Therefore, you might feel discomfort in your sinus or middle ear during the plane's ascent or descent. Some health experts recommend using decongestant nose drops or inhalers before a flight to avoid this problem.

Research

At least two-thirds of sinusitis cases caused by bacteria are due to two organisms that can also cause otitis media (middle ear infection) in children as well as pneumonia and acute exacerbations of chronic bronchitis. NIAID is supporting multiple studies to better understand the basis for infectivity of these organisms as well as identifying potential candidates for future vaccines, strategies that could eliminate these diseases.

A project supported by NIAID is developing an advanced "sinuscope" that will permit improved airway evaluation during a medical examination especially when surgical intervention is contemplated.

Scientific studies have shown a close relationship between having asthma and sinusitis. As many as 75 percent of people with asthma also get sinusitis. Some studies state that up to 80 percent of adults with chronic sinusitis also had allergic rhinitis. NIAID conducts and supports research on allergic diseases as well as bacteria and fungus that can cause sinusitis. This research is focused on developing better treatments and ways to prevent these diseases.

Scientists supported by NIAID and other institutions are investigating whether chronic sinusitis has genetic causes. They have found that certain alterations in the gene that causes cystic fibrosis may also increase the likelihood of developing chronic sinusitis. This research will give scientists new insights into the cause of the disease in some people and points to new strategies for diagnosis and treatment.

Another NIAID-supported research study has recently demonstrated that blood cells from patients with chronic sinusitis make chemicals that produce inflammation when exposed to fungal antigens, suggesting that fungi may play a role in many cases of chronic sinusitis. Further research, including clinical trials of antifungal drugs, will help determine whether, and for whom, this new treatment strategy holds promise.

Section 28.2

Sinus Headache

"Headache and Sinus Disease," by Howard Levine, M.D., Mt. Sinai Nasal-Sinus Center, Cleveland, OH. Copyright © 2005 American Rhinologic Society. All rights reserved. Reprinted with permission.

Headache is a common complaint that is often associated with sinusitis. However, the true cause for a headache may be difficult to determine because headaches have many causes. The United States Center for Disease Control reports that sinusitis affects over thirty million people and is the most common chronic disease in this country. Thus, many sinus sufferers will also suffer headaches. While headaches and sinusitis are common problems, sometimes headaches occur with sinusitis and sometimes they do not.

The Nasal Sinus Problem

Typically, a nasal and/or sinus problem will have congestion and stuffiness, often with nasal drainage. If an infection is present there will be discolored, thick drainage in the front of the nose and down the back of the throat. If a headache is present, it is usually a pressure sensation varying in intensity from almost nonexistent to somewhat severe.

Generally, a sinus headache will be located over the sinuses, (forehead, corners of the eye, and cheek areas). On occasion, the pain will be felt behind the eyes, in the back of the neck, or may extend into the upper teeth. Head movement usually worsens this headache.

The true cause for headache may be difficult to determine . . . sometimes headaches occur with sinusitis and sometimes not.

Non-Sinus Headaches

Non-sinus headaches may give these same symptoms, thus making it difficult to determine if the headache is truly from a sinus problem. For example, tension headaches will occur in the forehead and neck; migraine headaches often occur in and around the eyes.

It is unusual for a person with a sinus or nasal problem to have only a headache. A sinus headache is nearly always accompanied by nasal stuffiness, congestion, obstruction, or drainage. When headache is the only symptom, it is rarely sinus related.

Sinus Headaches

The main cause of nasal and sinus headaches is the nasal turbinates—nasal structures that swell and contract throughout the day, giving the feeling of nasal congestion and occasionally pressure. Worsened by irritants such as perfume, cigarette smoke, or allergens, the internal swelling causes facial pressure. When the turbinates swell, not only is the breathing passage blocked, but also normal sinus draining passages are blocked, creating a "back-up" situation.

Drainage remains "trapped" in the sinus cavity, causing the pain and pressure you feel over the sinuses. It may also cause an infection.

Oral decongestants (i.e., pseudoephedrine) or a nasal spray (i.e., Neo-Synephrine, oxymetazoline) will often give relief. However, these sprays should not be used for more than a few days since they can cause even more congestion when their effect wears off.

Caution is needed when using decongestant pills, especially if a person has a history of heart disease or high blood pressure. These adrenaline-like medications can cause a rapid heart rate or increased blood pressure.

If over-the-counter medical management for nasal congestion is not effective, a physician may choose to prescribe a steroid nasal spray.

If medical management fails or cannot be tolerated, surgery to reduce the turbinates is extremely successful.

Another cause for a sinus headache is the common cold, which may seem to be a sinus infection. If over-the-counter cold remedies fail and the symptoms continue beyond several days or if there are other debilitating medical problems, a physician should be called.

Section 28.3

Sinus Surgery

Sinus surgery has truly evolved in the last several years. This procedure was once performed through external incisions, required extensive packing, and caused significant patient discomfort and a lengthy recovery. With recent advances in technology including the nasal endoscope, this procedure is now incisionless and can often be performed with minimal packing, pain, and recovery.

The most common indication for endoscopic sinus surgery is a chronic sinus infection refractory to medical management. Less common indications include (but are not limited to): recurrent infections (rather than a single chronic infection), complications of sinus infections, nasal polyps or mucoceles, chronic sinus headaches, impaired sense of smell, tumors of the nasal and sinus cavities, cerebrospinal fluid leaks, nasolacrimal duct obstruction, choanal atresia, and the need to decompress the orbit. Prior to undergoing endoscopic sinus surgery, patients should talk with their physicians to make sure that all reasonable medical options have been exhausted. In addition, patients should avoid any medications that may exacerbate bleeding, such as aspirin and ibuprofen products, as well as certain vitamins and herbal remedies.

Endoscopic sinus surgery may be performed under local or general anesthesia. The procedure involves the use of a small telescope (nasal endoscope) placed into the nasal cavity to visualize the surgery. The goal of the surgery is to identify the narrow channels that connect the paranasal sinuses to the nasal cavity and to enlarge these areas, thereby improving drainage from the sinuses to the nose. Sometimes sinus surgery may require simultaneous repair of the nasal septum, which divides the two sides of the nose, or the turbinates, which filter and humidify air inside of the nose. The use of nasal packing will depend on the extent of surgery and physician preference. The recovery period will also vary depending on the extent of surgery but postoperative discomfort, congestion, and drainage should significantly improve after the first few postoperative days, with mild symptoms sometimes lingering several weeks after the surgery.

Endoscopic sinus surgery generally yields excellent results, and significant symptomatic improvement is achieved in the vast majority of patients. Adverse events are rare but may include postoperative bleeding, orbital complications, complications from the general anesthetic, cerebrospinal fluid leaks, and intracranial complications such as meningitis. However, it is important to realize that chronic sinus infections are located directly beneath the skull base and adjacent to the eye and the failure to treat this problem without surgery may lead to dire consequences such as intraorbital or intracranial spread of the infection.

Chapter 29

Snoring and Sleep Apnea

Chapter Contents

Section 29.1

Snoring

Basics

Snoring is noisy breathing during sleep. It is a common problem among all ages and both genders, and it affects approximately ninety million American adults—thirty-seven million on a regular basis. Snoring may occur nightly or intermittently. Persons most at risk are males and those who are overweight, but snoring is a problem of both genders, although it is possible that women do not present with this complaint as frequently as men. Snoring usually becomes more serious as people age. It can cause disruptions to your own sleep and your bed-partner's sleep. It can lead to fragmented and unrefreshing sleep, which translates into poor daytime function (tiredness and sleepiness). It does not seem to be associated with cardiovascular problems (hypertension, strokes, heart attacks), although this is still a matter that is under investigation.

While you sleep, the muscles of your throat relax, your tongue falls backward, and your throat becomes narrow and "floppy." As you breathe, the walls of the throat begin to vibrate—generally when you breathe in, but also, to a lesser extent, when you breathe out. These vibrations lead to the characteristic sound of snoring. The narrower your airway becomes, the greater the vibration and the louder your snoring. Sometimes the walls of the throat collapse completely so that it is completely occluded, creating a condition called apnea (cessation of breathing). This is a serious condition that requires medical attention.

There are several factors that facilitate snoring. First, the normal aging process leads to the relaxation of the throat muscles, thus resulting in snoring. Anatomical abnormalities of the nose and throat, such as enlarged tonsils or adenoids, nasal polyps, or deviated nasal septum cause exaggerated narrowing of the throat during sleep and thus lead to snoring. Functional abnormalities (e.g., inflammation of the nose and/or throat as may occur during respiratory infection or during allergy season) will result in snoring. Sleep position, such as sleeping on your back, may lead to snoring in some people. Alcohol is a potent muscle relaxant and its ingestion in the evening will cause snoring. Muscle relaxants taken in the evening may lead to or worsen snoring in some individuals. One of the most important risk factors is obesity, and in particular having a lot of fatty tissue around the neck.

Symptoms

People who snore make a vibrating, rattling, noisy sound while breathing during sleep. It may be a symptom of sleep apnea. Consult your doctor if you snore and have any of the following symptoms or signs:

- Excessive daytime sleepiness
- Morning headaches
- Recent weight gain
- Awakening in the morning not feeling rested
- Awaking at night feeling confused
- Change in your level of attention, concentration, or memory
- Observed pauses in breathing during sleep

Treatment

Snorers are generally unaware of their snoring, and must rely on the observations of their bed-partners. Some snorers may wake up at night choking and gasping for breath, but this occurs relatively infrequently. If you have been told that your snoring is disturbing to others, or you have some of the symptoms and signs listed above, consult your doctor. He or she will take your history, perform a physical exam and determine whether you require a consultation with a sleep specialist and a sleep test to determine if you have sleep apnea and to see how your snoring affects your sleep quality.

Depending on the results of the sleep study, you will be presented with a series of options to treat snoring. These will generally include 1) lifestyle modification (i.e., avoidance of risk factors mentioned above, sleep position training if applicable, treatment of allergies if applicable, etc.), 2) surgery (generally on the back of the throat and roof of the mouth, or the nose if applicable, using a variety of instruments including scalpel, laser, or microwaves), 3) appliances (mainly oral appliances constructed by a dentist experienced in treatment of snoring and sleep apnea, but also other appliances such as nasal dilators), and sometimes 4) CPAP (a continuous positive airway pressure appliance which blows room air into the back of the throat, thus preventing it from collapse). The latter method is the treatment of choice for sleep apnea. If you are diagnosed with this condition, it is imperative that you pursue treatment aggressively; untreated sleep apnea will lead to daytime dysfunction and puts you at a higher risk for vascular disease.

Your own doctor, or sleep specialist, will talk to you in detail about each of the above treatment approaches, their chances of success, possible complications, and costs. They will be able to advise you which of the above treatment approaches is the correct one for you.

Coping

People who suffer mild or occasional snoring, who wake up feeling refreshed, and who function well during the day may first try the following behavioral remedies, before consulting their doctor:

- Lose weight.
- Avoid tranquilizers, sleeping pills, and antihistamines before bedtime.
- Avoid alcohol for at least four hours and heavy meals or snacks for three hours before retiring.
- Establish regular sleeping patterns.
- Sleep on your side rather than your back.

Section 29.2

Sleep Apnea

Basics

Obstructive sleep apnea (OSA) is a disorder in which breathing is briefly and repeatedly interrupted during sleep. The word "apnea" literally means "without breath." Apnea is defined as a cessation of breath that lasts at least ten seconds. Obstructive apneas occur when the muscles in the back of the throat are not able to keep the throat open, despite efforts to breathe. This causes blockages in the airway and breathing interruptions, or apneas. Obstructive apneas can result in two problems: fragmented sleep and lowered levels of oxygen in the blood. The combination of sleep disturbance and oxygen starvation can result in multiple problems, including automobile accidents, hypertension, heart disease, and mood and memory problems. Sleep apnea can be life threatening and you should consult your doctor immediately if you feel you may suffer from it.

Although the connection between sleep apnea and heart disease is not entirely clear, we know that people with cardiovascular problems such as high blood pressure, heart attack, congestive heart failure, cardiac arrhythmia, and stroke have a high prevalence of sleep apnea. Sleep apnea also results in excessive daytime sleepiness that increases the likelihood of accidents, hinders productivity, and makes relationships more difficult.

More than eighteen million American adults have sleep apnea. It is very difficult at present to estimate the prevalence of childhood OSA because of widely varying monitoring techniques, but a minimum prevalence of 2 to 3 percent is likely, with prevalence as high as 10 to 20 percent in habitually snoring children. OSA occurs in all age groups and both sexes, but there are a number of factors that increase risk, including having a small upper airway (or large tongue, tonsils, or uvula); being overweight; having a recessed chin, small jaw, or a large overbite; a large neck size (seventeen inches or greater in a man, or sixteen inches or greater in a woman); smoking and alcohol use; being age forty or older; and ethnicity (African-Americans, Pacific-Islanders, and Hispanics). Also, OSA seems to run in some families, suggesting a possible genetic basis.

Symptoms

Chronic snoring is a strong indicator of sleep apnea and should be evaluated by a health professional. Since people with sleep apnea tend to be sleep deprived, they may suffer from sleeplessness and a wide range of other symptoms such as difficulty concentrating, depression, irritability, sexual dysfunction, learning and memory difficulties, and falling asleep while at work, on the phone, or driving. Left untreated, symptoms of sleep apnea can include disturbed sleep, excessive sleepiness during the day, high blood pressure, heart attack, congestive heart failure, cardiac arrhythmia, stroke, or depression.

Treatment

If you suspect you may have sleep apnea, the first thing to do is see your doctor. Bring with you a record of your sleep, fatigue levels throughout the day, and any other symptoms you might be having. Ask your bed partner if he or she notices that you snore heavily, choke, gasp, or stop breathing during sleep. Be sure to take an updated list of medications, including over-the-counter medications, with you any time you visit a doctor for the first time. You may want to call your medical insurance provider to find out if a referral is needed for a visit to a sleep center.

One of the most common methods used to diagnose sleep apnea is a sleep study, which may require an overnight stay at a sleep center. The sleep study monitors a variety of functions during sleep including sleep state, eye movement, muscle activity, heart rate, respiratory effort, airflow, and blood oxygen levels. This test is used both to diagnose sleep apnea and to determine its severity. Sometimes, treatment can be started during the first night in the sleep center.

The treatment of choice for obstructive sleep apnea is continuous positive airway pressure device (CPAP). CPAP is a mask that fits over the nose and/or mouth and gently blows air into the airway to help keep it open during sleep. This method of treatment is highly effective. Using the CPAP as recommended by your doctor is very important.

Second-line methods of treating sleep apnea include dental appliances, which reposition the lower jaw and tongue, and upper airway surgery to remove tissue in the airway. In general, these approaches are most helpful for mild disease or heavy snoring.

Lifestyle changes are effective ways of mitigating symptoms of sleep apnea. Here are some tips that may help reduce apnea severity:

- **Lose weight.** If you are overweight, this is the most important action you can take to cure your sleep apnea (CPAP only treats it; weight loss can cure it in the overweight person).

- **Avoid alcohol.** It causes frequent nighttime awakenings and makes the upper airway breathing muscles relax.

- **Quit smoking.** Cigarette smoking worsens swelling in the upper airway, making apnea (and snoring) worse.

- **Lie on Your Side.** Some patients with mild sleep apnea or heavy snoring have fewer breathing problems when they are lying on their sides instead of their backs.

Coping

The most important part of treatment for people with OSA is using the CPAP whenever they sleep. The health benefits of this therapy can be enormous, but only if used correctly. If you are having problems adjusting your CPAP or you're experiencing side effects of wearing the appliance, talk to the doctor who prescribed it and ask for assistance.

Chapter 30

Smell and Taste Disorders

Chapter Contents

Section 30.1

Smell Disorders

Reprinted from "Smell Disorders," National Institute on Deafness
and Other Communication Disorders, National Institutes of Health,
NIH Publication No. 01-3231, March 2002.

Every year, thousands of people develop problems with their sense of smell. In fact, more than two hundred thousand people visit a physician each year for help with smell disorders or related problems. If you experience a problem with your sense of smell, call your doctor. This section explains smell and smell disorders.

Many people who have smell disorders also notice problems with their sense of taste. If you would like more information about your sense of taste, the following section on taste disorders may answer some of your questions.

How does our sense of smell work?

The sense of smell is part of our chemical sensing system, or the chemosenses. Sensory cells in our nose, mouth, and throat have a role in helping us interpret smells, as well as taste flavors. Microscopic molecules released by the substances around us (foods, flowers, etc.) stimulate these sensory cells. Once the cells detect the molecules they send messages to our brains, where we identify the smell.

Olfactory, or smell nerve cells, are stimulated by the odors around us—the fragrance of a gardenia or the smell of bread baking. These nerve cells are found in a small patch of tissue high inside the nose, and they connect directly to the brain. Our sense of smell is also influenced by something called the common chemical sense. This sense involves nerve endings in our eyes, nose, mouth, and throat, especially those on moist surfaces. Beyond smell and taste, these nerve endings help us sense the feelings stimulated by different substances, such as the eye-watering potency of an onion or the refreshing cool of peppermint.

It's a surprise to many people to learn that flavors are recognized mainly through the sense of smell. Along with texture, temperature, and the sensations from the common chemical sense, the perception of flavor comes from a combination of odors and taste. Without the olfactory cells, familiar flavors like coffee or oranges would be harder to distinguish.

What are the smell disorders?

People who experience smell disorders experience either a loss in their ability to smell or changes in the way they perceive odors. As for loss of the sense of smell, some people have hyposmia, which is when their ability to detect odor is reduced. Other people can't detect odor at all, which is called anosmia. As for changes in the perception of odors, some people notice that familiar odors become distorted. Or, an odor that usually smells pleasant instead smells foul. Still other people may perceive a smell that isn't present at all.

What causes smell disorders?

Smell disorders have many causes, some clearer than others. Most people who develop a smell disorder have recently experienced an illness or an injury. Common triggers are upper respiratory infections and head injuries.

Among other causes of smell disorders are polyps in the nasal cavities, sinus infections, hormonal disturbances, or dental problems. Exposure to certain chemicals, such as insecticides and solvents, and some medicines has also been associated with smell disorders. People with head and neck cancers who receive radiation treatment are also among those who experience problems with their sense of smell.

How are smell disorders diagnosed?

Doctors and scientists have developed tests to determine the extent and nature of a person's smell disorder. Tests are designed to measure the smallest amount of odor patients can detect as well as their accuracy in identifying different smells. In fact, an easily administered "scratch and sniff" test allows a person to scratch pieces of paper treated to release different odors, sniff them, and try to identify each odor from a list of possibilities. In this way, doctors can easily determine whether patients have hyposmia, anosmia, or another kind of smell disorder.

Are smell disorders serious?

Yes. Like all of our senses, our sense of smell plays an important part in our lives. The sense of smell often serves as a first warning signal, alerting us to the smoke of a fire or the odor of a natural gas leak and dangerous fumes. Perhaps more important is that our chemosenses are sometimes a signal of serious health problems. Obesity, diabetes, hypertension, malnutrition, Parkinson disease, Alzheimer disease, multiple sclerosis, and Korsakoff psychosis are all accompanied or signaled by chemosensory problems like smell disorders.

Can smell disorders be treated?

Yes. Some people experience relief from smell disorders. Since certain medications can cause a problem, adjusting or changing that medicine may ease its effect on the sense of smell. Others recover their ability to smell when the illness causing their olfactory problem resolves. For patients with nasal obstructions such as polyps, surgery can remove the obstructions and restore airflow. Not infrequently, people enjoy a spontaneous recovery because olfactory neurons may regenerate following damage.

What research is being done?

The National Institute on Deafness and Other Communication Disorders (NIDCD) supports basic and clinical investigations of chemosensory disorders at institutions across the nation. Some of these studies are conducted at several chemosensory research centers, where scientists are making advances that help them understand our olfactory system and may lead to new treatments for smell disorders.

Some of the most recent research into our sense of smell is also the most exciting. Though a complete understanding of the uniquely sophisticated olfactory system is still in progress, recent studies on how receptors recognize odors, together with new technology, have revealed some long-hidden secrets to how the olfactory system manages to detect and discriminate between the many chemical compounds that form odors. Besides uncovering the physical mechanisms our bodies use to accomplish the act of identifying smell, these findings are helping scientists view the system as a model for other molecular sensory systems in the body. Further, scientists are confident that they are now laying the foundation to understanding the finest details about our sense of smell—research that may help them understand how smell affects and interacts with other physiological processes.

Since scientists began studying the olfactory system, much has been discovered about how our chemosenses work, especially in how they're affected by aging. Like other senses in our bodies, our sense of smell can be greatly affected simply by our growing older. In fact, scientists have found that the sense of smell begins to decline after age sixty. Women at all ages are generally more accurate than men in identifying odors, although smoking can adversely affect that ability in both men and women.

Another area of discovery has been the olfactory system's reaction to different medications. Like our sense of taste, our sense of smell can be damaged by certain medicine. Surprisingly, other medications, especially those prescribed for allergies, have been associated with an improvement of the sense of smell. Scientists are working to find out why this is so and develop drugs that can be used specifically to help restore the sense of smell to patients who've lost it. Also, smell cells (along with taste cells) are the only sensory cells that are regularly replaced throughout the lifespan. Scientists are examining these phenomena, which may provide ways to replace these and other damaged sensory and nerve cells.

NIDCD's research program goals for chemosensory sciences include the following:

- Promoting the regeneration of sensory and nerve cells

- Appreciating the effects of the environment (such as gasoline fumes, chemicals, and extremes of relative humidity and temperature) on smell and taste

- Preventing the effects of aging

- Preventing infectious agents and toxins from reaching the brain through the olfactory nerve

- Developing new diagnostic tests

- Understanding associations between chemosensory disorders and altered food intake in aging as well as in various chronic illnesses

- Improving treatment methods and rehabilitation strategies

What can I do to help myself?

The best thing you can do is see a doctor. Proper diagnosis by a trained professional, such as an otolaryngologist, is important. These physicians specialize in disorders of the head and neck, especially those related to the ear, nose, and throat. Diagnosis may lead to an effective treatment of the underlying cause of your smell disorder.

Many types of smell disorders are curable, and for those that are not, counseling is available to help patients cope.

Section 30.2

Taste Disorders

Reprinted from "Taste Disorders," National Institute on Deafness and Other Communication Disorders, National Institutes of Health, NIH Publication No. 01-3231A, March 2002.

If you experience a taste problem, it is important to remember that you are not alone. More than two hundred thousand people visit a physician for such a chemosensory problem each year. Many more taste disorders go unreported.

Many people who have taste disorders also notice problems with their sense of smell. If you would like more information about your sense of smell, the preceding section on smell disorders may answer some of your questions.

How does our sense of taste work?

Taste belongs to our chemical sensing system, or the chemosenses. The complex process of tasting begins when tiny molecules released by the substances around us stimulate special cells in the nose, mouth, or throat. These special sensory cells transmit messages through nerves to the brain, where specific tastes are identified.

Gustatory or taste cells react to food and beverages. These surface cells in the mouth send taste information to their nerve fibers. The taste cells are clustered in the taste buds of the mouth, tongue, and throat. Many of the small bumps that can be seen on the tongue contain taste buds.

Another chemosensory mechanism, called the common chemical sense, contributes to appreciation of food flavor. In this system, thousands of nerve endings—especially on the moist surfaces of the eyes, nose, mouth, and throat—give rise to sensations like the sting of ammonia, the coolness of menthol, and the irritation of chili peppers.

We can commonly identify at least five different taste sensations: sweet, sour, bitter, salty, and umami (the taste elicited by glutamate, which is found in chicken broth, meat extracts, and some cheeses). In the mouth, these tastes, along with texture, temperature, and the sensations from the common chemical sense, combine with odors to produce a perception of flavor. It is flavor that lets us know whether we are eating a pear or an apple. Some people are surprised to learn that flavors are recognized mainly through the sense of smell. If you hold your nose while eating chocolate, for example, you will have trouble identifying the chocolate flavor—even though you can distinguish the food's sweetness or bitterness. That is because the distinguishing characteristic of chocolate, for example, what differentiates it from caramel, is sensed largely by its odor.

What are the taste disorders?

The most common true taste complaint is phantom taste perceptions. Additionally, testing may demonstrate a reduced ability to taste sweet, sour, bitter, salty, and umami, which is called hypogeusia. Some people can detect no tastes, called ageusia. True taste loss is rare; perceived loss usually reflects a smell loss, which is often confused with a taste loss.

In other disorders of the chemical senses, the system may misread and/or distort an odor, a taste, or a flavor. Or a person may detect a foul taste from a substance that is normally pleasant tasting.

What causes taste disorders?

Some people are born with chemosensory disorders, but most develop them after an injury or illness. Upper respiratory infections are blamed for some chemosensory losses, and injury to the head can also cause taste problems.

Loss of taste can also be caused by exposure to certain chemicals such as insecticides and by some medicines. Taste disorders may result from oral health problems and some surgeries (e.g., third molar extraction and middle ear surgery). Many patients who receive radiation therapy for cancers of the head and neck develop chemosensory disorders.

How are taste disorders diagnosed?

The extent of a chemosensory disorder can be determined by measuring the lowest concentration of a chemical that a person can detect

401

or recognize. A patient may also be asked to compare the tastes of different chemicals or to note how the intensity of a taste grows when a chemical's concentration is increased.

Scientists have developed taste testing in which the patient responds to different chemical concentrations. This may involve a simple "sip, spit, and rinse" test, or chemicals may be applied directly to specific areas of the tongue.

Are taste disorders serious?

Yes. A person with a taste disorder is challenged not only by quality-of-life issues, but also deprived of an early warning system that most of us take for granted. Taste helps us detect spoiled food or beverages and, for some, the presence of food to which we're allergic. Perhaps more serious, loss of the sense of taste can also lead to depression and a reduced desire to eat.

Abnormalities in chemosensory function may accompany and even signal the existence of several diseases or unhealthy conditions, including obesity, diabetes, hypertension, malnutrition, and some degenerative diseases of the nervous system such as Parkinson disease, Alzheimer disease, and Korsakoff psychosis.

Can taste disorders be treated?

Yes. If a certain medication is the cause of a taste disorder, stopping or changing the medicine may help eliminate the problem. Some patients, notably those with respiratory infections or allergies, regain their sense of taste when the illness resolves. Often the correction of a general medical problem can also correct the loss of taste. Occasionally, recovery of the chemosenses occurs spontaneously.

What research is being done?

The NIDCD supports basic and clinical investigations of chemosensory disorders at institutions across the nation. Some of these studies are conducted at several chemosensory research centers, where scientists work together to unravel the secrets of taste disorders.

Some of the most recent research on our sense of taste focuses on identifying the key receptors in our taste cells and how they work in order to form a more complete understanding of the gustatory system, particularly how the protein mechanisms in G-protein-coupled receptors work. Advances in this area may have great practical uses, such as the creation of medicines and artificial food products that allow older adults with taste disorders to enjoy food again. Future research may examine how tastes change in both humans and animals. Some of this research will focus on adaptive taste changes over long periods in different animal species, while other research will examine why we accept or have an aversion to different tastes. Beyond this, scientists feel future gustatory research may also investigate how taste affects various processing activities in the brain. Specifically, how taste interacts with memory, influences hormonal feedback systems, and its role in the eating decisions and behavior.

Already, remarkable progress has been made in establishing the nature of changes that occur in taste senses with age. It is now known that age takes a much greater toll on smell than on taste. Also, taste cells (along with smell cells) are the only sensory cells that are regularly replaced throughout a person's lifespan—taste cells usually last about ten days. Scientists are examining these phenomena, which may provide ways to replace damaged sensory and nerve cells.

What can I do to help myself?

Proper diagnosis by a trained professional, such as an otolaryngologist, is important. These physicians specialize in disorders of the head and neck, especially those related to the ear, nose, and throat. Diagnosis may lead to treatment of the underlying cause of the disorder. Many types of taste disorders are curable, and for those that are not, counseling is available to help patients cope.

Section 30.3

Statistics on Taste and Smell

Excerpted and reprinted from "Statistics on Taste" and "Statistics on Smell," National Institute on Deafness and Other Communication Disorders, National Institutes of Health, June 2004.

Statistics on Taste

- Approximately 25 percent of Americans are nontasters, 50 percent are medium tasters, and 25 percent are "supertasters."

- More than 200,000 people visit a physician for chemosensory problems such as taste disorders each year. Many more taste disorders go unreported.

- Some people are surprised to learn that flavors are recognized mainly through the sense of smell. If you hold your nose while eating chocolate, for example, you will have trouble identifying the chocolate flavor—even though you can distinguish the food's sweetness or bitterness. That is because the distinguishing characteristic of chocolate (what differentiates it from caramel, for example) is sensed largely by its odor.

- Taste cells (along with smell cells) are the only sensory cells that are regularly replaced throughout a person's lifespan. Taste cells usually last about ten days.

Statistics on Smell

- According to estimates based on reported research, 1 to 2 percent of the North American population below the age of sixty-five experience smell loss to a significant degree. Smell loss is much greater in older populations, with nearly half of individuals sixty-five to eighty years old seemingly experiencing smell loss and nearly three-quarters of those over the age of eighty experiencing such loss. Note: These are the best estimates available from studies using actual smell tests. Surveys asking about smell ability without the administration of tests are likely to underestimate smell loss, since many individuals are not aware of their dysfunction unless it is marked. This phenomenon has been noted not only in "normal" populations, but also in individuals diagnosed with disorders associated with smell disorders such as Alzheimer disease and idiopathic Parkinson disease.

- More than 200,000 people visit a physician each year for help with smell disorders or related problems.

- Women at all ages are generally more accurate than men in identifying odors, although smoking can adversely affect that ability in both men and women.

- Smell cells (along with taste cells) are the only sensory cells that are regularly replaced throughout a person's lifespan.

Part Five

Disorders of the
Throat and Vocal Cords

Chapter 31

Sore Throat

Chapter Contents

Section 31.1

What Causes a Sore Throat?

What causes sore throats?

Sore throats can be caused by many things. Viruses (like those that cause colds) can lead to a sore throat. Bacteria can also cause a sore throat, as can smoking, breathing polluted air, drinking alcohol, and hay fever and other allergies.

What is tonsillitis?

Tonsillitis means swelling of the tonsils (at the back of your mouth on each side of your throat). It can cause a sore throat and other symptoms. Signs of strep throat and tonsillitis are often alike. Tonsillitis is usually caused by bacteria, though sometimes a virus may be involved.

Symptoms of Tonsillitis or Strep Throat

- Sore throat
- Fever
- Headache
- Vomiting
- White patches in your throat or on your tonsils
- Pain when you swallow
- Swollen, red tonsils
- Sore glands in your jaw and throat

If I have tonsillitis, will I need a tonsillectomy?

Tonsillectomy is a surgery used to remove tonsils. Most people who have tonsillitis don't need a tonsillectomy. You might need a tonsillectomy if you get severe tonsillitis a lot or if your tonsils are too large and cause problems with your breathing. Your doctor can tell you if a tonsillectomy is needed.

What is strep throat?

Strep throat is caused by a type of bacteria called Streptococcus. The pain of strep throat often feels much like sore throats caused by other bacteria or by viruses. What's important and different about strep throat is that if it isn't treated it can sometimes result in rheumatic fever, which can damage the valves of the heart.

What is mononucleosis?

Mononucleosis (mono) is a viral infection caused by the Epstein-Barr virus. One of the main signs of mono is a sore throat that may last for one to four weeks. Other signs include swollen glands in your neck, armpits, and groin; fever and chills; headache; and feeling tired.

What tests may be used to find the cause of my sore throat?

Your doctor may do a rapid strep test, a throat culture, or both. A rapid strep test will give results fast—usually within about fifteen minutes. But the test won't tell if your sore throat is caused by a bacterium other than Streptococcus or if it's caused by a virus. A throat culture takes longer—about twenty-four hours—but it's more accurate. If your doctor thinks you may have mono, he or she will probably do a blood test.

What is the treatment for a sore throat caused by bacteria?

If your sore throat is caused by Streptococcus, your family doctor will probably prescribe penicillin, taken by mouth for ten days. Another antibiotic, called erythromycin, can be used if you're allergic to penicillin. If your sore throat is caused by a different bacteria, your doctor may prescribe another type of antibiotic.

What is the treatment for a sore throat caused by a virus?

Antibiotics don't work against viruses. Infections caused by viruses usually just have to run their course. Most symptoms caused by a cold-type virus go away in a week to ten days.

Symptoms caused by mono can last for four weeks or more. If you have mono, your doctor will probably suggest that you get plenty of rest and that you not exercise too hard. You can take acetaminophen (brand name: Tylenol), ibuprofen (brand names: Advil, Motrin, Nuprin) or naproxen (brand name: Aleve) for the headache and other aches.

What about a sore throat that's caused by allergies?

If a sore throat is a symptom of hay fever or another allergy, your doctor can help you figure out how to avoid the things that trigger your allergies. Or you may need to take medicine for your allergies.

How can I avoid catching or passing a sore throat?

The best ways to avoid catching or passing the viruses and bacteria that can lead to a sore throat are to wash your hands regularly, avoid touching your eyes or mouth, and cover your mouth when coughing or sneezing.

Easing the Pain of a Sore Throat

- Take acetaminophen, ibuprofen, or naproxen.
- Gargle with warm salt water (1 teaspoon of salt per glass of water).
- Suck on throat lozenges or hard candy.
- Suck on flavored frozen desserts (such as Popsicles).
- Use a humidifier in your bedroom or other rooms you spend lots of time in.
- Drink lots of liquids.

Section 31.2

Strep Throat

From "Pediatric Common Questions, Quick Answers," by Donna M. D'Alessandro, M.D., Lindsay Huth, B.A., and Susan Kinzer, M.P.H., revised October 2004. © Donna M. D'Alessandro, M.D. All rights reserved. For additional information, visit http://www.virtualpediatrichospital.org.

What causes strep throat?

Strep throat is a throat infection caused by bacteria called streptococcus.

Who can get strep throat?

- Getting strep throat is common for school-age children and children in daycare.
- Strep throat is common in the winter months.

What are the symptoms of strep throat?

- Strep throat can cause a sore throat or a tickling feeling in the throat.
- Strep throat can cause pain when swallowing and bad breath.
- Strep throat can cause a fever, headache, earache, or stomachache.
- The tonsils may be swollen and bright red. Neck glands could be swollen.
- There might be yellow or white spots of pus on the back of the throat.
- The roof of the mouth may be red or have red spots.
- Infants may have a runny nose, crusty nose, and little appetite.

Is strep throat contagious?

- Yes. Strep throat is contagious.

413

- Strep bacteria are spread through coughing, sneezing, and direct contact.

- Children with strep throat are contagious until twenty-four hours after their first dose of antibiotics.

How is strep throat treated?

- The doctor will take a throat culture, a painless swab of the throat, to see if your child has strep.

- Test results will come back in one or two days.

- If the doctor uses a rapid strep test, it will take about ten minutes to get results.

- Strep throat is treated with antibiotics (usually penicillin) taken by shot or mouth.

- Antibiotics taken by mouth have to be taken for a full ten days to clear the infection.

- Acetaminophen (such as Tylenol, Panadol, or Liquiprin) or Ibuprofen can be given to ease aches, pain, and fever.

- Throat lozenges, hard candy, cool drinks, and ice cream can help ease throat pain.

- Your child should drink lots of fluids. Avoid acidic juices (orange juice) and spicy food.

- Older children can drink tea with honey or gargle warm salt water (one teaspoon of table salt in one cup water) to ease throat pain.

- A cool mist humidifier or a warm, damp towel can help throat pain and swollen glands.

How long does strep throat last?

- When strep throat is treated, pain lasts one to three days.

- Children can return to school or daycare twenty-four hours after the start of antibiotic treatment and if their temperature and energy are normal.

Can strep throat be prevented?

- You can prevent the spread of infection by washing dishes and glasses in hot soapy water.

- Wash your hands often, especially after caring for the sick person.
- Avoid close contact with the infected person.

When should I call the doctor?

- Go to the emergency room if your child has a hard time breathing or swallowing, or keeps drooling.
- Call the doctor if your child has a fever over 104 degrees F (or 40 degrees C) or a fever that lasts for many days.
- Call the doctor if your child can't open her mouth or drink liquids.
- Call the doctor if your child has joint pain or is very weak.
- Call the doctor if your child has a rash, earache, or glands that are swollen, red, or tender.

Quick Answers

- Strep throat is a throat infection caused by bacteria.
- Getting strep throat is common for school-age children and children in daycare.
- Strep throat can cause a sore throat, fever, headache, earache, and pain when swallowing.
- Strep bacteria are spread through coughing, sneezing, and direct contact.
- Strep throat is treated with antibiotics.
- Children can return to school or daycare twenty-four hours after the start of antibiotic treatment.
- One way to prevent the spread of infection is to wash hands and dishes with hot soapy water.
- Call the doctor if your child has a rash, earache, or glands that are swollen, red, or tender.

References

Casano, PJ. M.D. *Sore Throats: Causes and Cures*. American Academy of Otolaryngology: Head and Neck Surgery Public Service Brochure.

(cited 2001 July 27). Available from: URL: http://www.sinuscarecenter .com/throaaao.html

Marsocci SM, M.D., Pichichero ME M.D. Streptococcal Pharyngitis (Strep Throat, Strep Tonsillitis). *Pediatric Infectious Diseases Journal* 1992–2001 (cited 2001 July 27). URL: http://www.vh.org/Patients/ IHB/Peds/Infectious/Strep.html

Rutherford K M.D. KidsHealth. Strep Throat (Group A Streptococci Infections). 2001 May (cited 2001 July 27). URL: http://www.kids health.org/pageManager.jsp?dn=KidsHealth&lic=1&ps=107&cat _id=&article_set=941

Section 31.3

Strep Throat Test

Also known as: Throat culture, rapid strep test

Formal name: Group A streptococcus, Group A beta hemolytic streptococcus

Related tests: Influenza, blood cultures

Why get tested?

To determine if a sore throat (pharyngitis) is caused by a Group A streptococcal bacteria ("strep throat")

When to get tested?

If you have a sore throat and fever and your doctor thinks it may be due to a bacterial respiratory infection

Sample required?

A swab rubbed against your tonsils and the back of your throat.

What is being tested?

This test identifies the presence of the bacteria *Streptococcus pyogenes*, also known as group A beta-hemolytic streptococcus and group A streptococcus. Group A streptococci can infect the back of the throat (the pharynx) and cause "strep throat," the most common bacterial cause of pharyngitis (sore throat).

How is the sample collected for testing?

A doctor, nurse, or other healthcare professional uses a tongue depressor to hold down your tongue and then inserts a special swab into your mouth and rubs it against the back of your throat and tonsils. The swab may be used to do a rapid strep test in a doctor's office or clinic or it may be sent to a laboratory, where a rapid strep test and/or a throat culture is performed.

How is it used?

This test is used to determine whether a patient has pharyngitis that is due to a group A streptococcal infection.

Most sore throats are caused by a virus and may resolve without therapy within a few days. The bacteria group A streptococci cause pharyngitis in 5 to 15 percent of adults and 15 to 30 percent of children. It is important that these strep infections be promptly identified and treated with antibiotics. Strep throat is contagious and can spread to close contacts. If the infection is not treated, secondary complications may develop, such as rheumatic fever (which can damage the heart) and glomerulonephritis (which affects the kidneys). Because streptococcal infections are routinely diagnosed and treated, these complications have become much more rare in the United States, but they do still occur.

A rapid strep test and/or a throat culture can be used to diagnose group A streptococci as the cause of your sore throat and allow your doctor to prescribe the proper antibiotics for treatment.

If results of the rapid test, which takes ten to twenty minutes, are positive, further testing is not needed and your doctor will start you on antibiotic therapy. If the rapid strep test is negative, a culture to grow the bacteria should be done to confirm the results. A throat culture is more accurate than the rapid strep test, but it may take several days to get results.

When is it ordered?

Your doctor will typically order this test if you have a sore throat and a fever that might be due to an upper respiratory infection. Symptoms vary and may include:

- sore throat;
- fever;
- headache;
- tonsils that may appear red with white or yellow spots at the back of the throat;
- a swollen, tender neck;
- weakness; and
- loss of appetite.

What does the test result mean?

A positive throat culture or rapid test indicates the presence of group A streptococci, the bacteria that cause strep throat. A negative rapid test indicates that you probably do not have strep throat, but the possibility cannot be ruled out until the laboratory performs a culture. Note that recent antibiotic therapy or gargling with some mouthwashes may affect test results.

Is there anything else I should know?

Strep throat spreads from person-to-person through contact with respiratory secretions that contain the streptococcal bacteria. During flu season, the early symptoms of influenza (fever, chills, headache, sore throat, muscle pain) may mimic strep throat. Rarely, these same symptoms may be due to a more serious acute illness, septicemia (bacteria growing in the blood). To differentiate between strep and the flu, a rapid strep test and a rapid influenza test may both be done. If both tests are negative and the clinical signs warrant it, a complete blood count (CBC) may be ordered to evaluate the patient's white blood cells and blood cultures may be drawn to rule out sepsis. The treatment for each of these infections differs greatly and making a prompt diagnosis is imperative to starting the correct therapy.

Most patients with streptococcal pharyngitis will eventually recover without antibiotic treatment but will be contagious for a longer period of time and are at a greater risk of developing secondary complications.

Strep throat is most common in five- to ten- year olds. Up to 20 percent of school children may be "carriers," persons who have the bacteria but who have no symptoms. Carriers can still spread the infection to others.

Section 31.4

Epiglottitis

Epiglottitis is the swelling of the epiglottis. The epiglottis is a tongue-like flap of tissue that covers the opening to the trachea (windpipe). Epiglottitis is dangerous because a swollen epiglottis can make it difficult or impossible to breathe. See Figure 31.1.

Epiglottitis may occur any time of the year, but it often happens in winter and spring. Children of all ages as well as adults can be affected. A bacteria called Hib is often the cause of this infection. Thanks to the Hib vaccine, epiglottitis has become very uncommon.

What happens?

You may have noticed your child showing one or more of these signs and symptoms before coming to the hospital:

- a fever over 102°F
- trouble breathing
- wanting to sit up rather than lie down
- a very sore throat
- a soft voice
- drooling
- refusing to eat

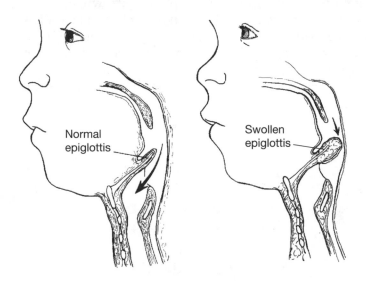

Figure 31.1. *Normal and swollen epiglottis (© 2006 Intermountain Healthcare, Inc. All Rights Reserved).*

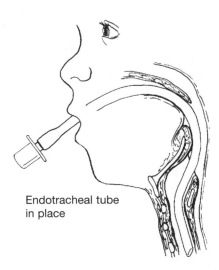

Figure 31.2. *Intubation to treat epiglottitis (© 2006 Intermountain Healthcare, Inc. All Rights Reserved).*

How do you treat epiglottitis?

Treatment will be immediate. The goal is to keep your child calm and open the airway from the mouth to the lungs. To do this, a tube will be placed through your child's mouth into the windpipe. This procedure is called intubation. See Figure 31.2.

Your child will be admitted to the Pediatric Intensive Care Unit (PICU) for continued treatment.

To fight the infection and keep your child calm, antibiotics and other medicines will be given until the swelling goes away. The swelling is usually gone in twelve to seventy-two hours.

Antibiotics are given for ten days. They may be given by IV (through a tiny tube into the vein). Once the swelling has gone down and the breathing tube is removed, the antibiotics can be taken by mouth. Your child will then be moved out of PICU to a different unit or home to finish the antibiotics. It is very important that all the antibiotics are taken.

How do you prevent epiglottitis?

Children of certain ages should receive the HIB vaccine to lessen the chance of getting epiglottitis. See your doctor to know whether your child needs this vaccine. Family members may need preventive treatment as well. Please talk about this with your family doctor.

Chapter 32

Tonsils and Adenoids

Chapter Contents

Section 32.1

Tonsils and Tonsillectomies

This information was provided by KidsHealth, one of the largest resources online for medically reviewed health information written for parents, kids, and teens. For more articles like this one, visit www.KidsHealth.org, or www.TeensHealth.org. © 2004 The Nemours Center for Children's Health Media, a division of The Nemours Foundation.

Everybody's heard of tonsils. But not everyone knows what tonsils do or why they may need to be removed. Knowing the facts can help alleviate the fears of both parents and children facing a tonsillectomy.

What are tonsils and tonsillitis?

Tonsils are glandular tissue located on both sides of the throat. The tonsils trap bacteria and viruses entering through the throat and produce antibodies to help fight infections.

Tonsillitis occurs when tonsils become infected and swell. If you look down your child's throat with a flashlight, the tonsils may be red and swollen or have a white or yellow coating on them. Other symptoms of tonsillitis may include:

- sore throat;
- pain or discomfort when swallowing;
- fever;
- raspy voice;
- swollen glands (lymph nodes) in the neck.

But enlarged or swollen tonsils are normal for many children. Don't rely on your own guesses when it comes to your child's health—you may not be able to judge whether your child's tonsils are infected. If you suspect tonsillitis, contact your child's doctor. Recurrent sore throats and infections should also be evaluated by your child's doctor, who may order a throat culture to check for strep throat.

What are tonsillectomies and what do they involve?

Because of success with antibiotics, surgery is no longer the standard treatment for tonsillitis that it was years ago. Left alone, your child's enlarged tonsils may eventually shrink on their own. However, your child's doctor may suggest removal of the tonsils, called a tonsillectomy, if your child has one or more of the following:

- persistent or recurrent tonsillitis
- recurrent sore throats
- recurrent throat infections
- swollen tonsils that make it hard to breath
- difficulty swallowing
- obstructive sleep apnea (a condition in which your child may stop breathing for a few seconds at a time during sleep because enlarged tonsils are partially blocking the airway)

Surgery, no matter how common or simple the procedure, is often frightening for both child and parent. You can help prepare your child for surgery by talking about what to expect. During the tonsillectomy:

- your child will receive general anesthesia. This means the surgery will be performed in an operating room so that an anesthesiologist can monitor your child.
- your child will be asleep for about twenty minutes.
- the surgeon can get to the tonsils through your child's open mouth—there's no need to cut your child's skin.
- the surgeon removes the tonsils with a series of incisions and then cauterizes (or seals) the blood vessels.

Your child will wake up in the recovery area. In most cases, the total time in the hospital is five to ten hours. However, children who have trouble breathing or show signs of bleeding will return immediately to the operating room. And kids under three years of age and kids with chronic disease, such as seizure disorders or cerebral palsy, will usually stay overnight for observation.

The typical recuperation after a tonsillectomy often involves a week or more of pain and discomfort due to the exposure of the throat muscles after the tonsils are removed. This can impact your child's ability to eat and drink and return to normal activities.

There is also a variation on traditional tonsillectomy techniques called intracapsular tonsillectomy. This procedure involves the controlled removal of all obstructing tonsil tissue—however, a small layer of tonsil tissue is purposely left in place to protect the underlying throat muscles. As a result, the recovery is much faster because most children experience less pain, don't need to use as much strong narcotic pain medications, and are more willing to eat and drink.

Since the residual tonsil tissue remains, there is a very slight chance that it can re-enlarge or become infected and require more tonsil surgery. This risk is small and occurs in less than 1 percent of children undergoing this procedure.

Section 32.2

Adenoids and Adenoidectomies

This information was provided by KidsHealth, one of the largest resources online for medically reviewed health information written for parents, kids, and teens. For more articles like this one, visit www.KidsHealth.org, or www.TeensHealth.org. © 2003 The Nemours Center for Children's Health Media, a division of The Nemours Foundation.

Adenoids and tonsils are often talked about together. But while they both work to help your body stay healthy, your adenoids and tonsils are actually separate things. So, just what are adenoids? What are they for? And why do kids sometimes have to get their adenoids removed?

What Are Adenoids?

The adenoids are lumpy clusters of spongy tissue that sit in the back of the nose above the roof the mouth. They sit high on each side of the throat behind the nose and the roof of the mouth. Adenoids get bigger after a kid is born and usually stop growing by the time a kid is between the ages of three and seven. Although you can easily see your tonsils by standing in front of a mirror and opening your mouth wide, you can't see your adenoids this way. A doctor has to use a small mirror or a special scope to get a peek at your adenoids. Sometimes a doctor may want you to get an x-ray of the adenoid area.

What Do Adenoids Do?

Like tonsils, adenoids help keep your body healthy by trapping harmful bacteria and viruses that you inhale. Adenoids also contain cells that make antibodies to help your body fight infections.

The infection-fighting job of adenoids happens in the first few years of a kid's life, a job that grows less important as you get older and your body develops other ways to fight germs. Some doctors believe that adenoids may not be important at all after kids reach their third birthday. In fact, adenoids usually shrink after about age five, and by the teenage years they often practically disappear.

When Adenoids Swell

Because adenoids trap germs that enter a kid's body, adenoid tissue sometimes temporarily swells as it tries to fight off an infection. Although adenoids may eventually return to their normal size without medical treatment, they often don't. Adenoids can even get so walloped by a bacterial invasion that they become infected themselves.

Swollen or enlarged adenoids are common. And often, if a kid's adenoids get infected or swollen, so do her tonsils. Your adenoids may be swollen or constantly infected if:

- you have a hard time breathing, or can breathe only through your mouth;
- your nose sounds "blocked," or like someone's pinching it when you talk;
- your breathing is noisy or "rattly" during the day;
- you snore a lot at night, or stop breathing for a few seconds when you're asleep;
- you have a hard time swallowing;
- you have a sore throat;
- you have swollen glands in your neck;
- you are having ear problems, or need a second or third set of ear tubes;
- you are having frequent sinus infections.

When infected adenoids swell, sometimes it's hard for a kid to hear things, sort of the way it sounds if you cup your hands over your ears. Sometimes adenoids can swell so much that they even affect the way teeth grow because the person is always keeping her mouth open (and teeth apart) to breathe.

What Will the Doctor Do?

Once upon a time, most doctors quickly recommended removing a kid's adenoids and tonsils when they became enlarged. Not anymore. Enlarged adenoids are actually normal for some kids. And because problems caused by adenoids usually go away by the teenage years, doctors don't like to take them out unless they absolutely have to.

If you have some of the symptoms of swollen adenoids, your mom or dad will probably take you to the doctor for a checkup. The doctor will ask you how things feel in your ears, nose, and throat, and then take a look at these parts. Your doctor will listen to your breathing by using a stethoscope. He or she may also feel your neck near your jaw. To get a really close look at things, your doctor may even want to take one or more x-rays.

Your doctor may use a small mirror or a bendable light to look at your adenoids. If he or she suspects infection, your doctor may prescribe antibiotics for you to take by mouth, or maybe an injection of penicillin.

When Adenoids Come Out

If enlarged or infected adenoids keep bothering your health and medicine doesn't help stop them from coming back, your doctor may finally recommend removing your adenoids. Although adenoids can be taken out without the tonsils, if you are having tonsil problems, the tonsils may need to be removed at the same time. This is called a tonsillectomy and adenoidectomy. A tonsillectomy and adenoidectomy is the most common operation that kids have.

Getting adenoids removed is especially important when repeated infections lead to sinus and ear infections. Badly swollen adenoids can interfere with ear pressure and fluid movement and this can sometimes lead to hearing loss. Kids whose infected adenoids cause frequent earaches and fluid buildup are candidates for an adenoidectomy with ear tube surgery.

If you are scheduled for surgery, you'll go to an operating room to have your adenoids, and maybe your tonsils, removed. Adenoids are removed through the mouth. But don't worry, you'll be given a medicine that makes you sleep during the operation, and removing your adenoids will not make you look any different. The cut area will be left to heal naturally. There are no stitches to worry about. Because your throat will be sore for a few days after surgery, you'll probably prefer eating a lot of soft foods, like ice cream, pudding, and soups. But you can eat whatever you want.

About a week after surgery, everything should return to normal. There is a small chance any tissue that's left behind can swell, but it rarely causes new problems. The good news is, you won't talk like someone's pinching your nose!

Chapter 33

Laryngeal Problems

Chapter Contents

Section 33.1

Laryngitis

This Information is reprinted with permission from the University of Rochester Health Service Health Promotion Office, Rochester, New York. © 2004 University of Rochester.

What Is Laryngitis?

Laryngitis is an inflammation of your voice box (larynx) due to overuse, irritation, or respiratory infection. The larynx is a framework of cartilage, muscle, and mucous membrane that forms the entrance of your windpipe (trachea). Inside the larynx are your vocal cords—two folds of mucous membrane covering muscle and cartilage.

Normally, your vocal cords open and close smoothly, forming sounds through their movement and vibration. But when air escapes between the cords when it is not supposed to, your voice sounds breathy, raspy and hoarse. Your voice may sound higher or lower than normal. The sound may be due to a weak or slightly paralyzed vocal cord on one side; polyps, which are small, soft growths; or nodules, which are harder growths.

Signs and Symptoms of Laryngitis

Laryngitis often makes you feel the need to constantly clear your throat. Other signs and symptoms may include the following:

- Hoarseness
- Weak voice
- Tickling sensation and rawness of your throat
- Sore throat
- Swollen vocal cords
- Dry throat
- Dry cough

432

Common Causes

Laryngitis occurs in two forms: acute and chronic. Acute laryngitis occurs suddenly and does not last long.

Laryngitis is chronic if the hoarseness in your throat lasts for a long time.

Causes of acute laryngitis may include these events:

- **Illness:** Usually, a viral infection such as a cold or the flu (influenza) causes acute laryngitis. A bacterial infection also may be the cause.

- **Irritation:** Excessive talking or singing, allergies, and breathing substances such as tobacco smoke and certain chemicals also can cause acute laryngitis.

Causes of chronic laryngitis may include the following:

- **Constant irritation:** Heavy smoking or excessive drinking of alcohol may inflame your vocal cords. Smoking also may cause polyps—small, soft growths on the mucous membrane covering your vocal cords. Polyps may interfere with the normal movement of your vocal cords.

- **Repeated overuse:** Excessive and repeated talking or singing can cause contact ulcers or the growth of polyps or nodules on your vocal cords. Nodules differ from polyps in that nodules occur on the layer that covers the mucous membrane. Nodules are also more like calluses and not as soft as polyps.

- **Aging:** As you age, your vocal cords can lose tension. With less tension, the cords no longer vibrate as they did before.

- **Nerve damage:** Injury to or pressure on the nerves supplying muscles that move your vocal cords—such as a blow to your larynx during an accident—can cause vocal cord paralysis.

Risk Factors

The following factors place you at greater risk of developing laryngitis:

- Overusing your voice by speaking too much, speaking too loudly, shouting, or singing

433

- Having respiratory infections, such as a cold, influenza, bronchitis, or sinusitis

- Exposure to irritating substances, such as cigarette smoke, excessive alcohol, stomach acid, or workplace chemicals

When to Seek Medical Advice

You can manage most acute cases of hoarseness or laryngitis, including those caused by viral infections or occasional overuse, with self-care steps, such as resting your voice, drinking plenty of fluids, and sucking on lozenges. If hoarseness lasts for more than two weeks, schedule an appointment with your primary care provider.

Screening and Diagnosis

Your primary care provider (PCP) may ask you to describe your signs and symptoms, how long you have had them, and whether any overuse of your vocal cords such as singing or shouting may have irritated your vocal cords. Your PCP may also ask whether you smoke and whether any other health conditions such as a cold, influenza, or allergies may be causing vocal irritation.

In addition, your PCP may want to listen to your voice and to look at your vocal cords. Your PCP can visually examine your vocal cords in a procedure called laryngoscopy by using a light and a tiny mirror to look into the back of your throat.

Treatment

The treatment your provider may recommend will depend on the cause of the laryngitis.

- If you have a respiratory infection such as a cold, your doctor may take a throat culture. For a bacterial infection such as strep throat, your provider may prescribe antibiotics.

- If polyps are the cause of your hoarse voice, your provider may recommend outpatient surgery to remove them.

- For chronic hoarseness due to a loosening of your vocal cords, surgically tightening the cords or injecting human collagen, a fibrous material, may stiffen a relaxed cord and return its normal function.

- For chronic hoarseness associated with other conditions, such as heartburn, smoking, or alcoholism, managing the underlying condition can help improve voice quality.

- For treatment of vocal cord paralysis, the approach depends on the underlying cause. But treatment may include injection of collagen into the tissues adjacent to the vocal cords or thyroplasty— surgery to improve the voice by altering the cartilage of the larynx.

Prevention

These tips can help you prevent dryness or irritation to your vocal cords:

- Do not smoke and avoid secondhand smoke.

- Drink plenty of water.

- Limit alcohol and caffeine to prevent a dry throat.

- Avoid clearing your throat.

Self-Care

If you have laryngitis, the following self-care steps may relieve irritation and hoarseness:

- Moisten your throat.

- Keep the air's humidity level high throughout your living space.

- Use an ultrasonic humidifier in your bedroom at night.

- Try eating soft, easy-to-swallow foods.

Coping Skills

A hoarse or weak voice associated with a cold usually will go away after two or three days. The following suggestions can help reduce strain or overuse:

- Avoid talking or singing too loudly or for too long. If you need to speak before large groups, try to use a microphone or megaphone.

ı

ɹur voice when you can.

ɔice training if you are a singer or if your voice quality is
___ant.

* Avoid whispering, which puts even more strain on your voice than normal speech.

Section 33.2

Gastroesophageal Reflux Disease and Reflux Laryngitis

What is acid reflux disease and what are the symptoms?

Gastroesophageal reflux disease, or GERD, is the recurring movement of stomach acid from the stomach back up into the esophagus (Gaynor, 1991). Stomach acid in the esophagus may cause heartburn or even chest pain; however, not all individuals will experience heartburn, as the esophagus is capable of withstanding a certain amount of acid exposure. On the other hand, the throat and voice box are not meant to withstand any exposure to acid. If acid actually refluxes into the lungs, chronic cough and pulmonary conditions can result, such as pneumonia or bronchitis.

Acid reflux into the larynx and throat is often referred to as "laryngopharyngeal reflux," or LPR. Symptoms of acid reflux into the larynx may include laryngitis, hoarseness, sensation of a lump in the throat, post-nasal drip, chronic throat clearing, excessive throat mucous, sore throat, cough, laryngospasm (spasm of the throat), and/or throat pain (Gaynor, 1990). With particular regard to singers and professional voice users, other symptoms may include increased time necessary to achieve adequate vocal warm-up, restricted vocal tone placement, and decreased pitch range (Ross, Noordzji, & Woo, 1998).

How does acid reflux happen?

Understanding how acid reflux occurs is crucial in understanding how to avoid it. At the end of the esophagus is a tight muscle, known as the "lower esophageal sphincter," or LES. This muscle is intended to relax only as food passes from the esophagus into the stomach. Reflux can occur when the pressure or tightness of this muscle is decreased. Certain substances and behaviors are linked to the lowering of pressure of the LES. According to Gaynor (1991), diets high in fat and carbohydrates, alcohol consumption, and the use of tobacco products may all result in a susceptibility to reflux. Carminatives (peppermint and spearmint) may also decrease LES pressure; therefore, conservative use of mint-flavored gums and candies may be well advised for individuals with reflux.

In the work of Wong, Hanson, Waring, & Shaw (2000), acid reflux was often found to occur with belching or when lying down after meals. To avoid this risk, individuals suffering from acid reflux should avoid carbonated beverages, which lead to belching, and should avoid eating two hours before lying down. Individuals with acid reflux may also have delayed emptying of the stomach in the lower intestinal tract, leaving increased amounts of food in the stomach. The more food there is in the stomach, the more time will be needed to allow for gastric emptying, and the higher the potential for more acid to be refluxed (Gaynor, 1991). To address this, it is often recommended that one have several small meals throughout the day rather than three large meals.

Certain behaviors also linked to lowered LES pressure include increased intra-abdominal pressure and bending over, creating an increased possibility for reflux (Gaynor, 1991). Forceful abdominal breathing during singing and strenuous workouts (which often involve bending over) can each contribute to lowered LES pressure. Since certain types of breathing and stretching both contribute to positive vocal use, singers and professional speakers suffering from GERD might discuss with their physician the merits of taking antacids prior to performances and/or physical workouts to neutralize any acid that might be refluxed.

How does acid reflux affect my voice?

Acid reflux into the larynx occurs when acid travels the length of the esophagus and spills over into the larynx. Any acidic irritation to the larynx may result in a hoarse voice. As the vocal cords begin to swell from the acidic irritation, their normal vibration is disrupted.

Even small amounts of exposure to acid may be related to significant laryngeal damage.

This disruption in the vibratory behavior of the vocal cords will often produce a change in your singing or speaking voice. When a singer or speaker encounters an undesirable vocal sound, the first impulse is to compensate by unknowingly changing the way in which one is singing or speaking. If the negative vocal results of acid reflux are addressed by a compensatory change in vocal technique, functionally abusive vocal behaviors often develop and can exacerbate the original symptoms through excessive muscular tension or even contribute to the development of vocal cord pathologies. For more detailed information on compensatory vocal behaviors, see an article by Dr. Jamie Koufman and Dr. Peter Belafsky entitled "The Demise of Behavioral Voice Disorders."

Reflux of acid into the larynx can have a detrimental effect on the voice for several reasons, as mentioned above. One unusual phenomenon has been observed whereby irritation found only in the lower esophagus can stimulate abnormal muscular contractions in the larynx such as coughing or throat clearing via shared nerved impulses between the esophagus and the larynx (Gaynor, 1991; Shaw & Searl, 1997; Wong, Hanson, Waring, & Shaw, 2000). As a result, individuals with acid reflux may have a persistent cough in the absence of any direct contact between stomach acid and the larynx. Persistent coughing can lead to vocal cord lesions, which in turn will negatively affect vocal quality and performance.

Individuals reflux stomach acid as a result of several factors, including hiatus hernia (malfunction of the stomach valve), obesity (being overweight), and poor eating habits. Poor eating habits, which can make reflux worse, include night eating, overeating, and consuming food or drinks that promote stomach acid production, such as spicy, fatty, or fried foods, acidic foods (tomato sauce, orange juice), soda, coffee, tea, chocolate, mints, and alcohol. In addition, using tobacco products in any form promotes stomach acid production.

How can I reduce my risk of acid reflux?

To reduce the likelihood of reflux, and to improve your condition, you may adhere to the following guidelines:

1.   No eating or drinking within three hours of bedtime or lying down to rest. This includes lying down anytime, such as an afternoon nap. Individuals suffering from reflux may have delayed

emptying of the stomach in the lower intestinal tract, leaving increased amounts of food in the stomach. The more food there is in the stomach, the higher the potential for more acid to be refluxed (Gaynor, 1991). As a result, added time will be needed to allow for gastric emptying. If circumstances dictate that one must eat late, the lighter and lower in fat the food, the quicker the stomach will empty into the intestinal tract.

2. Avoid overeating. Overfilling the stomach increases the likelihood of reflux. It is better to eat several small meals each day than to eat one or two big meals.

3. Avoid intra-abdominal pressure. Avoid tight-fitting clothing, bending over, or straining after eating (especially working out and lifting weights).

4. Reduce your intake of foods that increase stomach acid production. These include fatty, fried, spicy, or acidic foods, chocolate, caffeine, carbonated beverages, peppermint/ spearmint, and alcohol.

5. Elevate the head of your bed. Place cinder blocks under the legs at the head of your bed. This will put the bed at an incline of at least five inches.

6. Lose weight. You should lose weight if you are overweight; excess weight puts pressure on gastric contents.

7. Stop the use of any tobacco products. Good for you all around.

8. Take your medication. You may be placed on a medication to control your acid production. It is important to take these medicines as instructed; however, it has been shown that the medications most commonly prescribed for acid reflux, called proton pump inhibitors, are most effective if taken thirty to sixty minutes prior to your most substantial meal (usually dinner).

9. Use over-the-counter antacids. Over-the-counter antacids may be appropriate, especially if you will be singing or eating close to bedtime. If you are advised to take antacids, chewable antacids such as Rolaids and Tums are not recommended because they do not neutralize enough stomach acid to be effective. You may add a medication called an H_2 blocker to your daily routine,

such as Zantac or Pepcid, before singing or exercising and before bed. You may also use liquid antacids such as Maalox, Mylanta, Gelusil, Amphojel, or Gaviscon. Take these as instructed.

10. Chew your gum! New research from Great Britain shows post-meal gum chewing appeared to reduce acid in the esophagus and quell heartburn symptoms among people with chronic reflux problems. Why does it work? Gum stimulates saliva production, which theoretically works to neutralize acid remaining in the larynx and esophagus.

11. Sleep on your left side. The esophagus enters the stomach on your right side. Sleeping on your left side may help to prevent any food remaining in your stomach from pressing on the opening to the esophagus, which could cause reflux.

In summary, acid reflux affects many voice users, some of whom may be unaware that the source of their vocal difficulty is medical and can be addressed with the options listed above. If you think you may suffer from acid reflux, there is no danger in following the behavioral and dietary guidelines above, but a visit to a qualified medical professional is the only means of securing an accurate diagnosis. Some physicians who do not specialize in voice disorders may be unaware of the relationship between acid reflux and hoarseness, and the symptoms of acid reflux may be easily attributed to other illnesses or poor vocal techniques. Be sure to question your medical professional to be certain that the possible diagnosis of acid reflux is not overlooked.

References

Gaynor, E.B. (1991). Otolaryngologic manifestations of gastroesophageal reflux. *American Journal of Gastroenterology*, 86(7): 801–8.

Gaynor, E.B. (2000). Laryngeal complications of GERD. *Journal of Clinical Gastroenterology*, 30(3 Suppl), S31–34.

Ross, J.A., Noordzji, J.P., & Woo, P. (1998). Voice disorders in patients with suspected laryngo-pharyngeal reflux disease. *Journal of Voice*, 12(1), 84–88.

Shaw, G.Y. & Searl, J.P. (1997). Laryngeal manifestations of gastroesophageal reflux before and after treatment with omeprazole. *Southern Medical Journal*, 90(11), 1115–22.

Wong, R.K., Hanson, D.G., Waring, P.J., & Shaw, G. (2000). ENT manifestations of gastroesophageal reflux. *American Journal of Gastroenterology*, 95(8 Suppl), S15–22.

Section 33.3

Laryngeal Papillomatosis

Reprinted from "Laryngeal Papillomatosis," National Institute on Deafness and Other Communication Disorders, National Institutes of Health, NIH Publication No. 99-4543, June 1999. Revised by David A. Cooke, M.D., on March 30, 2006.

Laryngeal papillomatosis is a disease consisting of tumors that grow inside the larynx (voice box), vocal cords, or air passages leading from the nose into the lungs (respiratory tract). It is a rare disease caused by the human papilloma virus (HPV). Although scientists are uncertain how people are infected with HPV, they have identified more than sixty types of HPVs. Tumors caused by HPVs, called papillomas, are often associated with two specific types of the virus (HPV 6 and HPV 11). They may vary in size and grow very quickly. Eventually, these tumors may block the airway passage and cause difficulty breathing.

Laryngeal papillomatosis affects infants and small children as well as adults. Between 60 and 80 percent of cases occur in children, usually before the age of three. Because the tumors grow quickly, young children with the disease may find it difficult to breathe when sleeping, or they may experience difficulty swallowing. Adults with laryngeal papillomatosis may experience hoarseness, chronic coughing, or breathing problems.

There are several tests to diagnose laryngeal papillomatosis. Two routine tests are indirect and direct laryngoscopy. An indirect laryngoscopy is done in an office by a speech-language pathologist or by a doctor. To examine the larynx for tumors, the doctor places a small mirror in the back of the throat and angles the mirror down toward the larynx. A direct laryngoscopy is performed in the operating room under general anesthesia.

This procedure is usually used with children or adults during lengthy examinations to minimize discomfort. It involves looking directly at the larynx. Direct laryngoscopy allows the doctor to view the vocal folds and other parts of the larynx under high magnification and take samples of unusual tissue lesions that may be in the larynx or other parts of the throat.

Treatment

Many forms of treatment have been used to remove laryngeal papillomas, including surgery, chemotherapy, and antibiotic therapy. Currently, traditional surgical removal of the tumors and laser surgery, are both used. Traditional scalpel blades as well as newer devices known as microdebridement tools can cut away the tumors. Carbon dioxide laser surgery uses intense laser light to vaporize the papillomas. A second type of laser, the 585 nm pulsed dye laser, is also used in a similar fashion.

Once they have been removed, these tumors have a tendency to return unpredictably. It is not uncommon for patients to require repeat surgery. With some patients, surgery may be required every few weeks in order to keep the breathing passage open, while others may require surgery only once a year. In the most extreme cases, where tumor growth is aggressive, a tracheotomy may be performed. A tracheotomy is a surgical procedure where an incision is made in the front of the patient's neck and a breathing tube (trach tube) is inserted through a hole, called a stoma, into the trachea (windpipe). Rather than breathing through the nose and mouth, the patient will now breathe through the trach tube. Although the trach tube keeps the breathing passage open, doctors try to remove it as soon as it is feasible. However, there may be some patients who may be required to keep a trach tube indefinitely in order to keep the breathing passage open. In addition, because the trach tube re-routes all or some of the exhaled air away from the vocal cords, the patient may find it difficult to speak. With the help of a voice specialist or speech-language pathologist the patient will need to relearn how to use the voice.

Research

Scientists have developed a new technique using photodynamic therapy (PDT). With PDT, a physician injects a special dye that is sensitive to bright light into the blood stream. This dye collects in tumors but not healthy tissue, and when the dye is activated by a bright light of a specific wavelength, the tumors that have absorbed the dye are destroyed. In addition to eliminating the tumors using PDT, scientists have found that tumor regrowth is decreased with this technique, even for patients with the most severe form of the disease.

PDT was first developed to kill certain tumors in humans. Although treatment was promising, results were inconsistent and the technique was soon abandoned. However, recent research shows that treating patients with laryngeal papillomatosis using PDT appears to control tumor growth. The development of newer forms of the dye has contributed to the resurgence of this promising form of treatment that may prevent patients from having multiple surgical procedures.

Several medications have been used successfully to treat laryngeal papillomatosis, and a number of studies are underway to better determine how they compare to surgical methods. Cidofovir, an antiviral medication, appears promising in some studies. Alpha-Interferon, a drug that alters response of the immune system, has also been successful, although its side effects can be troublesome. A newer medication derived from vegetables, indole-3-carbinol (I3C), has complex hormonal effects that discourage papilloma growth. Very good results have been seen in trials to date, and it is well tolerated. Heat shock protein E7 (HspE7), a genetically engineered protein, is another promising agent currently under study.

It is likely that these medications will be used as combination therapy with surgical or laser approaches to help reduce risk of tumor recurrences.

Chapter 34

Swallowing Problems

Chapter Contents

Section 34.1

Dysphagia

Reprinted from "Dysphagia," National Institute on Deafness and Other Communication Disorders, National Institutes of Health, NIH Publication No. 99-4307, October 1998. Reviewed by David A. Cooke, M.D., on March 30, 2006.

What is dysphagia?

People with dysphagia have difficulty swallowing and may also experience pain while swallowing. Some people may be completely unable to swallow or may have trouble swallowing liquids, foods, or

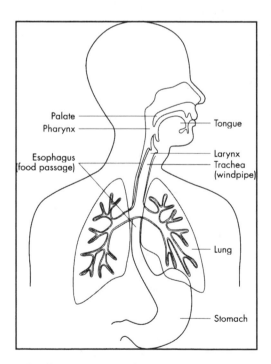

Figure 34.1. Profile showing location of pharynx, palate, esophagus, tongue, larynx, trachea, lungs, and stomach

saliva. Eating then becomes a challenge. Often, dysphagia makes it difficult to take in enough calories and fluids to nourish the body.

How do we swallow?

Swallowing is a complex process. Some fifty pairs of muscles and many nerves work to move food from the mouth to the stomach. This happens in three stages. First, the tongue moves the food around in the mouth for chewing. Chewing makes the food the right size to swallow and helps mix the food with saliva. Saliva softens and moistens the food to make swallowing easier. During this first stage, the tongue collects the prepared food or liquid, making it ready for swallowing.

The second stage begins when the tongue pushes the food or liquid to the back of the mouth, which triggers a swallowing reflex that passes the food through the pharynx (the canal that connects the mouth with the esophagus). During this stage, the larynx (voice box) closes tightly and breathing stops to prevent food or liquid from entering the lungs.

The third stage begins when food or liquid enters the esophagus, the canal that carries food and liquid to the stomach. This passage through the esophagus usually occurs in about three seconds, depending on the texture or consistency of the food.

How does dysphagia occur?

Dysphagia occurs when there is a problem with any part of the swallowing process. Weak tongue or cheek muscles may make it hard to move food around in the mouth for chewing. Food pieces that are too large for swallowing may enter the throat and block the passage of air.

Other problems include not being able to start the swallowing reflex (a stimulus that allows food and liquids to move safely through the pharynx) because of a stroke or other nervous system disorder. People with these kinds of problems are unable to begin the muscle movements that allow food to move from the mouth to the stomach. Another difficulty can occur when weak throat muscles cannot move all of the food toward the stomach. Bits of food can fall or be pulled into the windpipe (trachea), which may result in lung infection.

What are some problems caused by dysphagia?

Dysphagia can be serious. Someone who cannot swallow well may not be able to eat enough of the right foods to stay healthy or maintain an ideal weight.

Sometimes, when foods or liquids enter the windpipe of a person who has dysphagia, coughing or throat clearing cannot remove it. Food or liquid that stays in the windpipe may enter the lungs and create a chance for harmful bacteria to grow. A serious infection (aspiration pneumonia) can result.

Swallowing disorders may also include the development of a pocket outside the esophagus caused by weakness in the esophageal wall. This abnormal pocket traps some food being swallowed. While lying down or sleeping, a person with this problem may draw undigested food into the pharynx. The esophagus may be too narrow, causing food to stick. This food may prevent other food or even liquids from entering the stomach.

What causes dysphagia?

Dysphagia has many causes. Any condition that weakens or damages the muscles and nerves used for swallowing may cause dysphagia. For example, people with diseases of the nervous system, such as cerebral palsy or Parkinson disease, often have problems swallowing. Additionally, stroke or head injury may affect the coordination of the swallowing muscles or limit sensation in the mouth and throat. An infection or irritation can cause narrowing of the esophagus. People born with abnormalities of the swallowing mechanism may not be able to swallow normally. Infants who are born with a hole in the roof of the mouth (cleft palate) are unable to suck properly, which complicates nursing and drinking from a regular baby bottle.

In addition, cancer of the head, neck, or esophagus may cause swallowing problems. Sometimes the treatment for these types of cancers can cause dysphagia. Injuries of the head, neck, and chest may also create swallowing problems.

How is dysphagia treated?

There are different treatments for various types of dysphagia. First, doctors and speech-language pathologists who test for and treat swallowing disorders use a variety of tests that allow them to look at the parts of the swallowing mechanism. One test, called a fiber-optic laryngoscopy, allows the doctor to look down the throat with a lighted tube. Other tests, including video fluoroscopy, which takes videotapes of a patient swallowing, and ultrasound, which produces images of internal body organs, can painlessly take pictures of various stages of swallowing.

Once the cause of the dysphagia is found, surgery or medication may help. If treating the cause of the dysphagia does not help, the doctor may have the patient see a speech-language pathologist who is trained in testing and treating swallowing disorders. The speech-language pathologist will test the person's ability to eat and drink and may teach the person new ways to swallow.

Treatment may involve muscle exercises to strengthen weak facial muscles or to improve coordination. For others, treatment may involve learning to eat in a special way. For example, some people may have to eat with their head turned to one side or looking straight ahead. Preparing food in a certain way or avoiding certain foods may help other people. For instance, those who cannot swallow liquids may need to add special thickeners to their drinks. Other people may have to avoid hot or cold foods or drinks.

For some, however, consuming foods and liquids by mouth may no longer be possible. These individuals must use other methods to nourish their bodies. Usually this involves a feeding system, such as a feeding tube, that bypasses the part of the swallowing mechanism that is not working normally.

What research is being done on dysphagia?

Scientists are conducting research that will improve the ability of physicians and speech-language pathologists to evaluate and treat swallowing disorders. All aspects of the swallowing process are being studied in people of all ages, including those who do and do not have dysphagia. For example, scientists have found that there is great variation in tongue movement during swallowing. Knowing which tongue movements cause problems will help physicians and speech-language pathologists evaluate swallowing.

Research has also led to new, safe ways to study tongue and throat movements during the swallowing process. These methods will help physicians and speech pathologists safely reevaluate a patient's progress during treatment. Studies of treatment methods are helping scientists discover why some forms of treatment work with some people and not with others. For example, research has shown that, in most cases, a patient who has had a stroke should not drink with his or her head tipped back. Other research has shown that some patients with cancer who have had part or all of their tongue removed should drink with their head tipped back. This knowledge will help some patients avoid serious lung infections and help others avoid tube feedings.

Where can I get help?

If you have a swallowing problem, you may need to consult with an otolaryngologist (physician with special training in disorders of the ear, nose, and throat) or a speech-language pathologist trained in dysphagia. You may need to consult with a neurologist if a stroke or other neurologic disorder causes the swallowing problem. Other trained professionals who may provide treatment are occupational therapists and physical therapists.

Section 34.2

Achalasia

If you are like most people, you take your body for granted. As long as all is working well, you seldom think of it. One thing we all take for granted is the simple act of swallowing. You swallow your saliva. You swallow your food. You swallow fluids. Down they all go—while you pay attention to your busy day. You may swallow several times per minute—thousands of times a day, without ever thinking about it. What if every time you swallowed, it was an ordeal? You never knew if your food would go down—or come back up. Every time you ate, you were afraid. Eventually, you might quit eating out in public for fear of an attack. This is what happens to patients with achalasia, an uncommon motility disorder which affects swallowing.

How do we swallow?

To better understand achalasia, you need to learn how we normally swallow. The trick is to get the food to go down into the stomach and not regurgitate. Your esophagus, or food pipe, is not just a hollow lifeless tube. Rather, it is a made of several layers of muscle tissue that contract in a rhythmic fashion, like waves on a beach. These so-called peristaltic waves carry the food down to your stomach like a conveyor belt. That is why you can hang upside down and still eat a sandwich.

At the lower end of the esophagus is a one-way valve—named the lower esophageal sphincter, or LES. This valve is the guardian of the gate. It is normally tightly closed to prevent the backsplash of acidic stomach contents upward into your esophagus. When you swallow, the valve should relax and open briefly, allowing food to enter your stomach. It then snaps shut. When this valve is too weak, acid and food can reflux up into your esophagus, causing heartburn. This is a common problem, termed GERD, or gastroesophageal reflux disease.

What, if instead, the lower esophageal valve was too tight? When you try to swallow, it would not open completely and the food would not enter your stomach right away like it was supposed to do. The food would begin to accumulate in your lower esophagus. It might cause you to stop eating and even regurgitate undigested food. Not a pretty sight. Over time, the esophagus muscle would become stretched out and the esophagus might weaken. This is called aperistalsis. The walls of the esophagus no longer contract and push the food down into the stomach. The food would have to be propelled by gravity. When the esophageal wall muscles become weak and the valve below becomes too tight, this is called achalasia—a bad combination if swallowing is what you are trying to do. Doctors have known of this condition for over three hundred years, but it was first termed achalasia in 1927.

What causes achalasia?

Unfortunately, the cause of achalasia is not known. Biopsies have shown some damage to the nerves that control the esophagus and the LES. Why this happens to an individual is not known and cannot be predicted. It is not due to something one did or did not do. It is just a case of bad luck.

Who gets it?

Achalasia is more common in adults, but affects both sexes equally. Fortunately, it is quite uncommon, affecting only about one in ten thousand Americans. It is not inherited.

What are the symptoms?

Of course, the most frequent symptom is trouble with swallowing. The medical term for this symptom is dysphagia. This does not happen overnight, but gradually over a period of many months or years.

In fact, the average patient has symptoms for over two years before seeking medical attention. They complain about being slow eaters— always the last one to finish a meal, often consuming large amounts of fluid while eating. They may become full before the meal is over. Regurgitation of undigested food is quite common and it may even be found on the pillowcase in the morning. If food enters the lungs, it can cause severe coughing and even pneumonia. Repeated lung infections may lead to permanent lung injury. With such difficulty eating it is not unusual for these patients to lose considerable weight and become malnourished. Achalasia is not cancer, but untreated achalasia does increase the risk of squamous cell cancer of the esophagus about ten times above normal. It is important to treat this disease as early as possible, and aggressively.

How does the doctor know?

If you have trouble swallowing, your doctor may order several special tests to assess your swallowing function. These may include the following:

- **Barium esophagogram:** A simple x-ray of the esophagus, taken as you drink a barium milkshake. Barium shows up on x-ray so the x-ray doctor can see your esophagus in action. Sometimes, a simple chest x-ray will show a dilated esophagus and suggest this diagnosis. As the condition worsens, the esophagus dilates.

- **Esophageal manometry:** This important test is done by placing a thin catheter down the nose and into the esophagus. On the tip of the catheter is a pressure sensor that is connected to a computer. This allows measurement of strength and rhythm of esophageal contractions. Manometry also allows measurement of the pressure of the lower esophageal sphincter, both at rest and when you swallow. In patients with achalasia, manometry typically shows a weakened esophageal muscle and an overly tight LES with a high resting pressure that fails to relax with swallowing. There is also a spastic variant of this disease called vigorous achalasia, which can cause symptoms of chest pain and difficulty with swallowing.

- **Gastroscopy:** Many other conditions can cause difficulty with swallowing. Gastroscopy is a special "scope test" that is performed to rule out more common problems such as a ring of scar tissue, benign strictures, or cancer. This test is painlessly done under "twilight sleep" anesthesia and allows the doctor to directly examine the inside of the esophagus. A dilated esophagus with a tight LES is characteristic of achalasia.

What is the treatment?

Since there currently is no treatment to strengthen the dilated esophagus, treatment focuses on correcting the tight LES. Once the diagnosis has been confirmed, the patient has several options. The best treatment depends on the details of each individual case.

First, a trial of oral medications may be prescribed. These drugs are marketed to treat heart disease and high blood pressure, but seem to also temporarily relax the LES. Nitroglycerin, Isordil, Verapamil, and Nifedipine are a few of the drugs that have been successful in relaxing the LES, but have short-lived effectiveness. They may help in mild cases and are most helpful treating the chest pain seen in vigorous achalasia.

Botox is often tried, especially in patients who cannot tolerate surgery. Botox is a toxin produced by the bacterium Clostridium botulinum. It causes muscle paralysis and prevents spasm. Botox was originally introduced for the safe and effective treatment of muscle spasms. It was discovered that it is also useful in preventing spasm of the LES. It is injected directly into the LES muscle with a small needle during a gastroscopy examination, a painless outpatient procedure. This procedure is very safe. Botox does not paralyze the body as in food poisoning, or botulism. In the concentrations used, it only weakens the spot where it is injected—in this case the valve. Botox has not only been helpful, but has also been disappointing. The effect lasts only a few months and may become less effective with each additional treatment. It is also very expensive and you have to add the cost of the gastroscopy with each retreatment.

Forceful balloon dilation was the mainstay of treatment for achalasia for many years. In this procedure, a pneumatic balloon is passed down the esophagus, half above and half below the LES. The balloon is then rapidly inflated for about a minute. As the balloon expands, it forcefully stretches and weakens the LES. Forceful pneumatic dilatation can be very successful and may last for a decade or longer. The downside is that this balloon is much larger than the balloon dilators normally used to dilate an esophageal stricture or tight hiatal hernia. It has to be big enough to actually rip the tight LES valve and weaken it. As a consequence, this procedure is often quite painful and can even rupture the esophagus in about 5 percent of cases. This is a very serious complication that requires an emergency chest operation for repair.

The best way to permanently weaken an overly tight LES valve is to cut it. The procedure is called a surgical myotomy and has over a 90 percent success rate in alleviating the symptoms of achalasia. Surgery is not as successful in cases of vigorous achalasia. For many years, this has been performed through an open chest incision (Heller myotomy). In the past few years, there has been much interest in a laparoscopic technique which uses smaller incisions, allowing for a faster recovery and an earlier return to work. Most patients leave the hospital in just a few days and are able to return to work within two weeks.

Chapter 35

Voice and Vocal Cord Disorders

Chapter Contents

Section 35.1

Hoarseness

What is hoarseness?

Hoarseness is a general term that describes abnormal voice
changes. When hoarse, the voice may sound breathy, raspy, strained,
or there may be changes in volume (loudness) or pitch (how high or
low the voice is). The changes in sound are usually due to disorders
related to the vocal cords that are the sound-producing parts of the
voice box (larynx). While breathing, the vocal cords remain apart.
When speaking or singing, they come together, and as air leaves the
lungs, they vibrate, producing sound. Swelling or lumps on the vocal
cords prevent them from coming together properly and changes the
way the cords vibrate, which makes a change in the voice, altering
quality, volume, and pitch.

What are the causes of hoarseness?

Acute Laryngitis: There are many causes of hoarseness. Fortunately, most are not serious and tend to go away in a short period of
time. The most common cause is acute laryngitis, which usually occurs due to swelling from a common cold, upper respiratory tract viral
infection, or irritation caused by excessive voice use such as screaming at a sporting event or rock concert.

Vocal Nodules: More prolonged hoarseness is usually due to using your voice either too much, too loudly, or improperly over extended
periods of time. These habits can lead to vocal nodules (singers' nodes),
which are callous-like growths, or may lead to polyps of the vocal cords
(more extensive swelling). Both of these conditions are benign. Vocal
nodules are common in children and adults who raise their voice in
work or play.

Gastroesophageal Reflux: A common cause of hoarseness is gastroesophageal reflux, when stomach acid comes up the swallowing tube (esophagus) and irritates the vocal cords. Many patients with reflux-related changes of voice do not have symptoms of heartburn. Usually, the voice is worse in the morning and improves during the day. These people may have a sensation of a lump in their throat, mucus sticking in their throat, or an excessive desire to clear their throat.

Smoking: Smoking is another cause of hoarseness. Since smoking is the major cause of throat cancer, if smokers are hoarse, they should see an otolaryngologist.

Other Causes: Many unusual causes for hoarseness include allergies, thyroid problems, neurological disorders, trauma to the voice box, and occasionally, the normal menstrual cycle.

Who can treat my hoarseness?

Hoarseness due to a cold or flu may be evaluated by family physicians, pediatricians, and internists (who have learned how to examine the larynx). When hoarseness lasts longer than two weeks or has no obvious cause it should be evaluated by an otolaryngologist—head and neck surgeon (ear, nose, and throat doctor). Problems with the voice are best managed by a team of professionals who know and understand how the voice functions. These professionals are otolaryngologist—head and neck surgeons, speech/language pathologists, and teachers of singing, acting, or public speaking. Voice disorders have many different characteristics that may give professionals a clue to the cause.

How is hoarseness evaluated?

An otolaryngologist will obtain a thorough history of the hoarseness and your general health. Your doctor will usually look at the vocal cords with a mirror placed in the back of your throat, or a very small, lighted flexible tube (fiberoptic scope) may be passed through your nose in order to view your vocal cords. Videotaping the examination or using stroboscopy (slow motion assessment) may also help with the analysis.

These procedures are not uncomfortable and are well tolerated by most patients. In some cases, special tests (known as acoustic analysis) designed to evaluate the voice, may be recommended. These measure voice irregularities, how the voice sounds, airflow, and other characteristics that are helpful in establishing a diagnosis and guiding treatment.

When should I see an otolaryngologist (ENT doctor)?

- Hoarseness lasting longer than two weeks, especially if you smoke
- Pain not from a cold or flu
- Coughing up blood
- Difficulty swallowing
- Lump in the neck
- Loss or severe change in voice lasting longer than a few days

How are vocal disorders treated?

The treatment of hoarseness depends on the cause. Most hoarseness can be treated by simply resting the voice or modifying how it is used. The otolaryngologist may make some recommendations about voice use behavior, refer the patient to other voice team members, and in some instances recommend surgery if a lesion, such as a polyp, is identified. Avoidance of smoking or exposure to secondhand smoke (passive smoking) is recommended to all patients. Drinking fluids and possibly using medications to thin the mucus are also helpful.

Specialists in speech/language pathology (voice therapists) are trained to assist patients in behavior modification that may help eliminate some voice disorders. Patients who have developed bad habits, such as smoking or overuse of their voice by yelling and screaming, benefit most from this conservative approach. The speech/language pathologist may teach patients to alter their method of speech production to improve the sound of the voice and to resolve problems, such as vocal nodules. When a patients' problem is specifically related to singing, a singing teacher may help improve the patients' singing techniques.

What can I do to prevent and treat mild hoarseness?

- If you smoke, quit.
- Avoid agents that dehydrate the body, such as alcohol and caffeine.

- Avoid secondhand smoke.

- Drink plenty of water.

- Humidify your home.

- Watch your diet—avoid spicy foods.

- Try not to use your voice too long or too loudly.

- Use a microphone if possible in situations where you need to project your voice.

- Seek professional voice training.

- Avoid speaking or singing when your voice is injured or hoarse.

Section 35.2

Spasmodic Dysphonia

What is spasmodic dysphonia?

Spasmodic dysphonia (SD), a focal form of dystonia, is a neurological voice disorder that involves involuntary "spasms" of the vocal cords causing interruptions of speech and affecting the voice quality.

Is spasmodic dysphonia a form of dystonia?

Yes, spasmodic dysphonia is a focal form of dystonia. Dystonia is the general neurological term for a variety of problems characterized by excessive contraction of muscles with associated abnormal movements and postures. Other focal dystonias include blepharospasm (involving the eyelids), oromandibular dystonia, (involving the jaw and tongue), cervical dystonia or spasmodic torticollis (involving the neck), and writer's cramp (involving the hand). These forms of dystonia may appear in combination with spasmodic dysphonia.

459

Are there different types of spasmodic dysphonia?

The two types of recognized spasmodic dysphonia are adductor spasmodic dysphonia and abductor spasmodic dysphonia. Adductor SD causes an intermittent excessive closing of the vocal folds during vowel sounds in speech; while in abductor SD, there is a prolonged vocal-fold opening during voiceless consonants. The control problems of the vocal cords result in different speech symptoms in the two types of disorder. There are three subtypes of SD which have been identified by clinicians. One is a combination of adductor and abductor symptoms in which an individual may demonstrate both types of spasms as he/she speaks. In a second subtype, SD symptoms are accompanied by a voice tremor. A third subtype involves a primary voice tremor that is so severe the patient experiences adductor voice stoppages during the tremor.

What causes spasmodic dysphonia?

The cause of spasmodic dysphonia is unknown. The general medical consensus is that SD is a central nervous system disorder and a focal form of dystonia. Dystonia is the general neurological term for a variety of problems characterized by excessive contraction of muscles with associated abnormal movements and postures. Dystonia disorders are thought to originate in the area of the brain called the basal ganglia, which is the area that helps coordinate movements of the muscles throughout the body.

Who gets spasmodic dysphonia?

Spasmodic dysphonia does not discriminate. Anyone, regardless of race, age, or ethnicity, can manifest symptoms of SD. It is estimated that fifty thousand persons in North America are affected by SD, but this number may be higher due to ongoing misdiagnosis or undiagnosed cases of the disorder.

How is spasmodic dysphonia diagnosed?

Spasmodic dysphonia is reported to be one of the most frequently misdiagnosed conditions in speech-language pathology. Because there is no definitive test for SD, the diagnosis rests on the presence of characteristic clinical symptoms and signs in the absence of other conditions that may mimic spasmodic dysphonia.

Is there a cure for spasmodic dysphonia?

At this time, there is no cure for SD, but treatments are available. Research continues to better understand the cause(s) of SD.

Treatment

Are oral medications used in the treatment of spasmodic dysphonia?

Oral medications provide little relief in the symptoms of spasmodic dysphonia, but if other forms of dystonia are present, medications may help relieve those related symptoms. There are several possible categories of medications used in the treatment of dystonia including anticholinergics, benzodiazepines, and baclofen. The treatment of spasmodic dysphonia must be tailored to the individual patient.

Are botulinum toxin injections a safe and effective treatment?

Yes. Botulinum toxin, a biological product, is injected into specific muscles where it acts to reduce the involuntary contractions that cause the symptoms of spasmodic dysphonia. The injections weaken muscle activity sufficiently to reduce a spasm but not enough to cause paralysis. Local injections of botulinum toxin (BTX) into the vocal cord muscles have proven to be the most effective treatment for spasmodic dysphonia. The treatment weakens the vocal muscles so that spasms are greatly diminished and speech is greatly improved. The treatment can also reduce the breathiness and help decrease the effort required to speak.

What is the role of surgery in the treatment of spasmodic dysphonia?

Surgery for spasmodic dysphonia has recently been re-examined as a form of treatment for people for whom botulinum toxin injections are no longer providing relief of symptoms. Selective laryngeal adductor denervation-reinnervation surgery involves cutting the nerve to the affected vocal cord and re-innervating the muscle with another muscle to prevent muscle atrophy. This surgery is done almost exclusively by Dr. Gerald Berke at the University of California at Los Angeles with promising preliminary results. For some people who have

461

undergone the surgery, symptoms have returned and follow-up with botulinum toxin injections was needed. Studies are ongoing to determine the effectiveness of this surgery.

What role does speech therapy play in the treatment of spasmodic dysphonia?

General voice relaxation techniques and speech therapy may play an adjunct role in the treatment of spasmodic dysphonia. These include reducing one's vocal effort, loudness, intonation, and rate of utterance while increasing pause time between phrases. These techniques can only be reinforced and adapted if they do not intrude on the vocal naturalness.

How are complementary therapies helpful?

Traditional western practices have long been effective in diagnosing problems and assigning treatments but may do little to address how patients live on a daily basis. Medical fields are slowly incorporating a wider range of knowledge to include treatments outside of the traditional scope to better assist patients and to treat the "whole person"—mind, body, and spirit. Complementary therapy may play an active role in your treatment of SD, and it is intended to be used in conjunction with traditional therapies. To avoid any interactions and potential problems, it is important to have open communication among all physicians and practitioners who are working with you.

My insurance company won't cover my BOTOX® injection. What can I do?

Allergan, the manufacturer of BOTOX® (Botulinum Toxin Type A) Purified Neurotoxin Complex, sponsors a comprehensive reimbursement program for patients and providers called the BOTOX ADVANTAGE™ Program. The BOTOX ADVANTAGE™ Program includes a Reimbursement Hotline and Patient Assistance Program to assist patients who are receiving BOTOX® injections. The BOTOX® Reimbursement Hotline is designed to respond to your reimbursement questions and help access BOTOX®, even when you do not have insurance coverage. You can call 800-530-6680 or log onto www.botox .com.

Section 35.3

Vocal Fold Nodules, Polyps, and Cysts

"Benign Vocal Lesions: Nodules, Polyps, Cysts," by Ken W. Altman,
M.D., Ph.D., © 2002. Reprinted with permission from the author and
The Center for Voice at Northwestern University.

What Are Benign Vocal Lesions?

Benign vocal lesions are noncancerous growths of abnormal tissue on the vocal folds. They include "singer's" nodules, isolated polyps, polypoid degeneration (Reinke edema), and cysts. Since these lesions are not cancerous, they are usually not life threatening. However, lesions may affect voice quality and excessive growth may affect breathing patterns. A clinical diagnosis of nodules, polyps, or cysts does not rule out a malignancy (cancer) unless the lesion resolves with treatment or it is biopsied and is pathologically benign. The lesion may also be a benign neoplasm such as papilloma or leukoplakia that would not resolve with traditional treatment for nodules, polyps, or cysts.

What Causes These Lesions?

Each of these lesions has a potentially different cause, but there are common factors that contribute to their development. Generally, benign vocal lesions occur in response to injury, but are also well known to have multiple causes. The initial injury may be brought on by these causes:

- Chronic vocal use/misuse. For example, excessive loudness and use in a teacher, or singing excessively with poor breath support in a singer.

- Acute vocal misuse. For example, screaming at the football game, or an uncontrolled coughing spell during an upper respiratory infection.

- Trauma resulting from infection.

- Trauma from gastric reflux (GERD) injuring the laryngeal mucosa (protective cover of the vocal folds).

Other factors that contribute to chronic irritation of the larynx with excessive throat clearing can include the following:

- Post-nasal drip from resulting from allergic rhinitis
- Chronic sinusitis
- Exposure to chemical irritants such as that from tobacco use/abuse
- Pulmonary disease, which may lead to poor breath support during speech or cough-variant asthma
- Hypothyroidism, which may lead to an unusually low-pitched voice and speech/singing compensation for this low pitch may result in strain/misuse of the voice
- Poor vocal habits
- Medications that may affect the voice

How are Nodules, Polyps and Cysts Diagnosed?

The following are important:

- Time of onset of dysphonia (abnormal voice)
- Factors that accompanied the onset (such as an upper respiratory infection)
- Is hoarseness worse in morning, evening, or all day?
- The presence of vocal fatigue (voice tires easily with use)
- Pain or strain with continued voice use
- Singing range limitations
- Voice breaks or "drop-outs" while holding a note
- Past medical history
- List of medications (including homeopathic remedies), and medication allergies

Physical examination includes a complete head and neck exam by an otolaryngologist. Evaluation of the larynx requires one or more of the following:

- **Mirror exam:** a mirror is inserted into the back of the mouth, and the larynx is viewed with the use of a headlight. It provides good evaluation of mucosa color, but visualization is limited.

- **Flexible nasopharyngolaryngoscope (NPL):** after application of painless topical anesthesia, a flexible "telescope" is inserted through the nose, to the back of the throat, and down to visualize the larynx. The NPL is especially useful for particular laryngeal problems.

- **Rigid endoscopy:** a rod-like telescope with an angled tip allows the otolaryngologist to "look around the corner" to see the larynx. This exam provides excellent view and color evaluation, and is typically painless for the patient.

- **Videostroboscopy:** may be performed with either rigid or flexible telescopes. During this exam a microphone is placed on the patient's neck to pick up the voice frequency. A strobe light that is slightly desynchronized to the voice frequency is then flashed at the larynx. The vocal fold histology includes multiple layers with different mechanical properties, and a mucosal wave is produced during phonation. The desynchronized strobe light captures different stages of the laryngeal vibration and its image on video appears as a mucosal wave in slow motion. Videostroboscopy may be necessary to describe the nature of a lesion, with important effect on treatment course, indications for surgery, and prognosis.

Vocal Fold Nodules

Nodules occur more often in adult women, but also occur in male adolescents. Teachers, stock traders, and other vocal professionals who chronically use their voices in loud environments are particularly prone to development of nodules. Symptoms include chronic or recurrent hoarseness, loss of ability to sing high notes softly, frequent voice breaks, increased breathiness and vocal fatigue.

Nodules appear as bilateral symmetric swellings, usually at the junction of the anterior and mid-third portions of the vocal folds. Since the anterior two-thirds (membranous) portion of the vocal folds participate in phonation, shearing and collision forces occur maximally at the midpoint. Vascular congestion results with edema of the mucosa, and fluid in Reinke space, and thickening of the overlying epithelium.

Since nodules and polyps usually result from overuse and/or poor vocal technique, treatment centers on speech therapy and guidance, and sometimes requires a period of voice rest. Surgery is rarely indicated for vocal nodules.

Vocal Fold Polyps

Polyps occur more often in males (but may occur in either gender) after intense intermittent voice use/abuse, and there is often a history of aspirin or anticoagulant use.

Isolated vocal polyps are usually unilateral and either sessile (broad-based) or pedunculated (small stalk). They are thought to occur from breakage in a capillary (small blood vessel) in Reinke space, with leakage of blood, localized edema (swelling), and eventual organization into a fibrotic polyp.

Treatment centers on voice rest, medical treatment for sources of laryngeal irritation when indicated, and occasionally steroids to bring down the acute surrounding edema. Surgery is often indicated in cases that do not resolve with the above measures.

Polypoid Degeneration (Reinke Edema)

Reinke edema is a bilateral, diffuse swelling of Reinke space with excess gelatinous-like material that results in an irregular, sac-like appearance of the vocal folds. It is most commonly caused by tobacco/ smoke exposure, but may also be aggravated by gastric reflux, hormonal changes such as hypothyroidism, and chronic vocal abuse. Reinke edema produces a deep, husky-sounding voice.

If the edema is identified early, then stopping smoking (or other irritation) is often effective in resolving the polypoid edema. Surgery is sometimes effective in improving vocal quality, but rarely restores the voice to normal. Patients with Reinke edema require close follow-up by the otolaryngologist since the factors that contributed to the disorder (such as tobacco) may also contribute to the development of laryngeal carcinoma (cancer).

Vocal Fold Cysts

Patients with vocal cysts may have a history similar to those patients with vocal nodules. A large cyst may cause the patient to develop vocal strain or muscular tension to compensate for poor vibration and closure of the vocal folds. Also, unusual vibratory patterns with the cyst present may cause "diplophonia" (voice with two sounds). Vocal cysts occur more often in women, and may vary in size with the menstrual cycle in some patients. Cysts are almost always unilateral (appearing on only one side), but a large cyst may cause a "reactive" swelling on the opposite (contralateral) vocal fold.

Cysts are of two types: mucus retention and epithermoid.

- Mucus retention cysts result when a glandular duct becomes obstructed and retains secretions (usually after an upper respiratory infection with vocal overuse).

- Epidermoid cysts result either from minor glitches during embryologic development or from healing injured mucosa that buries skin. A ruptured cyst may result in a scar.

Treatment initially focuses on maximizing medical management of irritants, improving vocal habits, and vocal behavior modification through speech therapy. While some vocal professionals may clinically improve to be able to use their voice with minimal limitation, vocal cysts typically do not completely resolve and typically eventually require surgery.

Indications for Biopsy and Removal

- A lesion that is suspicious for cancer or a neoplastic process
- An enlarging lesion
- A lesion that failed medical and speech behavioral therapy
- The patient's vocal performance is impaired and surgery is likely to improve it

Important Points to Improve Rehabilitation from Surgery

- The patient should have realistic expectation of postsurgical improvement
- Good vocal habits
- Maximized medical treatment of related disorders
- Good speech behavior aided by speech therapist
- Period of strict postoperative voice rest
- Gradual return to maximal voice use
- Follow-up videostroboscopy to guide voice use with surgical recovery

467

Conclusions

Benign vocal lesions include vocal nodules, polyps, polypoid degeneration, and cysts. Each of these lesions has a different cause based on the vocal fold histology. Videostroboscopy may be used by an otolaryngologist to help diagnose these lesions. Surgical treatment, when indicated, should be precise with an adherence to the principles of advanced surgical technique.

Section 35.4

Vocal Cord Dysfunction (Paradoxical Vocal Cord Movement)

About Vocal Cord Dysfunction

What is vocal cord dysfunction?

In 1983, doctors at National Jewish Medical and Research Center described a condition that may be confused with asthma. This condition is called vocal cord dysfunction, or VCD. People with VCD will report asthma-like symptoms to their doctors.

What are the symptoms of vocal cord dysfunction?

Symptoms of VCD include:

- Shortness of breath;
- Hoarseness and/or wheezing;
- Chronic cough and/or throat clearing;

- Chest and throat tightness;
- "Just having trouble getting air in."

These symptoms are a result of an abnormal closing of the vocal cords (VCD) rather than inflammation of their airways (asthma).

Based on these symptoms, many people with VCD may be misdiagnosed with asthma and treated with asthma medications. Since VCD is not asthma, little or no improvement is seen in symptoms. If VCD is still not diagnosed, oral steroids (used in other chronic lung diseases like severe asthma) may be prescribed. Significant side effects can develop with long-term use of these medicines. Oral steroids are only recommended if it is shown that the benefits of their use outweigh the costs. Additionally, a misdiagnosis can also lead to frequent emergency room visits and hospitalizations—even intubation.

While it should be clear why a correct diagnosis of VCD is important, it is also critical to keep in mind that some people have both VCD and asthma, which complicates both the diagnosis and the treatment.

What happens with VCD?

To understand VCD, it is helpful to understand how the vocal cords function. The vocal cords are located at the top of the windpipe (trachea) and vibrate from exhaled air to produce noise and speech. Breathing in and out causes the vocal cords to open, allowing air to flow through the windpipe (trachea). However, with vocal cord dysfunction, the vocal cords close together, or constrict, during one or both parts of the breathing cycle. This leaves only a small opening for air to flow through the windpipe and causes asthma-like symptoms.

Management and Treatment of Vocal Cord Dysfunction (VCD)

How is VCD diagnosed?

Making a diagnosis of VCD can be very difficult. If the doctor suspects VCD she or he will ask many questions about symptoms. Common symptoms include a chronic cough, chronic throat clearing, shortness of breath, difficulty breathing, chest tightness, throat tightness, hoarseness, and wheezing. Many people diagnosed with VCD complain that they "just have trouble getting air in."

469

Are there any associations with other conditions?

Many people with VCD have problems with postnasal drip (from chronic nasal and/or sinus congestion) or gastroesophageal reflux disease. This relationship may be one of cause and effect because these two conditions can lead to chronic irritation of the throat that then causes the vocal cords to become hypersensitive to irritant stimuli.

What about breathing tests?

Breathing tests like spirometry can be useful in diagnosing VCD, but only if they are done when symptoms are occurring. In the absence of any other complicating condition like asthma, breathing tests for VCD will be normal. However, if spirometry is conducted when symptoms are present, and if the doctor obtains what is called a "flow volume loop," VCD will cause a flattening of the inspiratory (and/or expiratory) part of the loop.

What about laryngoscopy?

While spirometry is important and useful, a procedure called a laryngoscopy is the most important test in making the diagnosis of VCD. Using a flexible, fiber optic tube and tiny camera inserted into the back of the throat, a specialist can see how the vocal cords open and close. Like spirometry, this test should only be performed when symptoms are present because the vocal cords function normally in the absence of symptoms. Since people with VCD cannot trigger symptoms voluntarily, different tests to trigger symptoms may be required.

What can trigger VCD symptoms?

Possible triggers of VCD are often similar to asthma triggers. Triggers may include upper respiratory infections, air pollution, strong chemical fumes and odors, cigarette smoke, singing, laughing, emotional upset, post-nasal drip, gastroesophageal reflux disease, cold air, and exercise. Sometimes the trigger is not known.

How is VCD treated?

Once diagnosed with VCD, a specific treatment program can begin. If VCD is the only condition, asthma or other medications may be stopped. If both asthma and VCD are diagnosed, asthma medications may be continued, but are often decreased. Treatment for gastroesophageal reflux disease and post-nasal drip should be started if these are present.

What about speech therapy?

There are many special exercises and therapies that help control VCD. Speech therapy is a very important part of the treatment for VCD. Special exercises increase your awareness of abdominal breathing and relax your throat muscles. This enables you to have more control over your throat. Learning cough suppression and throat clearing techniques can also be extremely helpful. Practicing these techniques when symptom free insures effective use of them during an episode. All of the exercises are aimed at overcoming abnormal vocal cord movements and improving airflow into the lungs.

What about counseling?

Another important part of treatment is supportive counseling. Counseling can help adjust to a new diagnosis and a new treatment program. Counseling can also help identify and deal positively with stress that may be an underlying factor in VCD. Most people with VCD find counseling to be very beneficial.

Living with Vocal Cord Dysfunction

Living with the symptoms of vocal cord dysfunction: shortness of breath, hoarseness and/or wheezing, chronic cough and throat clearing, chest and throat tightness, or "just having trouble getting air in," can be frustrating at best, and even downright scary. The good news is that you don't have to live with these symptoms. VCD can be cured.

What can I do to alleviate symptoms of VCD in my daily life?

Probably the best thing you can do to cure VCD is to see a speech therapist. A speech therapist can help you in many ways:

*   Symptoms of VCD are often brought on by triggers. A speech therapist can help you recognize the early symptoms of an episode, as well as help you to identify the triggers. Early recognition of symptoms enables you start your preventative breathing techniques early. Identifying the triggers of your episodes will help you avoid these triggers and reduce the number of episodes.

471

- A speech therapist can teach you techniques to control abusive throat behaviors such as a chronic cough or chronic throat clearing. These abusive throat behaviors aggravate the vocal folds and make VCD worse.

- A speech therapist can teach you new breathing techniques like diaphragmatic breathing that can help make symptoms less severe during an episode. Stress reduction and relaxation techniques can also be learned to alleviate the anxiety that often accompanies or triggers an episode.

- A speech therapist will teach you about the anatomy and the functioning of the vocal folds. Learning about what happens to the vocal folds during an episode is helpful because it allows you to visualize what's going on inside your throat when practicing your new breathing techniques.

- A speech therapist can also recommend other sources of information and help. Doctors that specialize in asthma and other throat and lung problems may be able to help. Also, specialized counseling can help with behavioral or emotional problems.

The most important thing to know about living with VCD is that you don't have to. Talk to someone today and take back control of your breathing.

Section 35.5

Vocal Cord Paralysis

Reprinted from "Vocal Cord Paralysis," National Institute on Deafness and Other Communication Disorders, National Institutes of Health, NIH Publication No. 99-4306, June 1999. Reviewed by David A. Cooke, M.D., on March 30, 2006.

What is vocal cord paralysis?

Vocal cord paralysis is a voice disorder that occurs when one or both of the vocal cords (or vocal folds) do not open or close properly. Vocal cord paralysis is a common disorder, and symptoms can range from mild to life threatening.

The vocal cords are two elastic bands of muscle tissue located in the larynx (voice box) directly above the trachea (windpipe). The vocal cords produce voice when air held in the lungs is released and passed through the closed vocal cords, causing them to vibrate. When a person is not speaking, the vocal cords remain apart to allow the person to breathe.

Someone who has vocal cord paralysis often has difficulty swallowing and coughing because food or liquids slip into the trachea and lungs. This happens because the paralyzed cord or cords remain open, leaving the airway passage and the lungs unprotected.

What causes vocal cord paralysis?

Vocal cord paralysis may be caused by head trauma, a neurologic insult such as a stroke, a neck injury, lung or thyroid cancer, a tumor pressing on a nerve, or a viral infection. In older people, vocal cord paralysis is a common problem affecting voice production. People with certain neurologic conditions, such as multiple sclerosis or Parkinson disease, or people who have had a stroke may experience vocal cord paralysis. In many cases, however, the cause is unknown.

What are the symptoms?

People who have vocal cord paralysis experience abnormal voice changes, changes in voice quality, and discomfort from vocal straining.

For example, if only one vocal cord is damaged, the voice is usually hoarse or breathy. Changes in voice quality, such as loss of volume or pitch, may also be noticeable. Damage to both vocal cords, although rare, usually causes people to have difficulty breathing because the air passage to the trachea is blocked.

How is vocal cord paralysis diagnosed?

Vocal cord paralysis is usually diagnosed by an otolaryngologist—a doctor who specializes in ear, nose, and throat disorders. Noting the symptoms the patient has experienced, the otolaryngologist will ask how and when the voice problems started in order to help determine their cause. Next, the otolaryngologist listens carefully to the patient's voice to identify breathiness or harshness. Then, using an endoscope—a tube with a light at the end—the otolaryngologist looks directly into the throat at the vocal cords. A speech-language pathologist may also use an acoustic spectrograph, an instrument that measures voice frequency and clarity, to study the patient's voice and document its strengths and weaknesses.

How is vocal cord paralysis treated?

There are several methods for treating vocal cord paralysis, among them surgery and voice therapy. In some cases, the voice returns without treatment during the first year after damage. For that reason, doctors often delay corrective surgery for at least a year to be sure the voice does not recover spontaneously. During this time, the suggested treatment is usually voice therapy, which may involve exercises to strengthen the vocal cords or improve breath control during speech. Sometimes, a speech-language pathologist must teach patients to talk in different ways. For instance, the therapist might suggest that the patient speak more slowly or consciously open the mouth wider when speaking.

Surgery involves adding bulk to the paralyzed vocal cord or changing its position. To add bulk, an otolaryngologist injects a substance, commonly Teflon, into the paralyzed cord. Other substances currently used are collagen, a structural protein; silicone, a synthetic material; and body fat. The added bulk reduces the space between the vocal cords so the nonparalyzed cord can make closer contact with the paralyzed cord and thus improve the voice.

Sometimes an operation that permanently shifts a paralyzed cord closer to the center of the airway may improve the voice. Again, this operation allows the nonparalyzed cord to make better contact with the paralyzed cord. Adding bulk to the vocal cord or shifting its position can improve both voice and swallowing. After these operations, patients may also undergo voice therapy, which often helps to fine-tune the voice.

Treating people who have two paralyzed vocal cords may involve performing a surgical procedure called a tracheotomy to help breathing. In a tracheotomy, an incision is made in the front of the patient's neck and a breathing tube (tracheotomy tube) is inserted through a hole, called a stoma, into the trachea. Rather than breathing through the nose and mouth, the patient now breathes through the tube. Following surgery, the patient may need therapy with a speech-language pathologist to learn how to care for the breathing tube properly and how to reuse the voice.

What research is being done on vocal cord paralysis?

The National Institute on Deafness and Other Communication Disorders (NIDCD) supports research studies that may help provide new clinical measurements to diagnose vocal cord paralysis. For instance, computer software is being developed that can describe important aspects of the health of a person's larynx by analyzing the sounds it produces. By measuring instabilities in the motion of the vocal cords, the software may allow scientists and treatment clinics to relate these measurements to the study of the misuse of the voice and help diagnose disorders such as muscle paralysis and tissue loss.

Currently, the treatment for patients with damage to both vocal cords involves a tracheotomy, which may, however, cause voice production problems and decrease protection of the lungs in an effort to improve the airway. Recent studies show that another feasible approach to laryngeal rehabilitation may be using an electrical stimulation device to activate the reflexes of the paralyzed muscles that open the airway during breathing.

Where can I get help?

If you notice any unexplained voice changes or discomfort, you should consult an otolaryngologist or a speech-language pathologist for evaluation and possible treatment.

Section 35.6

Disorders of Vocal Abuse and Misuse

Reprinted from "Disorders of Vocal Abuse and Misuse," National Institute on Deafness and Other Communication Disorders, National Institutes of Health, NIH Publication No. 99-4375, May 1999. Reviewed by David A. Cooke, M.D., on March 30, 2006.

What are vocal abuse and misuse?

Vocal abuse is any behavior or occurrence that strains or injures the vocal folds (or vocal cords). This may include excessive talking, throat clearing, coughing, inhaling irritants, smoking, screaming, or yelling. Vocal misuse is improper voice usage such as speaking too loudly or at an abnormally high or low pitch. Frequent vocal abuse and misuse can damage the vocal folds and cause temporary or permanent changes in vocal function, voice quality, and possible loss of voice.

How is voice produced?

Voice is produced by vibration of the vocal folds. The vocal folds are two bands of smooth muscle tissue that lie opposite each other. They are located in the larynx or voice box. The larynx is positioned between the base of the tongue and the top of the trachea (windpipe), the passageway to the lungs.

When at rest, the vocal folds are open to allow an individual to breathe. To produce voice, the brain precisely coordinates a series of events. First, the folds come together in a firm but relaxed way. Once the folds are closed, air from the lungs passes through them, causing vibration and thus making sound. The sound from this vibration then travels through the throat, nose, and mouth (resonating cavities). The size and shape of these cavities, along with the size and shape of the vocal folds, help to determine voice quality.

Variety within an individual voice is the result of lengthening or shortening, tensing or relaxing the vocal folds. Moving the cartilages, or soft, flexible bone-like tissues to which the folds are attached, makes these adjustments possible. For example, shortening and relaxing the vocal folds makes a deep voice; lengthening and tensing them produces a high-pitched voice.

Who may be at risk for a disorder of vocal abuse or misuse?

Disorders of vocal abuse and misuse are the most prevalent and preventable of the types of voice disorders. Anyone, from infants to the elderly, who uses his or her voice excessively may develop a disorder related to vocal abuse. Lawyers, teachers, clergy, cheerleaders, and professional voice users such as singers and actors often develop these types of voice disorders. Much of the chronic hoarseness experienced by children is caused by vocal abuse or misuse.

What are some of the disorders of vocal abuse and misuse?

The most common disorders resulting from vocal abuse and misuse are laryngitis, vocal nodules, vocal polyps, and contact ulcers. Health professionals who have training in voice and voice disorders often refer to these conditions as "hyperfunctional voice disorders."

Laryngitis is an inflammation or swelling of the vocal folds. It may be caused by excessive use of the voice, by bacterial or viral infections, or by irritants such as inhaled chemicals or the backup of stomach acid into the throat (gastroesophageal reflux). The voice of someone with laryngitis will often sound raspy, breathy, and hoarse.

Vocal nodules, which are small, benign (noncancerous) growths on the vocal cords, are among the most common voice disorders directly related to vocal abuse. This condition is often called "singer's nodes" because it is a frequent problem among professional singers. Vocal nodules are callous-like growths that usually form in pairs, one on each vocal fold. They form at the area that receives the most pressure when the folds come together to vibrate. The nodules develop from damage caused by repeated pressure on the same area, much like a callous forms on areas of a person's feet that are irritated by tight shoes. The voice of a person who has vocal nodules usually sounds hoarse, low-pitched, and slightly breathy.

Vocal polyp. A vocal polyp, also called Reinke edema or polypoid degeneration, is a benign growth that is similar to a vocal nodule but is softer, more like a blister than a callous. It most often forms on only one vocal cord. A vocal polyp is often associated with long-term cigarette

477

smoking but may also be linked to hypothyroidism (decreased activity of the thyroid gland, which is involved in the growth and development of children and energy control in adults), gastroesophageal reflux, or chronic vocal misuse. People who develop a vocal polyp usually have a low-pitched, hoarse, breathy voice, similar to the voices of people who have vocal nodules.

Contact ulcers are a less common disorder of vocal abuse. They are experienced by people who use too much force when bringing the vocal folds together for speech. This excessive force causes ulcerated sores or a wearing away of tissue on or near the cartilages of the larynx that move to bring the vocal folds together. These ulcers are also found in people who have gastroesophageal reflux. People with this type of voice disorder often complain of their voice tiring easily and may feel pain in the throat, especially while talking.

How are disorders of vocal abuse and misuse diagnosed?

Anyone who experiences vocal change or hoarseness for more than two weeks should be examined by a physician, preferably an otolaryngologist (a physician/surgeon who specializes in diseases of the ears, nose, throat, and head and neck). While hoarseness is a common symptom of vocal abuse or misuse, it is also one of the first signs of cancer of the larynx. A physician's visit is especially important for people who smoke cigarettes, because smoking is closely associated with laryngeal cancer. The otolaryngologist will examine the individual's vocal folds and determine if a medical condition is causing the voice problem. As part of the voice examination, the otolaryngologist will often look directly at the vocal folds. This may be done by inserting a tiny mirror into the mouth to the back of the throat (laryngoscopy). The otolaryngologist may also examine the vocal folds by passing a small camera and light through the mouth or nose and into the throat (fiberoptic laryngoscopy). This method is often preferred because it allows viewing of vocal cord movement during speech.

Following an examination, the otolaryngologist may refer the individual to a speech-language pathologist, a health professional trained to evaluate and treat people who have voice, speech, language, or swallowing disorders that affect their ability to communicate. The speech-language pathologist will evaluate the pitch, loudness, and quality of the person's voice, and will also assess vocal techniques such as breathing and style of voicing. A voice recording is often made, and trial therapy techniques may be used to test their effectiveness at improving the voice.

478

How are disorders of vocal abuse and misuse treated?

Most disorders of vocal abuse and misuse are reversible. The best treatment is to identify and eliminate the vocal behavior that created the voice disorder. In many cases, a brief period of voice therapy is helpful so that the individual can learn good vocal techniques such as proper breath support for speech or eliminating forceful voicing.

In some instances, eliminating the abuse or misuse and voice therapy are not enough. In these cases, medication to block the production of stomach acid may be helpful. In some cases, an operation may be necessary to remove growths from the vocal folds. Since most disorders of vocal abuse and misuse easily recur following surgery if the vocal misuse continues, another period of voice therapy by a speech-language pathologist after surgery may help prevent recurrence of the problem.

Children with disorders of vocal abuse and misuse are often the most difficult to treat because it is not easy for them to change their vocal behaviors. Fortunately, most children outgrow these disorders by the time they are teenagers. For these reasons, many surgeons do not operate on children who have disorders of vocal abuse or misuse. A period of voice therapy, however, may help the child to learn proper voice behaviors.

What research is being conducted on disorders of vocal abuse and misuse?

Scientists are examining a multitude of issues related to vocal abuse and misuse. They are conducting in-depth studies of the tissues of the vocal folds to determine how various types of stress affect these delicate tissues. Scientists are especially interested in determining why vocal behaviors in some individuals lead to vocal nodules while similar behaviors in other individuals may lead to mild laryngitis, vocal polyps, or little or no voice change. They are also examining the tissue changes necessary for the development of laryngeal growths such as nodules and polyps, as well as laryngeal cancer, and how various treatments reverse those tissue changes. Speech-language pathologists are studying the effectiveness of behavioral techniques including use of machines to help people relearn proper vocal techniques such as good breath support or efficient use of the larynx. Studies that will improve the treatment of hyperfunctional voice disorders in children are also in progress. Of special interest is the long-term

479

impact of various treatments, especially medical and surgical treatments.

Section 35.7

Taking Care of Your Voice

Reprinted from "Taking Care of Your Voice," National Institute on Deafness and Other Communication Disorders, National Institutes of Health, NIH Publication No. 02-5160, September 2002.

What is voice?

We rely on our voices to inform, persuade, and connect with other people. Your voice is as unique as your fingerprint. Many people you know use their voices all day long, day in and day out. Singers, teachers, doctors, lawyers, nurses, sales people, and public speakers are among those who make great demands on their voices. Unfortunately, these individuals are most prone to experiencing voice problems. It is believed that 7.5 million people have diseases or disorders of voice. Some of these disorders can be avoided by taking care of your voice.

What are some causes of voice problems?

Causes of vocal problems may include upper respiratory infections, inflammation caused by acid reflux, vocal misuse and abuse, vocal nodules or laryngeal papillomatosis (growths), laryngeal cancer, neuromuscular diseases (such as spasmodic dysphonia or vocal cord paralysis), and psychogenic conditions due to psychological trauma. Keep in mind that most voice problems are reversible and can be successfully treated when diagnosed early.

How do you know when your voice is not healthy?

- Has your voice become hoarse or raspy?
- Have you lost your ability to hit some high notes when singing?
- Does your voice suddenly sound deeper?

- Does your throat often feel raw, achy, or strained?
- Has it become an effort to talk?
- Do you find yourself repeatedly clearing your throat?

If you answered "yes" to any of these questions, you may be experiencing a voice problem. You should consult a doctor. An otolaryngologist is a physician or surgeon who specializes in diseases or disorders of the ears, nose, and throat. He or she can determine the underlying cause of your voice problem. The professional who can help you with improving the use of your voice and avoiding vocal abuse is a speech-language pathologist.

How can I prevent voice problems?

- Limit your intake of drinks that include alcohol or caffeine. These act as diuretics (substances that increase urination) and cause the body to lose water. This loss of fluids dries out the voice. Alcohol also irritates the mucous membranes that line the throat.

- Drink plenty of water. Six to eight glasses a day is recommended.

- Don't smoke and avoid secondhand smoke. Cancer of the vocal folds is seen most often in individuals who smoke.

- Practice good breathing techniques when singing or talking. It is important to support your voice with deep breaths from the diaphragm, the wall that separates your chest and abdomen. Singers and speakers are often taught exercises that improve this breath control. Talking from the throat, without supporting breath, puts a great strain on the voice.

- Avoid eating spicy foods. Spicy foods can cause stomach acid to move into the throat or esophagus (reflux).

- Use a humidifier in your home. This is especially important in winter or in dry climates. Thirty percent humidity is recommended.

- Try not to overuse your voice. Avoid speaking or singing when your voice is hoarse.

- Wash your hands often to prevent colds and flu.

- Include plenty of whole grains, fruits, and vegetables in your diet. These foods contain vitamins A, E, and C. They also help keep the mucus membranes that line the throat healthy.

481

- Do not cradle the phone when talking. Cradling the phone between the head and shoulder for extended periods of time can cause muscle tension in the neck.

- Exercise regularly. Exercise increases stamina and muscle tone. This helps provide good posture and breathing, which are necessary for proper speaking.

- Get enough rest. Physical fatigue has a negative effect on voice.

- Avoid talking in noisy places. Trying to talk above noise causes strain on the voice.

- Avoid mouthwash or gargles that contain alcohol or irritating chemicals. If you still wish to use a mouthwash that contains alcohol, limit your use to oral rinsing. If gargling is necessary, use a saltwater solution.

- Avoid using mouthwash to treat persistent bad breath. Halitosis (bad breath) may be the result of a problem that mouthwash can't cure, such as low-grade infections in the nose, sinuses, tonsils, gums, or lungs, as well as from gastric reflux from the stomach.

- Consider using a microphone. In relatively static environments such as exhibit areas, classrooms, or exercise rooms, a lightweight microphone and an amplifier-speaker system can be of great help.

- Consider voice therapy. A speech-language pathologist who is experienced in treating voice problems can provide education on healthy use of the voice and instruction in proper voice techniques.

What research on voice is NIDCD supporting?

The National Institute on Deafness and Other Communication Disorders (NIDCD) supports and conducts research and research training on the normal and disordered processes of hearing, balance, smell, taste, voice, speech, and language. NIDCD also supports the development of assistive or augmentative devices that improve communication for individuals who have communication challenges. Within the research support for voice is a range of activity from the molecular mechanisms of disease processes, such as papilloma virus, to clinical research that identifies strategies for diagnosis, treatment, or cure of voice disorders.

An active area of research is examining the dose of vibrational exposure that human vocal folds receive during phonation. At the cellular level, the effect of gene expression and protein production are being studied as a function of this vibrational dose. Results may lead to engineered vocal fold tissues that can withstand vibrational stress.

Other studies of voice disorders focus on determining the nature, causes, diagnosis, and prevention of these disorders. These studies may lead to the development of treatments and interventions that will improve the quality of life for those who are already challenged by severe voice disorders. Substantial progress has been made in the development of augmentative communication devices to facilitate the expressive communication of persons with severe communication disabilities. An investigation of conversational performance by users of augmentative communicative devices is in progress. Other funded research evaluates whether a low-cost, laser-activated keyboard for accessing personal computers is feasible. With access to personal computers, individuals with disabilities can immediately use software programs and speech synthesizers for augmentative communication. There is ongoing research on the mechanisms of laryngeal papillomatosis and of laryngeal cancer.

Because teachers are among the individuals with a high incidence of vocal disorders, NIDCD is supporting the development of an educational website for teachers to support healthy behaviors and protection of their voices.

Section 35.8

Statistics on Voice Disorders

Excerpted from "Statistics on Voice, Speech, and Language,"
National Institute on Deafness and Other Communication Disorders,
National Institutes of Health, June 18, 2004.

Statistics

- Approximately 7.5 million people in the United States have trouble using their voices.

- Spasmodic dysphonia (a voice disorder caused by involuntary movements of one or more muscles of the larynx or voice box) can affect anyone. The first signs of this disorder are found most often in individuals between thirty and fifty years of age. More women appear to be affected by spasmodic dysphonia than men.

- Laryngeal papillomatosis is a rare disease consisting of tumors that grow inside the larynx (voice box), vocal cords, or the air passages leading from the nose into the lungs. It is caused by the human papilloma virus (HPV). Although scientists are uncertain how people are infected with HPV, they have identified more than sixty types of HPVs. Between 60 and 80 percent of laryngeal papillomatosis cases occur in children, usually before the age of three.

- A cleft palate is the fourth most common birth defect, affecting approximately one of every seven hundred live births. Velocardiofacial syndrome (which can include a cleft palate, as well as heart defects, a characteristic facial appearance, minor learning problems, and speech and feeding problems) occurs in approximately 5 to 8 percent of children born with a cleft palate. It is estimated that over 130,000 individuals in the United States have this syndrome.

Summary Report

Voice (or vocalization) is the sound produced by humans and other vertebrates using the lungs and the vocal folds in the larynx, or voice

484

box. Voice is not always produced as speech, however. Infants babble and coo; animals bark, moo, whinny, growl, and meow; and adult humans laugh, sing, and cry. Voice is generated by airflow from the lungs as the vocal folds are brought close together. When air is pushed past the vocal folds with sufficient pressure, the vocal folds vibrate. If the vocal folds in the larynx did not vibrate normally, speech could be produced only as a whisper. Your voice is as unique as your fingerprint. It helps define your personality, mood, and health.

Approximately 7.5 million people in the United States have trouble using their voices. Disorders of the voice involve problems with pitch, loudness, and quality. Pitch is the highness or lowness of a sound based on the frequency of the sound waves. Loudness is the perceived volume (or amplitude) of the sound, while quality refers to the character or distinctive attributes of a sound. Many people who have normal speaking skills have great difficulty communicating when their vocal apparatus fails. This can occur if the nerves controlling the larynx are impaired because of an accident, a surgical procedure, a viral infection, or cancer.

Part Six

Cancers of the
Ears, Nose, and Throat

Chapter 36

Head and Neck Cancer: Questions and Answers

What is cancer?

Cancer is a group of many related diseases that begin in cells, the body's basic unit of life. Normally, cells grow and divide to form new cells in an orderly way. They perform their functions for a while, and then they die. Sometimes, however, cells do not die. Instead, they continue to divide and create new cells that the body does not need. The extra cells form a mass of tissue, called a growth or tumor. There are two types of tumors: benign and malignant. Benign tumors are not cancer. They do not invade nearby tissue or spread to other parts of the body. Malignant tumors are cancer. Their growth invades normal structures near the tumor and spreads to other parts of the body. Metastasis is the spread of cancer beyond one location in the body.

What kinds of cancers are considered cancers of the head and neck?

Most head and neck cancers begin in the cells that line the mucosal surfaces in the head and neck area, e.g., mouth, nose, and throat. Mucosal surfaces are moist tissues lining hollow organs and cavities of the body open to the environment. Normal mucosal cells look like scales (squamous) under the microscope, so head and neck cancers are often referred to as squamous cell carcinomas. Some head and

Reprinted from "Head and Neck Cancer: Questions and Answers," National Cancer Institute, National Institutes of Health, March 9, 2005.

neck cancers begin in other types of cells. For example, cancers that begin in glandular cells are called adenocarcinomas.

Cancers of the head and neck are further identified by the area in which they begin:

- **Oral cavity:** The oral cavity includes the lips, the front two-thirds of the tongue, the gingiva (gums), the buccal mucosa (lining inside the cheeks and lips), the floor (bottom) of the mouth under the tongue, the hard palate (bony top of the mouth), and the small area behind the wisdom teeth.

- **Salivary glands:** The salivary glands produce saliva, the fluid that keeps mucosal surfaces in the mouth and throat moist. There are many salivary glands; the major ones are in the floor of the mouth, and near the jawbone.

- **Paranasal sinuses and nasal cavity:** The paranasal sinuses are small hollow spaces in the bones of the head surrounding the nose. The nasal cavity is the hollow space inside the nose.

- **Pharynx:** The pharynx is a hollow tube about five inches long that starts behind the nose and leads to the esophagus (the tube that goes to the stomach) and the trachea (the tube that goes to the lungs). The pharynx has three parts:

  - **Nasopharynx:** The nasopharynx, the upper part of the pharynx, is behind the nose.

  - **Oropharynx:** The oropharynx is the middle part of the pharynx. The oropharynx includes the soft palate (the back of the mouth), the base of the tongue, and the tonsils.

  - **Hypopharynx:** The hypopharynx is the lower part of the pharynx.

- **Larynx:** The larynx, also called the voice box, is a short passageway formed by cartilage just below the pharynx in the neck. The larynx contains the vocal cords. It also has a small piece of tissue, called the epiglottis, which moves to cover the larynx to prevent food from entering the air passages.

- **Lymph nodes in the upper part of the neck:** Sometimes, squamous cancer cells are found in the lymph nodes of the upper neck when there is no evidence of cancer in other parts of the head and neck. When this happens, the cancer is called metastatic squamous neck cancer with unknown (occult) primary.

Cancers of the brain, eye, and thyroid as well as those of the scalp, skin, muscles, and bones of the head and neck are not usually grouped with cancers of the head and neck.

How common are head and neck cancers?

Head and neck cancers account for approximately 3 to 5 percent of all cancers in the United States. These cancers are more common in men and in people over age fifty. It is estimated that about thirty-nine thousand men and women in this country will develop head and neck cancer in 2005.

What causes head and neck cancers?

Tobacco (including smokeless tobacco, sometimes called "chewing tobacco" or "snuff") and alcohol use are the most important risk factors for head and neck cancers, particularly those of the oral cavity, oropharynx, hypopharynx, and larynx. Eighty-five percent of head and neck cancers are linked to tobacco use. People who use both tobacco and alcohol are at greater risk for developing these cancers than people who use either tobacco or alcohol alone.

Other risk factors for cancers of the head and neck include the following:

- **Oral cavity:** Sun exposure (lip); possibly human papillomavirus (HPV) infection.

- **Salivary glands:** Radiation to the head and neck. This exposure can come from diagnostic x-rays or from radiation therapy for noncancerous conditions or cancer.

- **Paranasal sinuses and nasal cavity:** Certain industrial exposures, such as wood or nickel dust inhalation. Tobacco and alcohol use may play less of a role in this type of cancer.

- **Nasopharynx:** Asian, particularly Chinese, ancestry; Epstein-Barr virus infection; occupational exposure to wood dust; and consumption of certain preservatives or salted foods.

- **Oropharynx:** Poor oral hygiene; HPV infection and the use of mouthwash that has a high alcohol content are possible, but not proven, risk factors.

- **Hypopharynx:** Plummer-Vinson (also called Paterson-Kelly) syndrome, a rare disorder that results from iron and other nutritional

491

deficiencies. This syndrome is characterized by severe anemia and leads to difficulty swallowing due to webs of tissue that grow across the upper part of the esophagus.

- **Larynx:** Exposure to airborne particles of asbestos, especially in the workplace.

Immigrants from Southeast Asia who use paan (betel quid) in the mouth should be aware that this habit has been strongly associated with an increased risk for oral cancer. Also, consumption of mate, a tea-like beverage habitually consumed by South Americans, has been associated with an increased risk of cancers of the mouth, throat, esophagus, and larynx.

People who are at risk for head and neck cancers should talk with their doctor about ways they can reduce their risk. They should also discuss how often to have checkups.

What are common symptoms of head and neck cancers?

Symptoms of several head and neck cancer sites include a lump or sore that does not heal, a sore throat that does not go away, difficulty swallowing, and a change or hoarseness in the voice. Other symptoms may include the following:

- **Oral cavity:** A white or red patch on the gums, tongue, or lining of the mouth; a swelling of the jaw that causes dentures to fit poorly or become uncomfortable; and unusual bleeding or pain in the mouth.

- **Nasal cavity and sinuses:** Sinuses that are blocked and do not clear, chronic sinus infections that do not respond to treatment with antibiotics, bleeding through the nose, frequent headaches, swelling or other trouble with the eyes, pain in the upper teeth, or problems with dentures.

- **Salivary glands:** Swelling under the chin or around the jawbone; numbness or paralysis of the muscles in the face; or pain that does not go away in the face, chin, or neck.

- **Oropharynx and hypopharynx:** Ear pain.

- **Nasopharynx:** Trouble breathing or speaking, frequent headaches, pain or ringing in the ears, or trouble hearing.

- **Larynx:** Pain when swallowing, or ear pain.

- **Metastatic squamous neck cancer:** Pain in the neck or throat that does not go away.

These symptoms may be caused by cancer or by other, less serious conditions. It is important to check with a doctor or dentist about any of these symptoms.

How are head and neck cancers diagnosed?

To find the cause of symptoms, a doctor evaluates a person's medical history, performs a physical examination, and orders diagnostic tests. The exams and tests conducted may vary depending on the symptoms. Examination of a sample of tissue under the microscope is always necessary to confirm a diagnosis of cancer.

Some exams and tests that may be useful are described below:

- **Physical examination** may include visual inspection of the oral and nasal cavities, neck, throat, and tongue using a small mirror and/or lights. The doctor may also feel for lumps on the neck, lips, gums, and cheeks.

- **Endoscopy** is the use of a thin, lighted tube called an endoscope to examine areas inside the body. The type of endoscope the doctor uses depends on the area being examined. For example, a laryngoscope is inserted through the mouth to view the larynx; an esophagoscope is inserted through the mouth to examine the esophagus; and a nasopharyngoscope is inserted through the nose so the doctor can see the nasal cavity and nasopharynx.

- **Laboratory tests** examine samples of blood, urine, or other substances from the body.

- **X-rays** create images of areas inside the head and neck on film.

- **CT (or CAT) scan** is a series of detailed pictures of areas inside the head and neck created by a computer linked to an x-ray machine.

- **Magnetic resonance imaging (or MRI)** uses a powerful magnet linked to a computer to create detailed pictures of areas inside the head and neck.

- **PET scan** uses sugar that is modified in a specific way so it is absorbed by cancer calls and appears as dark areas on the scan.

- **Biopsy** is the removal of tissue. A pathologist studies the tissue under a microscope to make a diagnosis. A biopsy is the only sure way to tell whether a person has cancer.

If the diagnosis is cancer, the doctor will want to learn the stage (or extent) of disease. Staging is a careful attempt to find out whether the cancer has spread and, if so, to which parts of the body. Staging may involve an examination under anesthesia (in the operating room), x-rays and other imaging procedures, and laboratory tests. Knowing the stage of the disease helps the doctor plan treatment.

What health professionals treat patients with head and neck cancers?

Patients with head and neck cancers are best treated by a team of specialists. The specialists vary, depending on the location and extent of the cancer. The medical team may include oral surgeons; ear, nose, and throat surgeons (also called otolaryngologists); pathologists; medical oncologists; radiation oncologists; prosthodontists; dentists; plastic surgeons; dietitians; social workers; nurses; physical therapists; and speech-language pathologists (sometimes called speech therapists).

How are head and neck cancers treated?

The treatment plan for an individual patient depends on a number of factors, including the exact location of the tumor, the stage of the cancer, and the person's age and general health. The patient and the doctor should consider treatment options carefully. They should discuss each type of treatment and how it might change the way the patient looks, talks, eats, or breathes.

- **Surgery:** The surgeon may remove the cancer and some of the healthy tissue around it. Lymph nodes in the neck may also be removed (lymph node dissection), if the doctor suspects that the cancer has spread. Surgery may be followed by radiation treatment. Head and neck surgery often changes the patient's ability to chew, swallow, or talk. The patient may look different after surgery, and the face and neck may be swollen. The swelling usually goes away within a few weeks. However, lymph node dissection can slow the flow of lymph, which may collect in the tissues; this swelling may last for a long time. After a laryngectomy (surgery to remove the larynx), parts of the neck and throat may feel numb because nerves have been cut. If lymph nodes in the neck were removed, the shoulder and neck may be weak and stiff. Patients should report any side effects to their doctor or nurse, and discuss what approach to take. Information about rehabilitation can be found below.

- **Radiation therapy, also called radiotherapy:** This treatment involves the use of high-energy x-rays to kill cancer cells. Radiation may come from a machine outside the body (external radiation therapy). It can also come from radioactive materials placed directly into or near the area where the cancer cells are found (internal radiation therapy or radiation implant). In addition to its desired effect on cancer cells, radiation therapy often causes unwanted effects. Patients who receive radiation to the head and neck may experience redness, irritation, and sores in the mouth; a dry mouth or thickened saliva; difficulty in swallowing; changes in taste; or nausea. Other problems that may occur during treatment are loss of taste, which may decrease appetite and affect nutrition, and earaches (caused by hardening of the ear wax). Patients may also notice some swelling or drooping of the skin under the chin and changes in the texture of the skin. The jaw may feel stiff and patients may not be able to open their mouth as wide as before treatment. Patients should report any side effects to their doctor or nurse and ask how to manage these effects.

- **Chemotherapy, also called anticancer drugs:** This treatment is used to kill cancer cells throughout the body. The side effects of chemotherapy depend on the drugs that are given. In general, anticancer drugs affect rapidly growing cells, including blood cells that fight infection, cells that line the mouth and the digestive tract, and cells in hair follicles. As a result, patients may have side effects such as lower resistance to infection, sores in the mouth and on the lips, loss of appetite, nausea, vomiting, diarrhea, and hair loss. They may also feel unusually tired and experience skin rash and itching, joint pain, loss of balance, and swelling of the feet or lower legs. Patients should talk with their doctor or nurse about the side effects they are experiencing, and how to handle them.

Are clinical trials (research studies) available for patients with head and neck cancers?

Clinical trials are research studies conducted with people who volunteer to take part. Participation in clinical trials is an option for many patients with head and neck cancers.

Treatment trials are designed to find more effective cancer treatments and better ways to use current treatments. In some studies, all patients receive the new treatment. In others, doctors compare different therapies by giving the new treatment to one group of patients and standard therapy to another group. Doctors are studying new types and schedules for delivering radiation therapy, new anticancer drugs, new drug combinations, and new ways of combining treatments. They are also studying ways to treat head and neck cancers using biological therapy (a type of treatment that stimulates the immune system to fight cancer) by itself or in combination with anticancer drugs or radiation therapy.

Scientists are also conducting clinical trials to find better ways to reduce the side effects of chemotherapy and radiation therapy for head and neck cancers. These clinical trials, called supportive care trials, explore ways to improve the comfort and quality of life of cancer patients and cancer survivors.

People interested in taking part in a clinical trial should talk with their doctor.

What rehabilitation or support options are available for patients with head and neck cancers?

Rehabilitation is a very important part of treatment for patients with head and neck cancer. The goals of rehabilitation depend on the extent of the disease and the treatment a patient has received. The health care team makes every effort to help the patient return to normal activities as soon as possible.

Depending on the location of the cancer and the type of treatment, rehabilitation may include physical therapy, dietary counseling, speech therapy, and/or learning how to care for a stoma after a laryngectomy. A stoma is an opening into the windpipe through which a patient breathes after a laryngectomy.

Sometimes, especially with cancer of the oral cavity, a patient may need reconstructive and plastic surgery to rebuild the bones or tissues of the mouth. If this is not possible, a prosthodontist may be able to make a prosthesis (an artificial dental and/or facial part) to restore satisfactory swallowing and speech. Patients will receive special training to use the device.

Patients who have trouble speaking after treatment, or who have lost their ability to speak, may need speech therapy. Often, a speech-language pathologist will visit the patient in the hospital to plan therapy and teach speech exercises or alternative methods of speaking. Speech therapy usually continues after the patient returns home.

Eating may be difficult after treatment for head and neck cancer. Some patients receive nutrients directly into a vein (IV) after surgery, or need a feeding tube until they can eat on their own. A feeding tube is a flexible plastic tube that is passed into the stomach through the nose or an incision (cut) in the abdomen. A nurse or speech-language pathologist can help patients learn how to swallow again after surgery.

Is follow-up treatment necessary? What does it involve?

Regular follow-up care is very important after treatment for head and neck cancer to make sure the cancer has not returned, or that a second primary (new) cancer has not developed. Depending on the type of cancer, medical checkups could include exams of the stoma, mouth, neck, and throat. Regular dental exams may also be necessary. From time to time, the doctor may perform a complete physical exam, blood tests, x-rays, and CT, PET, or MRI scans. The doctor may continue to monitor thyroid and pituitary gland function, especially if the head or neck was treated with radiation. Also, the doctor is likely to counsel patients to stop smoking. Research has shown that continued smoking may reduce the effectiveness of treatment and increase the chance of a second primary cancer.

What can people who have had head and neck cancer do to reduce the risk of developing a second primary (new) cancer?

People who have been treated for head and neck cancer have an increased chance of developing a new cancer, usually in the head and neck, esophagus, or lungs. The chance of a second primary cancer varies depending on the original diagnosis, but is higher for people who smoke and drink alcohol. Patients who do not smoke should never start. Those who smoke should do their best to quit. Studies have shown that continuing to smoke or drink (or both) increases the chance of a second primary cancer for up to twenty years after the original diagnosis.

Some research has shown that isotretinoin (13-cis-retinoic acid), a substance related to vitamin A, may reduce the risk of the tumor recurring (coming back) in patients who have been successfully treated for cancers of the oral cavity, oropharynx, and larynx. However, treatment with isotretinoin has not yet been shown to improve survival or to prevent future cancers.

Chapter 37

Oropharyngeal Cancer

Cancer of the oropharynx is a disease in which cancer cells are found in the tissues of the oropharynx. The oropharynx is the middle part of the throat (also called the pharynx). The pharynx is a hollow tube about five inches long that starts behind the nose and goes down to the neck to become part of the esophagus (the tube that goes to the stomach). Air and food pass through the pharynx on the way to the windpipe (trachea) or the esophagus. The oropharynx includes the base of the tongue, the tonsils, the soft palate (the back of the mouth), and the walls of the pharynx.

Cancer of the oropharynx most commonly starts in the cells that line the oropharynx.

A doctor should be seen if a person has a sore throat that does not go away, trouble swallowing, weight loss, a lump in the back of the mouth or throat, a change in the voice, or pain in the ear.

If there are symptoms, a doctor will examine the throat using a mirror and lights. The doctor will also feel the throat for lumps. If tissue that is not normal is found, the doctor will need to cut out a small piece and look at it under the microscope to see if there are any cancer cells. This is called a biopsy.

The chance of recovery (prognosis) depends on where the cancer is in the throat, whether the cancer is just in the throat or has spread to other tissues (the stage), and the patient's general state of health.

Reprinted from PDQ® Cancer Information Summary. National Cancer Institute; Bethesda, MD. Oropharyngeal Cancer (PDQ®): Treatment: Patient. Updated 06/2005. Available at http://cancer.gov. Accessed October 24, 2005.

After the treatment, a doctor should be seen regularly because there is a chance of having a second primary cancer in the head or neck region. Smoking or drinking alcohol after treatment increases the chance of developing a second primary cancer.

Stages of Cancer of the Oropharynx

Once cancer of the oropharynx is found, more tests will be done to find out if cancer cells have spread to other parts of the body. This is called staging. A doctor needs to know the stage of the disease to plan treatment. Imaging tests may be done, including special x-rays and an MRI (magnetic resonance imaging) scan, which uses a magnet, radio waves, and a computer to make a picture of the inside of the body. The following stages are used for cancer of the oropharynx.

Stage 0: Cancer is found only in cells lining the oropharynx. Stage 0 cancer is also called carcinoma in situ.

Stage I: The cancer is two centimeters (about ¾ inch) or smaller and has not spread outside the oropharynx.

Stage II: The cancer is larger than two centimeters, but not larger than four centimeters (about 1½ inches), and has not spread outside the oropharynx.

Stage III: Stage III is either of the following:

- The cancer is larger than four centimeters and has not spread outside the oropharynx.

- The cancer is any size and has spread to only one lymph node on the same side of the neck as the cancer. (Lymph nodes are small, bean-shaped structures found throughout the body. They help fight infection and disease.) The lymph node that contains cancer is three centimeters (just over one inch) or smaller.

Stage IVA: Stage IVA is either of the following:

- The cancer has spread to tissues near the oropharynx, including the voice box, roof of the mouth, lower jaw, muscle of the tongue, or central muscles of the jaw. Cancer may have spread to one or more nearby lymph nodes, none larger than six centimeters (almost 2½ inches).

500

- The cancer is any size, is only in the oropharynx, and has spread to one lymph node that is larger than three centimeters but no larger than six centimeters, or to more than one lymph node, none larger than six centimeters.

Stage IVB: Stage IVB is either of the following:

- The cancer is found in a lymph node that is larger than six centimeters and may have spread to other tissues around the oropharynx.

- Cancer surrounds the main artery in the neck or has spread to bones in the jaw or skull, to muscle in the side of the jaw, or to the upper part of the throat behind the nose; the cancer may have spread to nearby lymph nodes.

Stage IVC: In stage IVC, cancer has spread to other parts of the body; the tumor may be any size and may have spread to lymph nodes.

Recurrent: Recurrent disease means that the cancer has come back (recurred) after it has been treated. It may come back in the oropharynx or in another part of the body.

Treatment Option Overview

How Cancer of the Oropharynx Is Treated

There are treatments for all patients with cancer of the oropharynx. Three kinds of treatment are used:

- Surgery (taking out the cancer)

- Radiation therapy (using high-dose x-rays or other high-energy rays to kill cancer cells)

- Chemotherapy (using drugs to kill cancer cells)

Surgery is a common treatment of cancer of the oropharynx. A doctor may remove the cancer and some of the healthy tissue around the cancer. If cancer has spread to lymph nodes, the lymph nodes will be removed (lymph node dissection). A new type of surgery called micrographic surgery is being tested in clinical trials for early cancers of the oropharynx. Micrographic surgery removes the cancer and as little normal tissue as possible. During this surgery, the doctor removes the

501

cancer and then uses a microscope to look at the cancerous area to make sure there are no cancer cells remaining.

Radiation therapy uses high-energy x-rays to kill cancer cells and shrink tumors. Radiation may come from a machine outside the body (external radiation therapy) or from putting materials that produce radiation (radioisotopes) through thin plastic tubes in the area where the cancer cells are found (internal radiation therapy). Fractionated radiation therapy is given in several smaller, equal doses over a period of several days. External radiation to the thyroid or the pituitary gland may change the way the thyroid gland works. The doctor may test the thyroid gland before and after therapy to make sure it is working properly. Giving drugs with the radiation therapy to make the cancer cells more sensitive to radiation (radiosensitization) is being tested in clinical trials. If smoking is stopped before radiation therapy is started, there is a better chance of surviving longer.

Chemotherapy uses drugs to kill cancer cells. Chemotherapy may be taken by pill, or it may be put into the body by a needle in the vein or muscle. Chemotherapy is called a systemic treatment because the drug enters the bloodstream, travels through the body, and can kill cancer cells throughout the body.

People with oropharyngeal cancer have a higher risk of getting other cancers in the head and neck area. Clinical trials of chemoprevention therapy are testing whether certain drugs can prevent second cancers from developing in the mouth, throat, windpipe, nose, or esophagus (the tube that connects the throat to the stomach).

Hyperthermia therapy (warming the body to kill cancer cells) is being tested in clinical trials. Hyperthermia therapy uses a special machine to heat the body for a certain period of time to kill cancer cells. Because cancer cells are often more sensitive to heat than normal cells, the cancer cells die and the cancer shrinks.

Because the oropharynx helps in breathing, eating, and talking, patients may need special help adjusting to the side effects of the cancer and its treatment. A doctor will consult with several kinds of doctors who can help determine the best treatment. Trained medical staff can also help patients recover from treatment and adjust to new ways of eating and talking. Plastic surgery, or help learning to eat and speak, may be needed if a large part of the oropharynx is taken out.

Treatment by Stage

Treatment of cancer of the oropharynx depends on where the cancer is in the oropharynx; the stage of the disease; the effect of treatment on the patient's ability to talk, eat, and breathe normally; and the patient's age and overall health.

Standard treatment may be considered because of its effectiveness in patients in past studies, or participation in a clinical trial may be considered. Not all patients are cured with standard therapy and some standard treatments may have more side effects than are desired. For these reasons, clinical trials are designed to find better ways to treat cancer patients and are based on the most up-to-date information. Clinical trials are ongoing in many parts of the country for patients with cancer of the oropharynx.

Stage I Oropharyngeal Cancer: Treatment may be one of the following:

- Radiation therapy or surgery

- A clinical trial of fractionated radiation therapy

Stage II Oropharyngeal Cancer: Treatment will be surgery to remove the cancer or radiation therapy.

Stage III Oropharyngeal Cancer: Treatment may be one of the following:

- Surgery to remove the cancer followed by radiation therapy with or without chemotherapy

- Radiation therapy, which may be fractionated radiation therapy

- Radiation therapy combined with chemotherapy

- A clinical trial of chemotherapy followed by surgery or radiation therapy

- A clinical trial of chemotherapy combined with radiation therapy

- A clinical trial of new ways of giving radiation therapy

Stage IV Oropharyngeal Cancer: If the cancer can be removed by surgery, treatment may be one of the following:

- Surgery to remove the cancer followed by radiation therapy with or without chemotherapy

- Radiation therapy

- A clinical trial of chemotherapy combined with radiation therapy
- A clinical trial of new ways of giving radiation therapy

If the cancer cannot be removed by surgery, treatment may be one of the following:

- Radiation therapy with or without chemotherapy
- A clinical trial of chemotherapy followed by surgery or radiation therapy
- A clinical trial of chemotherapy with radiation therapy and drugs to make the cancer cells more sensitive to radiation therapy (radiosensitizers)
- A clinical trial of chemotherapy and fractionated radiation therapy given at the same time
- A clinical trial of new ways of giving radiation therapy
- A clinical trial of hyperthermia therapy combined with radiation therapy

Following treatment, it is important to have careful head and neck examinations to look for recurrence. Checkups will be done monthly in the first year, every two months in the second year, every three months in the third year, and every six months thereafter.

Recurrent Oropharyngeal Cancer: Treatment may be one of the following:

- Surgery to remove the cancer
- Radiation therapy
- A clinical trial of chemotherapy
- A clinical trial of hyperthermia therapy plus radiation therapy

Following treatment, it is important to have careful head and neck examinations to look for recurrence. Checkups will be done monthly in the first year, every two months in the second year, every three months in the third year, and every six months thereafter.

Chapter 38

Nasopharyngeal Cancer

General Information about Nasopharyngeal Cancer

Nasopharyngeal cancer is a disease in which malignant (cancer) cells form in the tissues of the nasopharynx.

The nasopharynx is the upper part of the pharynx (throat) behind the nose. The pharynx is a hollow tube about five inches long that starts behind the nose and ends at the top of the trachea (windpipe) and esophagus (the tube that goes from the throat to the stomach). Air and food pass through the pharynx on the way to the trachea or the esophagus. The nostrils lead into the nasopharynx. An opening on each side of the nasopharynx leads into an ear. Nasopharyngeal cancer most commonly starts in the squamous cells that line the oropharynx (the part of the throat behind the mouth).

Ethnic background and exposure to the Epstein-Barr virus can affect the risk of developing nasopharyngeal cancer.

Risk factors may include the following:

- Chinese or Asian ancestry

- Exposure to the Epstein-Barr virus: The Epstein-Barr virus has been associated with certain cancers, including nasopharyngeal cancer and some lymphomas.

Reprinted from PDQ® Cancer Information Summary. National Cancer Institute; Bethesda, MD. Nasopharyngeal Cancer (PDQ®): Treatment: Treatment-Patient. Updated 06/2005. Available at http:cancer.gov. Accessed October 24, 2005.

Possible signs of nasopharyngeal cancer include trouble breathing, speaking, or hearing.

These and other symptoms may be caused by nasopharyngeal cancer. Other conditions may cause the same symptoms. A doctor should be consulted if any of the following problems occur:

- A lump in the nose or neck
- A sore throat
- Trouble breathing or speaking
- Nosebleeds
- Trouble hearing
- Pain or ringing in the ears
- Headaches

Tests that examine the nose and throat are used to detect (find) and diagnose nasopharyngeal cancer.

The following tests and procedures may be used:

- **Physical exam of the throat:** An exam in which the doctor feels for swollen lymph nodes in the neck and looks down the throat with a small, long-handled mirror to check for abnormal areas.

- **Nasoscopy:** A procedure to look inside the nose for abnormal areas. A nasoscope (a thin, lighted tube) is inserted through the nose. Tissue samples may be taken for biopsy.

- **Neurological exam:** A series of questions and tests to check the brain, spinal cord, and nerve function. The exam checks a person's mental status, coordination, and ability to walk normally, and how well the muscles, senses, and reflexes work. This may also be called a neuro exam or a neurologic exam.

- **Head and chest x-rays:** An x-ray of the skull and organs and bones inside the chest. An x-ray is a type of energy beam that can go through the body and onto film, making a picture of areas inside the body.

- **MRI (magnetic resonance imaging):** A procedure that uses a magnet, radio waves, and a computer to make a series of detailed pictures of areas inside the body. This procedure is also called nuclear magnetic resonance imaging (NMRI).

- **CT scan (CAT scan):** A procedure that makes a series of detailed pictures of areas inside the body, taken from different angles. The pictures are made by a computer linked to an x-ray machine. A dye may be injected into a vein or swallowed to help the organs or tissues show up more clearly. This procedure is also called computed tomography, computerized tomography, or computerized axial tomography.

- **Laboratory tests:** Medical procedures that test samples of tissue, blood, urine, or other substances in the body. These tests help to diagnose disease, plan and check treatment, or monitor the disease over time.

- **Biopsy:** The removal of cells or tissues so they can be viewed under a microscope by a pathologist to check for signs of cancer.

Certain factors affect prognosis (chance of recovery) and treatment options.

The prognosis (chance of recovery) and treatment options depend on the following:

- The stage of the cancer (whether it affects part of the nasopharynx, involves the whole nasopharynx, or has spread to other places in the body)

- The type of nasopharyngeal cancer

- The size of the tumor

- The patient's age and general health

Stages of Nasopharyngeal Cancer

After nasopharyngeal cancer has been diagnosed, tests are done to find out if cancer cells have spread within the nasopharynx or to other parts of the body.

The process used to find out whether cancer has spread within the nasopharynx or to other parts of the body is called staging. The information gathered from the staging process determines the stage of the disease. It is important to know the stage in order to plan treatment. The results of the tests used to diagnose nasopharyngeal cancer are often also used to stage the disease.

Stage 0 (Carcinoma in Situ): In stage 0 nasopharyngeal cancer, cancer is found only in the lining of the nasopharynx. Stage 0 cancer is also called carcinoma in situ.

Stage I: In stage I nasopharyngeal cancer, cancer is found only in the nasopharynx.

Stage II: Stage II nasopharyngeal cancer is divided into stage IIA and stage IIB as follows:

- Stage IIA: Cancer has spread from the nasopharynx to the oropharynx (the middle part of the throat that includes the soft palate, the base of the tongue, and the tonsils), and/or to the nasal cavity.

- Stage IIB: Cancer is found in the nasopharynx and has spread to lymph nodes on one side of the neck, or has spread to the area surrounding the nasopharynx and may have spread to lymph nodes on one side of the neck. The involved lymph nodes are six centimeters or smaller.

Stage III: In stage III nasopharyngeal cancer, the cancer:

- is found in the nasopharynx and has spread to lymph nodes on both sides of the neck and the lymph nodes are six centimeters or smaller; or

- has spread into the soft tissues (oropharynx and/or nasal cavity) and to lymph nodes on both sides of the neck and the lymph nodes are six centimeters or smaller; or

- has spread beyond the soft tissues into areas around the pharynx and to lymph nodes on both sides of the neck and the lymph nodes are six centimeters or smaller; or

- has spread to nearby bones or sinuses and may have spread to lymph nodes on one or both sides of the neck and the involved lymph nodes are six centimeters or smaller.

Stage IV: Stage IV nasopharyngeal cancer is divided into stage IVA, stage IVB, and stage IVC as follows:

- Stage IVA: Cancer has spread beyond the nasopharynx and may have spread to the cranial nerves, the hypopharynx (bottom part of the throat), areas in and around the side of the skull or jawbone, and/or the bone around the eye. Cancer may also have spread to lymph nodes on one or both sides of the neck, and the involved lymph nodes are six centimeters or smaller.

- Stage IVB: Cancer has spread to lymph nodes above the collarbone and/or the involved lymph nodes are larger than six centimeters.

- Stage IVC: Cancer has spread beyond nearby lymph nodes to other parts of the body.

Recurrent Nasopharyngeal Cancer: Recurrent nasopharyngeal cancer is cancer that has recurred (come back) after it has been treated. The cancer may come back in the nasopharynx or in other parts of the body.

Treatment Option Overview

Different types of treatment are available for patients with nasopharyngeal cancer. Some treatments are standard (the currently used treatment), and some are being tested in clinical trials. Before starting treatment, patients may want to think about taking part in a clinical trial. A treatment clinical trial is a research study meant to help improve current treatments or obtain information on new treatments for patients with cancer. When clinical trials show that a new treatment is better than the standard treatment, the new treatment may become the standard treatment.

Clinical trials are taking place in many parts of the country. Choosing the most appropriate cancer treatment is a decision that ideally involves the patient, family, and health care team.

Radiation Therapy

Radiation therapy is a cancer treatment that uses high-energy x-rays or other types of radiation to kill cancer cells. There are two types of radiation therapy. External radiation therapy uses a machine outside the body to send radiation toward the cancer. Internal radiation therapy uses a radioactive substance sealed in needles, seeds, wires, or catheters that are placed directly into or near the cancer. The way the radiation therapy is given depends on the type and stage of the cancer being treated.

External radiation therapy to the thyroid or the pituitary gland may change the way the thyroid gland works. The doctor may test the thyroid gland before and after therapy to make sure it is working properly. Having a dentist evaluate dental health and correct any existing problems is particularly important before beginning radiation therapy.

Chemotherapy

Chemotherapy is a cancer treatment that uses drugs to stop the growth of cancer cells, either by killing the cells or by stopping the cells from dividing. When chemotherapy is taken by mouth or injected into a vein or muscle, the drugs enter the bloodstream and can reach cancer cells throughout the body (systemic chemotherapy). When chemotherapy is placed directly into the spinal column, an organ, or a body cavity such as the abdomen, the drugs mainly affect cancer cells in those areas (regional chemotherapy). The way the chemotherapy is given depends on the type and stage of the cancer being treated.

Surgery

Surgery is removing the cancer in an operation. Surgery is sometimes used for nasopharyngeal cancer that does not respond to radiation therapy. If cancer has spread to the lymph nodes, the doctor may remove lymph nodes and other tissues in the neck.

New types of treatment are being tested in clinical trials. These include the following:

Biologic Therapy

Biologic therapy is a treatment that uses the patient's immune system to fight cancer. Substances made by the body or made in a laboratory are used to boost, direct, or restore the body's natural defenses against cancer. This type of cancer treatment is also called biotherapy or immunotherapy.

Intensity-Modulated Radiation Therapy

Intensity-modulated radiation therapy (IMRT) is a type of three-dimensional radiation therapy that uses computer-generated images to show the size and shape of the tumor.

Treatment Options by Stage

Stage I Nasopharyngeal Cancer: Treatment of stage I nasopharyngeal cancer is usually radiation therapy to the tumor and lymph nodes in the neck.

Stage II Nasopharyngeal Cancer: Treatment of stage II nasopharyngeal cancer may include the following:

- Chemotherapy combined with radiation therapy
- Radiation therapy to the tumor and lymph nodes in the neck

Stage III Nasopharyngeal Cancer: Treatment of stage III nasopharyngeal cancer may include the following:

- Chemotherapy combined with radiation therapy
- Radiation therapy to the tumor and lymph nodes in the neck
- Radiation therapy followed by surgery to remove cancer-containing lymph nodes in the neck that persist or come back after radiation therapy
- A clinical trial of chemotherapy before, combined with, or after radiation therapy

Stage IV Nasopharyngeal Cancer: Treatment of stage IV nasopharyngeal cancer may include the following:

- Chemotherapy combined with radiation therapy
- Radiation therapy to the tumor and lymph nodes in the neck
- Radiation therapy followed by surgery to remove cancer-containing lymph nodes in the neck that persist or come back after radiation therapy
- Chemotherapy for cancer that has metastasized (spread) to other parts of the body
- A clinical trial of chemotherapy before, combined with, or after radiation therapy
- A clinical trial of new radiation therapy such as intensity-modulated radiation therapy

Recurrent Nasopharyngeal Cancer: Treatment of recurrent nasopharyngeal cancer may include the following:

- External radiation therapy plus internal radiation therapy
- Surgery
- Chemotherapy
- A clinical trial of biologic therapy and/or chemotherapy

This summary refers to specific treatments under study in clinical trials, but it may not mention every new treatment being studied.

Chapter 39

Paranasal Sinus and Nasal Cavity Cancer

Cancer of the paranasal sinus and nasal cavity is a disease in which cancer (malignant) cells are found in the tissues of the paranasal sinuses or nasal cavity. The paranasal sinuses are small hollow spaces around the nose. The sinuses are lined with cells that make mucus, which keeps the nose from drying out; the sinuses are also a space through which the voice can echo to make sounds when a person talks or sings. The nasal cavity is the passageway just behind the nose through which air passes on the way to the throat during breathing. The area inside the nose is called the nasal vestibule.

There are several paranasal sinuses, including the frontal sinuses above the nose, the maxillary sinuses in the upper part of either side of the upper jawbone, the ethmoid sinuses just behind either side of the upper nose, and the sphenoid sinus behind the ethmoid sinus in the center of the skull.

Cancer of the paranasal sinus and nasal cavity most commonly starts in the cells that line the oropharynx. Much less often, cancer of the paranasal sinus and nasal cavity starts in the color-making cells called melanocytes, and is called a melanoma. If the cancer starts in the muscle or connecting tissue, it is called a sarcoma. Another type of cancer that can occur here, but grows more slowly, is called an

Reprinted from PDQ® Cancer Information Summary. National Cancer Institute; Bethesda, MD. Paranasal Sinus and Nasal Cavity Cancer (PDQ®): Treatment-Patient. Updated 07/2005. Available at: http://cancer.gov. Accessed October 4, 2005.

inverting papilloma. Cancers called midline granulomas may also occur in the paranasal sinuses or nasal cavity, and they cause the tissue around them to break down.

A doctor should be seen for any of the following problems:

- Blocked sinuses that do not clear
- A sinus infection
- Nosebleeds
- A lump or sore that doesn't heal inside the nose
- Frequent headaches or sinus pain
- Swelling or other trouble with the eyes
- Pain in the upper teeth
- Dentures that no longer fit well

If there are symptoms, a doctor will examine the nose using a mirror and lights. The doctor may order a CT scan (a special x-ray that uses a computer) or an MRI scan (an x-ray-like procedure that uses magnetic energy) to make a picture of the inside of parts of the body. A special instrument (called a rhinoscope or a nasoscope) may be put into the nose to see inside. If tissue that is not normal is found, the doctor will need to cut out a small piece and look at it under the microscope to see if there are any cancer cells. This is called a biopsy. Sometimes the doctor will need to cut into the sinus to do a biopsy.

The chance of recovery (prognosis) depends on where the cancer is in the sinuses, whether the cancer is just in the area where it started or has spread to other tissues (the stage), and the patient's general state of health.

Stages of Cancer of the Paranasal Sinus and Nasal Cavity

Once cancer of the paranasal sinus and nasal cavity is found, more tests will be done to find out if cancer cells have spread to other parts of the body. This is called staging. It is important to know the stage of the disease to plan treatment. Staging systems have been established for the most common paranasal sinus cavity cancers.

Stages of Cancer of Maxillary Sinus

The following stages are used for maxillary sinus cancer:

Stage 0: In stage 0, cancer is found in the innermost lining of the maxillary sinus only. Stage 0 cancer is also called carcinoma in situ.

Stage I: In stage I, cancer is found in the mucous membranes of the maxillary sinus.

Stage II: In stage II, cancer has spread to bone around the maxillary sinus, including the roof of the mouth and the nose, but not to bones at the back of the maxillary sinus or the base of the skull.

Stage III: In stage III, cancer is found in any of the following places:

- Bone at the back of the maxillary sinus
- Tissues under the skin
- The eye socket
- The base of the skull
- The ethmoid sinuses

or

Cancer is found in one lymph node on the same side of the neck as the cancer, and the lymph node is three centimeters or smaller; cancer also is found in any of the following places:

- The maxillary sinus
- Bones around the maxillary sinus
- Tissues under the skin
- The eye socket
- The base of the skull
- The ethmoid sinuses

Stage IV: Stage IV is divided into stages IVA, IVB, and IVC.

Stage IVA: In stage IVA, cancer has spread to either one lymph node on the same side of the neck as the cancer and the lymph node is larger than three centimeters but smaller than six centimeters; or, cancer has spread to more than one lymph node anywhere in the neck, and all are 6 centimeters or smaller; cancer is also found in any of the following areas:

- The maxillary sinus
- Bones around the maxillary sinus
- Tissues under the skin
- The eye socket
- The base of the skull
- The ethmoid sinuses

or

Cancer is found in one or more lymph nodes in the neck, none larger than six centimeters, and in any of the following areas:

- The front of the eye
- The skin of the cheek
- The base of the skull
- Behind the jaw
- The bone between the eyes
- The sphenoid or frontal sinuses

Stage IVB: In stage IVB, cancer has spread to either:

- one or more lymph nodes larger than six centimeters; or
- the back of the eye, the brain, the base and middle parts of the skull, nerves in the head, and/or the upper part of the throat behind the nose; cancer may also be found in one or more lymph nodes.

Stage IVC: In stage IVC, cancer has spread to other parts of the body.

Stages of Cancer of Nasal Cavity and Ethmoid Sinus

The following stages are used for nasal cavity and ethmoid sinus cancer:

Stage 0: In stage 0, cancer is found in the innermost lining of the nasal cavity or ethmoid sinus only. Stage 0 cancer is also called carcinoma in situ.

Stage I: In stage 1, cancer is found in only one area (of either the nasal cavity or the ethmoid sinus) and may have spread into bone.

Stage II: In stage II, cancer is found in two areas (of either the nasal cavity or the ethmoid sinus) or has spread to a nearby area; cancer may have spread into bone.

Stage III: In stage III, cancer is found in any of the following places:

- The eye socket
- The maxillary sinus
- The roof of the mouth
- The bone between the eyes

or

Cancer is found in a single lymph node on the same side of the neck as the cancer and the lymph node is three centimeters or smaller; cancer also is found in any of the following places:

- The nasal cavity or ethmoid sinus
- The eye socket
- The maxillary sinus
- The roof of the mouth
- The bone between the eyes

Stage IV: Stage IV is divided into stages IVA, IVB, and IVC.

Stage IVA: In stage IVA, cancer has spread to either one lymph node on the same side of the neck as the cancer and the lymph node is larger than three centimeters but smaller than six centimeters; or, cancer has spread to more than one lymph node anywhere in the neck, and all are six centimeters or smaller; cancer is also found in any of the following places:

- The nasal cavity or ethmoid sinus
- The eye socket
- The maxillary sinus
- The roof of the mouth
- The bone between the eyes

or

Cancer is found in one or more lymph nodes in the neck, and the lymph nodes are six centimeters or smaller; cancer is also found in any of the following areas:

- The front of the eye
- The skin of the nose or cheek
- Front parts of the skull
- The base of the skull
- The sphenoid or frontal sinuses

Stage IVB: In stage IVB, cancer is found in any of the following areas:

- The back of the eye
- The brain
- The middle parts of the skull
- Nerves in the head
- The upper part of the throat behind the nose
- The base of the skull

Cancer may also be found in one or more lymph nodes.

or

Cancer is found in a lymph node that is larger than six centimeters.

Stage IVC: In stage IVC, cancer has spread to other parts of the body.

Recurrent: Recurrent disease means that the cancer has come back (recurred) after it has been treated. It may come back in the paranasal sinuses or nasal cavity or in another part of the body.

Treatment Option Overview

There are treatments for all patients with cancer of the paranasal sinus and nasal cavity. Three kinds of treatment are used:

- Surgery (taking out the cancer)

- Radiation therapy (using high-dose x-rays or other high-energy rays to kill cancer cells)
- Chemotherapy (using drugs to kill cancer cells)

Surgery is commonly used to remove cancers of the paranasal sinus or nasal cavity. Depending on where the cancer is and how far it has spread, a doctor may need to cut out bone or tissue around the cancer. If cancer has spread to lymph nodes in the neck, the lymph nodes may be removed (lymph node dissection).

Radiation therapy is also a common treatment of cancer of the paranasal sinus and nasal cavity. Radiation therapy uses high-energy x-rays to kill cancer cells and shrink tumors. Radiation may come from a machine outside the body (external radiation therapy) or from putting materials that produce radiation (radioisotopes) through thin plastic tubes in the area where the cancer cells are found (internal radiation therapy). External radiation to the thyroid or the pituitary gland may change the way the thyroid gland works. The doctor may wish to test the thyroid gland before and after therapy to make sure it is working properly.

Chemotherapy uses drugs to kill cancer cells. Chemotherapy may be taken by pill, or it may be put into the body by a needle in a vein or muscle. Chemotherapy is called a systemic treatment because the drug enters the bloodstream, travels through the body, and can kill cancer cells throughout the body.

Because the paranasal sinuses and nasal cavity help in talking and breathing, and are close to the face, patients may need special help adjusting to the side effects of the cancer and its treatment. A doctor will consult with several kinds of doctors who can help determine the best treatment. Trained medical staff can also help in recovery from treatment. Patients may need plastic surgery if a large amount of tissue or bone around the paranasal sinuses or nasal cavity is taken out.

Treatment by Stage

Treatment of cancer of the paranasal sinus and nasal cavity depends on where the cancer is, the stage of the disease, and the patient's age and overall health.

Standard treatment may be considered because of its effectiveness in patients in past studies, or participation in a clinical trial may be considered. Not all patients are cured with standard therapy and some standard treatments may have more side effects than are desired. For these reasons, clinical trials are designed to find better ways to treat cancer patients and are based on the most up-to-date information. Clinical trials are ongoing in some parts of the country for patients with cancer of the paranasal sinus and nasal cavity.

Stage I Paranasal Sinus and Nasal Cavity Cancer: Treatment depends on the type of cancer and where the cancer is found.

If cancer is in the maxillary sinus, treatment will probably be surgery to remove the cancer. Radiation therapy may be given after surgery.

If cancer is in the ethmoid sinus, treatment may be one of the following:

- Radiation therapy, if the cancer cannot be removed with surgery
- Surgery followed by radiation therapy

If cancer is in the sphenoid sinus, treatment is the same as for nasopharyngeal cancer and will probably be radiation therapy with or without chemotherapy.

If cancer is in the nasal cavity, treatment may be surgery, radiation therapy, or both.

If the cancer is an inverting papilloma, treatment will probably be surgery. If the cancer comes back after surgery, patients may receive more surgery or radiation therapy.

If the cancer is a melanoma or sarcoma, treatment will probably be surgery. For certain types of sarcoma, a combination of surgery, radiation therapy, and chemotherapy may be given.

If the cancer is a midline granuloma, treatment will probably be radiation therapy.

If cancer is in the nose (nasal vestibule), treatment may be surgery or radiation therapy.

Stage II Paranasal Sinus and Nasal Cavity Cancer: Treatment depends on the type of cancer and where the cancer is found.

If cancer is in the maxillary sinus, treatment will probably be surgery to remove the cancer. Radiation therapy is given before or after surgery.

If cancer is in the ethmoid sinus, treatment may be one of the following:

- External-beam radiation therapy
- Surgery followed by radiation therapy

If cancer is in the sphenoid sinus, treatment is the same as for nasopharyngeal cancer and will probably be radiation therapy with or without chemotherapy.

If cancer is in the nasal cavity, treatment may be one of the following:

- Surgery and/or radiation therapy
- Radiation with or without chemotherapy

If the cancer is an inverting papilloma, treatment will probably be surgery. If the cancer comes back after surgery, patients may receive more surgery or radiation therapy.

If the cancer is a melanoma or sarcoma, treatment will probably be surgery. For certain types of sarcoma, a combination of surgery, radiation therapy, and chemotherapy may be given.

If the cancer is a midline granuloma, treatment will probably be radiation therapy.

If the cancer is in the nose (nasal vestibule), treatment may be surgery or radiation therapy.

Stage III Paranasal Sinus and Nasal Cavity Cancer: Treatment depends on the type of cancer and where the cancer is found.

If cancer is in the maxillary sinus, treatment may be one of the following:

- Surgery to remove the cancer. Radiation therapy is given before or after surgery.
- A clinical trial of a special type of radiation therapy given before or after surgery.

If cancer is in the ethmoid sinus, treatment may be one of the following:

- Surgery followed by radiation therapy
- A clinical trial of chemotherapy before surgery or radiation therapy
- A clinical trial of chemotherapy after surgery or after a combination of treatments

If cancer is in the sphenoid sinus, treatment is the same as for nasopharyngeal cancer and will probably be radiation therapy with or without chemotherapy.

If cancer is in the nasal cavity, treatment may be one of the following:

- Surgery
- Radiation therapy with or without chemotherapy
- Surgery plus radiation therapy
- A clinical trial of chemotherapy before surgery or radiation therapy
- A clinical trial of chemotherapy after surgery or after a combination of treatments

If the cancer is an inverting papilloma, treatment will probably be surgery. If the cancer comes back after surgery, patients may receive more surgery or radiation therapy.

If the cancer is a melanoma or sarcoma, treatment will probably be surgery. Radiation therapy may be given if the cancer cannot be removed with surgery. For certain types of sarcoma, a combination of surgery, radiation therapy, and chemotherapy may be given.

If the cancer is a midline granuloma, treatment will probably be radiation therapy.

If the cancer is in the nose (nasal vestibule), treatment may be one of the following:

- External-beam and/or internal radiation therapy
- Surgery if the cancer comes back following treatment
- A clinical trial of chemotherapy before surgery or radiation therapy
- A clinical trial of chemotherapy after surgery or after a combination of treatments

Stage IV Paranasal Sinus and Nasal Cavity Cancer: Treatment depends on the type of cancer and where the cancer is found.

If cancer is in the maxillary sinus, treatment will probably be one of the following:

- Radiation therapy
- A clinical trial of chemotherapy before surgery or radiation therapy
- A clinical trial of radiation therapy

If cancer is in the ethmoid sinus, treatment may be one of the following:

- Surgery followed by radiation therapy
- Radiation therapy followed by surgery
- Chemotherapy and radiation therapy given at the same time
- A clinical trial of chemotherapy before surgery or radiation therapy

If cancer is in the sphenoid sinus, treatment is the same as for nasopharyngeal cancer and may be one of the following:

- Radiation therapy with or without chemotherapy
- A clinical trial of chemotherapy before surgery or radiation therapy

If cancer is in the nasal cavity, treatment may be one of the following:

- Surgery
- Radiation therapy with or without chemotherapy
- Surgery plus radiation therapy
- A clinical trial of chemotherapy before surgery or radiation therapy

If the cancer is an inverting papilloma, treatment may be one of the following:

- Surgery. If the cancer comes back after surgery, patients may receive more surgery or radiation therapy.
- A clinical trial of chemotherapy before surgery or radiation therapy

If the cancer is a melanoma or sarcoma, treatment may be one of the following:

- Surgery
- Radiation therapy
- Chemotherapy

- A clinical trial of chemotherapy before surgery or radiation therapy

If the cancer is a midline granuloma, treatment may be one of the following:

- Radiation therapy
- A clinical trial of chemotherapy before surgery or radiation therapy

If the cancer is in the nose (nasal vestibule), treatment may be one of the following:

- External-beam and/or internal radiation therapy
- Surgery if the cancer comes back following treatment
- A clinical trial of chemotherapy before surgery or radiation therapy

Recurrent Paranasal Sinus and Nasal Cavity Cancer: Treatment depends on the type of cancer, where the cancer is found, and the type of treatment the patient received before.

If cancer is in the maxillary sinus, treatment will probably be one of the following:

- Radiation therapy alone or after extensive surgery (if limited surgery was done for the original cancer)
- Surgery (if radiation therapy was given for the original cancer)
- Chemotherapy. Clinical trials are testing new chemotherapy drugs.

If cancer is in the ethmoid sinus, treatment may be one of the following:

- Radiation therapy alone or after extensive surgery (if limited surgery was done for the original cancer)
- Surgery (if radiation therapy was given for the original cancer)
- Chemotherapy. Clinical trials are testing new chemotherapy drugs.

If cancer is in the sphenoid sinus, treatment will probably be radiation therapy. Chemotherapy is given if radiation therapy does not work.

If cancer is in the nasal cavity, treatment may be one of the following:

- Radiation therapy alone or after extensive surgery (if limited surgery was done for the original cancer)
- Surgery (if radiation therapy was given for the original cancer)
- Chemotherapy. Clinical trials are testing new chemotherapy drugs.

If the cancer is an inverting papilloma, treatment will probably be surgery. If the cancer comes back after surgery, patients may receive more surgery or radiation therapy.

If the cancer is a melanoma or sarcoma, treatment may be surgery or chemotherapy.

If the cancer is a midline granuloma, treatment will probably be radiation therapy.

If the cancer is in the nose (nasal vestibule), treatment may be one of the following:

- Surgery (if radiation therapy was given for the original cancer)
- Radiation therapy alone or after extensive surgery (if limited surgery was done for the original cancer)
- Chemotherapy. Clinical trials are testing new chemotherapy drugs.

Chapter 40

What You Need to Know about Esophageal Cancer

Introduction

The diagnosis of cancer of the esophagus brings with it many questions and a need for clear, understandable answers. This chapter provides information about the symptoms, diagnosis, and treatment of cancer of the esophagus, and it describes some of the possible causes (risk factors) of this disease. Having this important information may make it easier for patients and their families to handle the challenges they face.

The Esophagus

The esophagus is a hollow tube that carries food and liquids from the throat to the stomach. When a person swallows, the muscular walls of the esophagus contract to push food down into the stomach. Glands in the lining of the esophagus produce mucus, which keeps the passageway moist and makes swallowing easier. The esophagus is located just behind the trachea (windpipe). In an adult, the esophagus is about ten inches long.

Understanding the Cancer Process

Cancer is a disease that affects cells, the body's basic unit of life. To understand any type of cancer, it is helpful to know about normal cells and what happens when they become cancerous.

Reprinted from "What You Need to Know about Esophageal Cancer," National Cancer Institute, National Institutes of Health, September 16, 2002.

The body is made up of many types of cells. Normally, cells grow, divide, and produce more cells when they are needed. This process keeps the body healthy and functioning properly. Sometimes, however, cells keep dividing when new cells are not needed. The mass of extra cells forms a growth or tumor. Tumors can be benign or malignant.

- **Benign tumors** are not cancer. They usually can be removed and, in most cases, they do not come back. Cells in benign tumors do not spread to other parts of the body. Most important, benign tumors are rarely a threat to life.

- **Malignant tumors** are cancer. Cells in malignant tumors are abnormal and divide without control or order. These cancer cells can invade and destroy the tissue around them. Cancer cells can also break away from a malignant tumor and enter the bloodstream or lymphatic system (the tissues and organs that produce, store, and carry white blood cells that fight infection and other diseases). This process, called metastasis, is how cancer spreads from the original (primary) tumor to form new (secondary) tumors in other parts of the body.

Cancer that begins in the esophagus (also called esophageal cancer) is divided into two major types, squamous cell carcinoma and adenocarcinoma, depending on the type of cells that are malignant. Squamous cell carcinomas arise in squamous cells that line the esophagus. These cancers usually occur in the upper and middle part of the esophagus. Adenocarcinomas usually develop in the glandular tissue in the lower part of the esophagus. The treatment is similar for both types of esophageal cancer.

If the cancer spreads outside the esophagus, it often goes to the lymph nodes first. (Lymph nodes are small, bean-shaped structures that are part of the body's immune system.) Esophageal cancer can also spread to almost any other part of the body, including the liver, lungs, brain, and bones.

Risk Factors

The exact causes of cancer of the esophagus are not known. However, studies show that any of the following factors can increase the risk of developing esophageal cancer:

- **Age:** Esophageal cancer is more likely to occur as people get older; most people who develop esophageal cancer are over age sixty.

- **Sex:** Cancer of the esophagus is more common in men than in women.

- **Tobacco Use:** Smoking cigarettes or using smokeless tobacco is one of the major risk factors for esophageal cancer.

- **Alcohol Use:** Chronic and/or heavy use of alcohol is another major risk factor for esophageal cancer. People who use both alcohol and tobacco have an especially high risk of esophageal cancer. Scientists believe that these substances increase each other's harmful effects.

- **Barrett Esophagus:** Long-term irritation can increase the risk of esophageal cancer. Tissues at the bottom of the esophagus can become irritated if stomach acid frequently "backs up" into the esophagus—a problem called gastric reflux. Over time, cells in the irritated part of the esophagus may change and begin to resemble the cells that line the stomach. This condition, known as Barrett's esophagus, is a premalignant condition that may develop into adenocarcinoma of the esophagus.

- **Other Types of Irritation:** Other causes of significant irritation or damage to the lining of the esophagus, such as swallowing lye or other caustic substances, can increase the risk of developing esophageal cancer.

- **Medical History:** Patients who have had other head and neck cancers have an increased chance of developing a second cancer in the head and neck area, including esophageal cancer.

Having any of these risk factors increases the likelihood that a person will develop esophageal cancer. Still, most people with one or even several of these factors do not get the disease. And most people who do get esophageal cancer have none of the known risk factors.

Identifying factors that increase a person's chances of developing esophageal cancer is the first step toward preventing the disease. We already know that the best ways to prevent this type of cancer are to quit (or never start) smoking cigarettes or using smokeless tobacco and to drink alcohol only in moderation. Researchers continue to study the causes of esophageal cancer and to search for other ways to prevent it. For example, they are exploring the possibility that increasing one's intake of fruits and vegetables, especially raw ones, may reduce the risk of this disease.

Researchers are also studying ways to reduce the risk of esophageal cancer for people with Barrett esophagus.

The best ways to prevent cancer of the esophagus are to quit (or never start) using tobacco and to limit the use of alcohol.

Recognizing Symptoms

Early esophageal cancer usually does not cause symptoms. However, as the cancer grows, symptoms may include the following:

- Difficult or painful swallowing
- Severe weight loss
- Pain in the throat or back, behind the breastbone, or between the shoulder blades
- Hoarseness or chronic cough
- Vomiting
- Coughing up blood

These symptoms may be caused by esophageal cancer or by other conditions. It is important to check with a doctor.

Diagnosing Esophageal Cancer

To help find the cause of symptoms, the doctor evaluates a person's medical history and performs a physical exam. The doctor usually orders a chest x-ray and other diagnostic tests. These tests may include the following:

- **A barium swallow (also called an esophagram)** is a series of x-rays of the esophagus. The patient drinks a liquid containing barium, which coats the inside of the esophagus. The barium makes any changes in the shape of the esophagus show up on the x-rays.

- **Esophagoscopy (also called endoscopy)** is an examination of the inside of the esophagus using a thin lighted tube called an endoscope. An anesthetic (substance that causes loss of feeling or awareness) is usually used during this procedure. If an abnormal area is found, the doctor can collect cells and tissue through the endoscope for examination under a microscope. This is called a biopsy. A biopsy can show cancer, tissue changes that may lead to cancer, or other conditions.

Staging the Disease

If the diagnosis is esophageal cancer, the doctor needs to learn the stage (or extent) of disease. Staging is a careful attempt to find out whether the cancer has spread and, if so, to what parts of the body. Knowing the stage of the disease helps the doctor plan treatment. Listed below are descriptions of the four stages of esophageal cancer:

- **Stage I:** The cancer is found only in the top layers of cells lining the esophagus.

- **Stage II:** The cancer involves deeper layers of the lining of the esophagus, or it has spread to nearby lymph nodes. The cancer has not spread to other parts of the body.

- **Stage III:** The cancer has invaded more deeply into the wall of the esophagus or has spread to tissues or lymph nodes near the esophagus. It has not spread to other parts of the body.

- **Stage IV:** The cancer has spread to other parts of the body. Esophageal cancer can spread almost anywhere in the body, including the liver, lungs, brain, and bones.

Some tests used to determine whether the cancer has spread include the following:

- **CAT (or CT) scan (computed tomography):** A computer linked to an x-ray machine creates a series of detailed pictures of areas inside the body.

- **Bone scan:** This technique, which creates images of bones on a computer screen or on film, can show whether cancer has spread to the bones. A small amount of radioactive substance is injected into a vein; it travels through the bloodstream and collects in the bones, especially in areas of abnormal bone growth. An instrument called a scanner measures the radioactivity levels in these areas.

- **Bronchoscopy:** The doctor puts a bronchoscope (a thin, lighted tube) into the mouth or nose and down through the windpipe to look into the breathing passages.

Treatment

Treatment for esophageal cancer depends on a number of factors, including the size, location, and extent of the tumor, and the general health of the patient. Patients are often treated by a team of specialists,

531

which may include a gastroenterologist (a doctor who specializes in diagnosing and treating disorders of the digestive system), surgeon (a doctor who specializes in removing or repairing parts of the body), medical oncologist (a doctor who specializes in treating cancer), and radiation oncologist (a doctor who specializes in using radiation to treat cancer). Because cancer treatment may make the mouth sensitive and at risk for infection, doctors often advise patients with esophageal cancer to see a dentist for a dental exam and treatment before cancer treatment begins.

Many different treatments and combinations of treatments may be used to control the cancer and/or to improve the patient's quality of life by reducing symptoms.

- **Surgery** is the most common treatment for esophageal cancer. Usually, the surgeon removes the tumor along with all or a portion of the esophagus, nearby lymph nodes, and other tissue in the area. (An operation to remove the esophagus is called an esophagectomy.) The surgeon connects the remaining healthy part of the esophagus to the stomach so the patient is still able to swallow. Sometimes, a plastic tube or part of the intestine is used to make the connection. The surgeon may also widen the opening between the stomach and the small intestine to allow stomach contents to pass more easily into the small intestine. Sometimes surgery is done after other treatment is finished.

- **Radiation therapy,** also called radiotherapy, involves the use of high-energy rays to kill cancer cells. Radiation therapy affects cancer cells in the treated area only. The radiation may come from a machine outside the body (external radiation) or from radioactive materials placed in or near the tumor (internal radiation). A plastic tube may be inserted into the esophagus to keep it open during radiation therapy. This procedure is called intraluminal intubation and dilation. Radiation therapy may be used alone or combined with chemotherapy as primary treatment instead of surgery, especially if the size or location of the tumor would make an operation difficult. Doctors may also combine radiation therapy with chemotherapy to shrink the tumor before surgery. Even if the tumor cannot be removed by surgery or destroyed entirely by radiation therapy, radiation therapy can often help relieve pain and make swallowing easier.

- **Chemotherapy** is the use of anticancer drugs to kill cancer cells. The anticancer drugs used to treat esophageal cancer travel throughout the body. Anticancer drugs used to treat esophageal cancer are usually given by injection into a vein (IV). Chemotherapy may be combined with radiation therapy as primary treatment (instead of surgery) or to shrink the tumor before surgery.

- **Laser therapy** is the use of high-intensity light to destroy tumor cells. Laser therapy affects the cells only in the treated area. The doctor may use laser therapy to destroy cancerous tissue and relieve a blockage in the esophagus when the cancer cannot be removed by surgery. The relief of a blockage can help to reduce symptoms, especially swallowing problems.

- **Photodynamic therapy (PDT),** a type of laser therapy, involves the use of drugs that are absorbed by cancer cells; when exposed to a special light, the drugs become active and destroy the cancer cells. The doctor may use PDT to relieve symptoms of esophageal cancer such as difficulty swallowing.

Clinical trials (research studies) to evaluate new ways to treat cancer are an important option for many patients with esophageal cancer. In some studies, all patients receive the new treatment. In others, doctors compare different therapies by giving the new treatment to one group of patients and the usual (standard) therapy to another group. Through research, doctors learn new, more effective ways to treat cancer.

Side Effects of Treatment

The side effects of cancer treatment depend on the type of treatment and may be different for each person. Doctors and nurses can explain the possible side effects of treatment, and they can suggest ways to help relieve symptoms that may occur during and after treatment.

- Surgery for esophageal cancer may cause short-term pain and tenderness in the area of the operation, but this discomfort or pain can be controlled with medicine. Patients are taught special breathing and coughing exercises to keep their lungs clear.

- Radiation therapy affects normal as well as cancerous cells. Side effects of radiation therapy depend mainly on the dose and the part of the body that is treated. Common side effects of radiation therapy to the esophagus are a dry, sore mouth and throat; difficulty swallowing; swelling of the mouth and gums; dental cavities;

fatigue; skin changes at the site of treatment; and loss of appetite.

- Chemotherapy, like radiation therapy, affects normal as well as cancerous cells. Side effects depend largely on the specific drugs and the dose (amount of drug administered). Common side effects of chemotherapy include nausea and vomiting, poor appetite, hair loss, skin rash and itching, mouth and lip sores, diarrhea, and fatigue. These side effects generally go away gradually during the recovery periods between treatments or after treatment is over.

- Laser therapy can cause short-term pain where the treatment was given, but this discomfort can be controlled with medicine.

- Photodynamic therapy makes the skin and eyes highly sensitive to light for six weeks or more after treatment. Other temporary side effects of PDT may include coughing, trouble swallowing, abdominal pain, and painful breathing or shortness of breath.

Nutrition for Cancer Patients

Eating well during cancer treatment means getting enough calories and protein to control weight loss and maintain strength. Eating well often helps people with cancer feel better and have more energy.

However, many people with esophageal cancer find it hard to eat well because they have difficulty swallowing. Patients may not feel like eating if they are uncomfortable or tired. Also, the common side effects of treatment, such as poor appetite, nausea, vomiting, dry mouth, or mouth sores, can make eating difficult. Foods may taste different.

After surgery, patients may receive nutrients directly into a vein. (This way of getting nourishment into the body is called an IV.) Some may need a feeding tube (a flexible plastic tube that is passed through the nose to the stomach or through the mouth to the stomach) until they are able to eat on their own.

Patients with esophageal cancer are usually encouraged to eat several small meals and snacks throughout the day, rather than try to eat three large meals. When swallowing is difficult, many patients can still manage soft, bland foods moistened with sauces or gravies. Puddings, ice cream, and soups are nourishing and are usually easy to swallow. It may be helpful to use a blender to process solid foods. The doctor, dietitian, nutritionist, or other health care provider can advise patients about these and other ways to maintain a healthy diet.

The Importance of Follow-up Care

Follow-up care after treatment for esophageal cancer is important to ensure that any changes in health are found. If the cancer returns or progresses or if a new cancer develops, it can be treated as soon as possible. Checkups may include physical exams, x-rays, or lab tests. Between scheduled appointments, patients should report any health problems to their doctor as soon as they appear.

Providing Emotional Support

Living with a serious disease is challenging. Apart from having to cope with the physical and medical challenges, people with cancer face many worries, feelings, and concerns that can make life difficult. They may find they need help coping with the emotional as well as the practical aspects of their disease. In fact, attention to the emotional burden of having cancer is often a part of a patient's treatment plan. The support of the health care team (doctors, nurses, social workers), support groups, and patient-to-patient networks can help people feel less isolated and distressed, and improve the quality of their lives. Cancer support groups provide a setting in which cancer patients can talk about living with cancer with others who may be having similar experiences. Patients may want to speak to a member of their health care team about finding a support group.

Questions for Your Doctor

This chapter is designed to help you get information you need from your doctor so that you can make informed decisions about your health care. In addition, asking your doctor the following questions will help you further understand your condition. To help you remember what the doctor says, you may take notes or ask whether you may use a tape recorder. Some people also want to have a family member or friend with them when they talk to the doctor—to take part in the discussion, to take notes, or just to listen.

Diagnosis

- What tests can diagnose esophageal cancer? Are they painful?
- How soon after the tests will I learn the results?

Treatment

- What treatments are recommended for me?

535

- What clinical trials are appropriate for my type of cancer?
- Will I need to be in the hospital to receive my treatment? For how long?
- How might my normal activities change during my treatment?

Side Effects

- What side effects should I expect? How long will they last?
- Whom should I call if I am concerned about a side effect?
- What will be done if I have pain?

Follow-up

- After treatment, how often do I need to be checked? What type of follow-up care should I have?
- What type of nutritional support will I need? Where can I get it?
- Will I eventually be able to resume my normal activities?

The Health Care Team

- Who will be involved with my treatment and rehabilitation? What is the role of each member of the health care team in my care?
- What has been your experience in caring for patients with esophageal cancer?

Resources

- Are there support groups in the area with people I can talk to?
- Are there organizations where I can get more information about cancer, specifically esophageal cancer?
- Are there websites I can visit that have accurate information about cancer, especially esophageal cancer?

Chapter 41

Hypopharyngeal Cancer

General Information about Hypopharyngeal Cancer

Hypopharyngeal cancer is a disease in which malignant (cancer) cells form in the tissues of the hypopharynx.

The hypopharynx is the bottom part of the pharynx (throat). The pharynx is a hollow tube about five inches long that starts behind the nose, goes down the neck, and ends at the top of the trachea (windpipe) and esophagus (the tube that goes from the throat to the stomach). Air and food pass through the pharynx on the way to the trachea or the esophagus.

Most hypopharyngeal cancers form in squamous cells, the thin, flat cells lining the inside of the hypopharynx. The hypopharynx has three different areas. Cancer may be found in one or more of these areas.

Use of tobacco products and heavy drinking can affect the risk of developing hypopharyngeal cancer.

Risk factors include the following:

- Smoking tobacco

- Chewing tobacco

- Heavy alcohol use

Reprinted from PDQ® Cancer Information Summary. National Cancer Institute; Bethesda, MD. Hypopharyngeal Cancer (PDQ®): Treatment-Patient. Updated 08/2005. Available at: http://cancer.gov. Accessed October 23, 2005.

- Eating a diet without enough nutrients
- Having Plummer-Vinson syndrome

Possible signs of hypopharyngeal cancer include a sore throat and ear pain.

These and other symptoms may be caused by hypopharyngeal cancer. Other conditions may cause the same symptoms. A doctor should be consulted if any of the following problems occur:

- A sore throat that does not go away
- Ear pain
- A lump in the neck
- Painful or difficult swallowing
- A change in voice

Tests that examine the throat and neck are used to help detect (find) and diagnose hypopharyngeal cancer.

The following tests and procedures may be used:

- **Physical exam of the throat:** An exam in which the doctor feels for swollen lymph nodes in the neck and looks down the throat with a small, long-handled mirror to check for abnormal areas.

- **Endoscopy:** A procedure used to look at areas in the throat that cannot be seen with a mirror during the physical exam of the throat. An endoscope (a thin, lighted tube) is inserted through the nose or mouth to check the throat for anything that seems unusual. Tissue samples may be taken for biopsy.

- **CT scan (CAT scan):** A procedure that makes a series of detailed pictures of areas inside the body, taken from different angles. The pictures are made by a computer linked to an x-ray machine. A dye may be injected into a vein or swallowed to help the organs or tissues show up more clearly. This procedure is also called computed tomography, computerized tomography, or computerized axial tomography.

- **MRI (magnetic resonance imaging):** A procedure that uses a magnet, radio waves, and a computer to make a series of detailed pictures of areas inside the body. This procedure is also called nuclear magnetic resonance imaging (NMRI).

- **Head, neck, and chest x-rays:** An x-ray of the head, neck, and organs and bones inside the chest. An x-ray is a type of energy beam that can go through the body and onto film, making a picture of areas inside the body.

- **Barium esophagogram:** An x-ray of the esophagus. The patient drinks a liquid that contains barium (a silver-white metallic compound). The liquid coats the esophagus and x-rays are taken.

- **Esophagoscopy:** A procedure to look inside the esophagus to check for abnormal areas. An esophagoscope (a thin, lighted tube) is inserted through the mouth or nose and down the throat into the esophagus. Tissue samples may be taken for biopsy.

- **Bronchoscopy:** A procedure to look inside the trachea and large airways in the lung for abnormal areas. A bronchoscope (a thin, lighted tube) is inserted through the nose or mouth into the trachea and lungs. Tissue samples may be taken for biopsy.

- **Biopsy:** The removal of cells or tissues so they can be viewed under a microscope to check for signs of cancer.

Certain factors affect prognosis (chance of recovery) and treatment options.

- The stage of the cancer (whether it affects part of the hypopharynx, involves the whole hypopharynx, or has spread to other places in the body). Hypopharyngeal cancer is usually detected in later stages because early symptoms rarely occur.

- The patient's age, gender, and general health

- The location of the cancer

- Whether the patient smokes during radiation therapy

Treatment options depend on the following:

- The stage of the cancer

- Keeping the patient's ability to talk, eat, and breathe as normal as possible

- The patient's general health

Patients who have had hypopharyngeal cancer are at an increased risk of developing a second cancer in the head or neck. Frequent and careful follow-up is important.

Stages of Hypopharyngeal Cancer

After hypopharyngeal cancer has been diagnosed, tests are done to find out if cancer cells have spread within the hypopharynx or to other parts of the body.

The process used to find out if cancer has spread within the hypopharynx or to other parts of the body is called staging. The information gathered from the staging process determines the stage of the disease. It is important to know the stage of the disease in order to plan treatment. The results of some of the tests used to diagnose hypopharyngeal cancer are often also used to stage the disease.

The following stages are used for hypopharyngeal cancer:

Stage 0 (Carcinoma in Situ): In stage 0, cancer is found only in the lining of the hypopharynx. Stage 0 cancer is also called carcinoma in situ.

Stage I: In stage I, the tumor is found in one area of the hypopharynx only and is two centimeters or smaller.

Stage II: In stage II, the tumor is either:

- larger than two centimeters but not larger than four centimeters and has not spread to the larynx (voice box); or

- found in more than one area of the hypopharynx or in nearby tissues.

Stage III: In stage III, one of the following is found:

- The tumor is in only one area of the hypopharynx and is two centimeters or smaller; cancer has also spread to a single lymph node on the same side of the neck and the lymph node is three centimeters or smaller.

- Cancer is in more than one area of the hypopharynx, is in nearby tissues, or is larger than two centimeters but not larger than four centimeters and is not in the larynx; cancer has also spread to a single lymph node on the same side of the neck and the lymph node is three centimeters or smaller.

- The tumor is larger than four centimeters or has spread to the larynx; cancer may have spread to a single lymph node on the same side of the neck and the lymph node is three centimeters or smaller.

Stage IV: Stage IV is divided into stage IVA, IVB, and IVC as follows:

- In stage IVA, the tumor:
  - can be any size and has spread to nearby soft tissue, connective tissue, the thyroid, or the esophagus; cancer may be found either in one lymph node on the same side of the neck (the lymph node is three centimeters or smaller) or in one or more lymph nodes anywhere in the neck (all of these lymph nodes are six centimeters or smaller); or
  - is in only one area of the hypopharynx, is two centimeters or smaller, and has also spread to one or more lymph nodes anywhere in the neck (all of these lymph nodes are six centimeters or smaller); or
  - is in more than one area of the hypopharynx, is in nearby tissues, or is larger than two centimeters but not larger than four centimeters and has not spread to the larynx; cancer has spread to one or more lymph nodes anywhere in the neck (all of these lymph nodes are six centimeters or smaller); or
  - is larger than four centimeters or has spread to the larynx; cancer has also spread to one or more lymph nodes anywhere in the neck (all of these lymph nodes are six centimeters or smaller).
- In stage IVB, the tumor either:
  - has spread to nearby soft tissue, connective tissue, blood vessels, the thyroid, or the esophagus, and may have spread to lymph nodes of any size; or
  - is any size and has spread to lymph nodes that are larger than six centimeters.
- In stage IVC, cancer has spread beyond the hypopharynx to other parts of the body.

Recurrent Hypopharyngeal Cancer: Recurrent hypopharyngeal cancer is cancer that has recurred (come back) after it has been treated. The cancer may come back in the hypopharynx or in other parts of the body.

Treatment Option Overview

Different types of treatment are available for patients with hypopharyngeal cancer. Some treatments are standard (the currently used treatment), and some are being tested in clinical trials. Before starting treatment, patients may want to think about taking part in a clinical trial. A treatment clinical trial is a research study meant to help improve current treatments or obtain information on new treatments for patients with cancer. When clinical trials show that a new treatment is better than the standard treatment, the new treatment may become the standard treatment.

Clinical trials are taking place in many parts of the country. Choosing the most appropriate cancer treatment is a decision that ideally involves the patient, family, and health care team.

Three types of standard treatment are used:

Surgery

Surgery (removing the cancer in an operation) is a common treatment for all stages of hypopharyngeal cancer. The following surgical procedures may be used:

- **Laryngopharyngectomy:** Surgery to remove the larynx (voice box) and part of the pharynx (throat).

- **Partial laryngopharyngectomy:** Surgery to remove part of the larynx and part of the pharynx. A partial laryngopharyngectomy prevents loss of the voice.

- **Neck dissection:** Surgery to remove lymph nodes and other tissues in the neck.

Even if the doctor removes all the cancer that can be seen at the time of the surgery, some patients may be given chemotherapy or radiation therapy after surgery to kill any cancer cells that are left. Treatment given after the surgery, to increase the chances of a cure, is called adjuvant therapy.

Radiation therapy

Radiation therapy is a cancer treatment that uses high-energy x-rays or other types of radiation to kill cancer cells. There are two types of radiation therapy. External radiation therapy uses a machine outside the body to send radiation toward the cancer. Internal radiation therapy uses a radioactive substance sealed in needles, seeds, wires, or catheters that are placed directly into or near the cancer. The way the radiation therapy is given depends on the type and stage of the cancer being treated.

Radiation therapy may be more effective in patients who have stopped smoking before beginning treatment. External radiation therapy to the thyroid or the pituitary gland may change the way the thyroid gland works. The thyroid gland may be tested before and after therapy to make sure it is working properly.

Chemotherapy

Chemotherapy is a cancer treatment that uses drugs to stop the growth of cancer cells, either by killing the cells or by stopping the cells from dividing. When chemotherapy is taken by mouth or injected into a vein or muscle, the drugs enter the bloodstream and can reach cancer cells throughout the body (systemic chemotherapy). When chemotherapy is placed directly into the spinal column, an organ, or a body cavity such as the abdomen, the drugs mainly affect cancer cells in those areas (regional chemotherapy). The way the chemotherapy is given depends on the type and stage of the cancer being treated.

Chemotherapy may be used to shrink the tumor before surgery or radiation therapy. This is called neoadjuvant chemotherapy.

New types of treatment are being tested in clinical trials.

Treatment Options by Stage

Stage I Hypopharyngeal Cancer: Treatment of stage I hypopharyngeal cancer may include the following:

- Laryngopharyngectomy and neck dissection with or without high-dose radiation therapy to the lymph nodes of the neck

- Partial laryngopharyngectomy with or without high-dose radiation therapy to the lymph nodes on both sides of the neck

Stage II Hypopharyngeal Cancer: Treatment of stage II hypopharyngeal cancer may include the following:

- Laryngopharyngectomy and neck dissection. High-dose radiation therapy to the lymph nodes of the neck may be given before or after surgery.

- Partial laryngopharyngectomy. High-dose radiation therapy to the lymph nodes of the neck may be given before or after surgery.

- Chemotherapy given during or after radiation therapy or after surgery

- A clinical trial of chemotherapy followed by radiation therapy or surgery

Stage III Hypopharyngeal Cancer: Treatment of stage III hypopharyngeal cancer may include the following:

- Radiation therapy before or after surgery

- Chemotherapy given during or after radiation therapy or after surgery

- A clinical trial of chemotherapy followed by surgery and/or radiation therapy

- A clinical trial of chemotherapy given at the same time as radiation therapy

- A clinical trial of surgery followed by chemotherapy given at the same time as radiation therapy

Treatment and follow-up of stage III hypopharyngeal cancer is complex and is ideally overseen by a team of specialists with experience and expertise in treating this type of cancer. If all or part of the hypopharynx is removed, the patient may need plastic surgery and other special help with breathing, eating, and talking.

Stage IV Hypopharyngeal Cancer: Treatment of stage IV hypopharyngeal cancer that can be treated with surgery may include the following:

- Radiation therapy before or after surgery

- A clinical trial of chemotherapy followed by surgery and/or radiation therapy

- A clinical trial of surgery followed by chemotherapy given at the same time as radiation therapy

Surgical treatment and follow-up of stage IV hypopharyngeal cancer is complex and is ideally overseen by a team of specialists with experience and expertise in treating this type of cancer. If all or part of the hypopharynx is removed, the patient may need plastic surgery and other special help with breathing, eating, and talking.

Treatment of stage IV hypopharyngeal cancer that cannot be treated with surgery may include the following:

- Radiation therapy

- Chemotherapy given at the same time as radiation therapy

- A clinical trial of radiation therapy with chemotherapy

Follow-up to check for recurrence should include careful head and neck exams once a month in the first year after treatment ends, every two months in the second year, every three months in the third year, and every six months thereafter.

Recurrent Hypopharyngeal Cancer: Treatment of recurrent hypopharyngeal cancer may include the following:

- Surgery

- Radiation therapy

- Chemotherapy

- A clinical trial of chemotherapy

This summary refers to specific treatments under study in clinical trials, but it may not mention every new treatment being studied.

Follow-up to check for recurrence should include careful head and neck exams once a month in the first year after treatment ends, every two months in the second year, every three months in the third year, and every six months thereafter.

Chapter 42

What You Need to Know about Cancer of the Larynx

The Larynx

The larynx is an organ at the front of your neck. It is also called the voice box. It is about two inches long and two inches wide. It is above the windpipe (trachea). Below and behind the larynx is the esophagus.

The larynx has two bands of muscle that form the vocal cords. The cartilage at the front of the larynx is sometimes called the Adam's apple.

The larynx has three main parts:

- The top part of the larynx is the supraglottis.

- The glottis is in the middle. Your vocal cords are in the glottis.

- The subglottis is at the bottom. The subglottis connects to the windpipe.

The larynx plays a role in breathing, swallowing, and talking. The larynx acts like a valve over the windpipe. The valve opens and closes to allow breathing, swallowing, and speaking:

- **Breathing:** When you breathe, the vocal cords relax and open. When you hold your breath, the vocal cords shut tightly.

Reprinted from "What You Need to Know about Cancer of the Larynx," National Cancer Institute, National Institutes of Health, May 5, 2003.

- **Swallowing:** The larynx protects the windpipe. When you swallow, a flap called the epiglottis covers the opening of your larynx to keep food out of your lungs. The food passes through the esophagus on its way from your mouth to your stomach.

- **Talking:** The larynx produces the sound of your voice. When you talk, your vocal cords tighten and move closer together. Air from your lungs is forced between them and makes them vibrate. This makes the sound of your voice. Your tongue, lips, and teeth form this sound into words.

What Is Cancer?

Cancer begins in cells, the building blocks that make up tissues. Tissues make up the organs of your body. Normally, cells grow and divide to form new cells as your body needs them. When cells grow old, they die, and new cells take their place.

Sometimes this orderly process goes wrong. New cells form when the body does not need them, and old cells do not die when they should. These extra cells can form a mass of tissue called a growth or tumor. Growths on the larynx also may be called nodules or polyps. Not all growths are cancer. Growths can be benign or malignant.

Benign growths are not cancer:

- They are rarely life-threatening.

- Usually, benign tumors can be removed, and they seldom grow back.

- Cells from benign tumors do not spread to tissues around them or to other parts of the body.

Malignant growths are cancer:

- They are generally more serious and may be life-threatening.

- Malignant tumors usually can be removed, but they can grow back.

- Cells from malignant tumors invade and damage nearby tissues and organs. Also, cancer cells can break away from a malignant tumor and enter the bloodstream or lymphatic system. That is how cancer cells spread from the original cancer (the primary tumor) to form new tumors in other organs. The spread of cancer is called metastasis. Different types of cancer tend to spread to different parts of the body.

Cancer of the larynx also may be called laryngeal cancer. It can develop in any part of the larynx. Most cancers of the larynx begin in the glottis. The inner walls of the larynx are lined with cells called squamous cells. Almost all laryngeal cancers begin in these cells. These cancers are called squamous cell carcinomas.

If cancer of the larynx spreads (metastasizes), the cancer cells often spread to nearby lymph nodes in the neck. The cancer cells can also spread to the back of the tongue, other parts of the throat and neck, the lungs, and other parts of the body. When this happens, the new tumor has the same kind of abnormal cells as the primary tumor in the larynx. For example, if cancer of the larynx spreads to the lungs, the cancer cells in the lungs are actually laryngeal cancer cells. The disease is called metastatic cancer of the larynx, not lung cancer. It is treated as cancer of the larynx, not lung cancer. Doctors sometimes call the new tumor "distant" disease.

Cancer of the Larynx: Who's at Risk?

No one knows the exact causes of cancer of the larynx. Doctors cannot explain why one person gets this disease and another does not. We do know that cancer is not contagious. You cannot "catch" cancer from another person.

People with certain risk factors are more likely to get cancer of the larynx. A risk factor is anything that increases your chance of developing this disease.

Studies have found the following risk factors:

- **Age:** Cancer of the larynx occurs most often in people over the age of fifty-five.

- **Gender:** Men are four times more likely than women to get cancer of the larynx.

- **Race:** African Americans are more likely than whites to be diagnosed with cancer of the larynx.

- **Smoking:** Smokers are far more likely than nonsmokers to get cancer of the larynx. The risk is even higher for smokers who drink alcohol heavily. People who stop smoking can greatly decrease their risk of cancer of the larynx, as well as cancer of the lung, mouth, pancreas, bladder, and esophagus. Also, quitting smoking reduces the chance that someone with cancer of the larynx will get a second cancer in the head and neck region. (Cancer of the larynx is part of a group of cancers called head and neck cancers.)

- **Alcohol:** People who drink alcohol are more likely to develop laryngeal cancer than people who don't drink. The risk increases with the amount of alcohol that is consumed. The risk also increases if the person drinks alcohol and also smokes tobacco.

- **A personal history of head and neck cancer:** Almost one in four people who have had head and neck cancer will develop a second primary head and neck cancer.

- **Occupation:** Workers exposed to sulfuric acid mist or nickel have an increased risk of laryngeal cancer. Also, working with asbestos can increase the risk of this disease. Asbestos workers should follow work and safety rules to avoid inhaling asbestos fibers.

Other studies suggest that having certain viruses or a diet low in vitamin A may increase the chance of getting cancer of the larynx. Another risk factor is having gastroesophageal reflux disease (GERD), which causes stomach acid to flow up into the esophagus.

Most people who have these risk factors do not get cancer of the larynx. If you are concerned about your chance of getting cancer of the larynx, you should discuss this concern with your health care provider. Your health care provider may suggest ways to reduce your risk and can plan an appropriate schedule for checkups.

Symptoms

The symptoms of cancer of the larynx depend mainly on the size of the tumor and where it is in the larynx. Symptoms may include the following:

- Hoarseness or other voice changes
- A lump in the neck
- A sore throat or feeling that something is stuck in your throat
- A cough that does not go away
- Problems breathing
- Bad breath

- An earache
- Weight loss

These symptoms may be caused by cancer or by other, less serious problems. Only a doctor can tell for sure.

Diagnosis

If you have symptoms of cancer of the larynx, the doctor may do some or all of the following exams:

- **Physical exam:** The doctor will feel your neck and check your thyroid, larynx, and lymph nodes for abnormal lumps or swelling. To see your throat, the doctor may press down on your tongue.

- **Indirect laryngoscopy:** The doctor looks down your throat using a small, long-handled mirror to check for abnormal areas and to see if your vocal cords move as they should. This test does not hurt. The doctor may spray a local anesthesia in your throat to keep you from gagging. This exam is done in the doctor's office.

- **Direct laryngoscopy:** The doctor inserts a thin, lighted tube called a laryngoscope through your nose or mouth. As the tube goes down your throat, the doctor can look at areas that cannot be seen with a mirror. A local anesthetic eases discomfort and prevents gagging. You may also receive a mild sedative to help you relax. Sometimes the doctor uses general anesthesia to put a person to sleep. This exam may be done in a doctor's office, an outpatient clinic, or a hospital.

- **CT scan:** An x-ray machine linked to a computer takes a series of detailed pictures of the neck area. You may receive an injection of a special dye so your larynx shows up clearly in the pictures. From the CT scan, the doctor may see tumors in your larynx or elsewhere in your neck.

- **Biopsy:** If an exam shows an abnormal area, the doctor may remove a small sample of tissue. Removing tissue to look for cancer cells is called a biopsy. For a biopsy, you receive local or general anesthesia, and the doctor removes tissue samples through a laryngoscope. A pathologist then looks at the tissue under a microscope to check for cancer cells. A biopsy is the only sure way to know if a tumor is cancerous.

551

If you need a biopsy, you may want to ask the doctor the following questions:

- What kind of biopsy will I have? Why?

- How long will it take? Will I be awake? Will it hurt?

- How soon will I know the results?

- Are there any risks? What are the chances of infection or bleeding after the biopsy?

- If I do have cancer, who will talk with me about treatment? When?

Staging

To plan the best treatment, your doctor needs to know the stage, or extent, of your disease. Staging is a careful attempt to learn whether the cancer has spread and, if so, to what parts of the body. The doctor may use x-rays, CT scans, or magnetic resonance imaging to find out whether the cancer has spread to lymph nodes, other areas in your neck, or distant sites.

Treatment

People with cancer of the larynx often want to take an active part in making decisions about their medical care. It is natural to want to learn all you can about your disease and treatment choices. However, shock and stress after a diagnosis of cancer can make it hard to remember what you want to ask the doctor. Here are some ideas that might help:

- Make a list of questions.

- Take notes at the appointment.

- Ask the doctor if you may use a tape recorder during the appointment.

- Ask a family member or friend to come to the appointment with you.

Your doctor may refer you to a specialist who treats cancer of the larynx, such as a surgeon, otolaryngologist (an ear, nose, and throat doctor), radiation oncologist, or medical oncologist. You can also ask your doctor for a referral. Treatment usually begins within a few weeks of the diagnosis. Usually, there is time to talk to your doctor about treatment choices, get a second opinion, and learn more about the disease before making a treatment decision.

Getting a Second Opinion

Before starting treatment, you might want a second opinion about your diagnosis and treatment plan. Some insurance companies require a second opinion; others may cover a second opinion if you or your doctor requests it. There are a number of ways to find a doctor for a second opinion:

- Your doctor may refer you or you may ask for a referral to one or more specialists. At cancer centers, several specialists often work together as a team. The team may include a surgeon, radiation oncologist, medical oncologist, speech pathologist, and nutritionist. At some cancer centers, you may be able to see them all on the same day.

- A local medical society, a nearby hospital, or a medical school can often provide the names of specialists in your area.

- The American Board of Medical Specialties (ABMS) has a list of doctors who have met certain education and training requirements and have passed specialty examinations. The Official ABMS Directory of Board Certified Medical Specialists lists doctors' names along with their specialty and their educational background. The directory is available in most public libraries. Also, ABMS offers this information on the Internet at http://www.abms.org.

Preparing for Treatment

The doctor can describe your treatment choices and the results you can expect for each treatment option. You will want to consider how treatment may change the way you look, breathe, and talk. You and your doctor can work together to develop a treatment plan that meets your needs and personal values.

The choice of treatment depends on a number of factors, including your general health, where in the larynx the cancer began, the size of the tumor, and whether the cancer has spread.

If you smoke, a good way to prepare for treatment is to stop smoking. Studies show that treatment is more likely to be successful for people who don't smoke. Your doctor may be able to suggest ways to help you stop smoking.

You may want to talk with the doctor about taking part in a clinical trial, a research study of new treatment methods. Clinical trials are an important option. Patients who join trials have the first chance to benefit from new treatments that have shown promise in earlier research.

These are questions you may want to ask your doctor before treatment begins:

- Where is my cancer and has it spread?

- What are my treatment choices? Which do you recommend for me? Why?

- What are the benefits of each treatment?

- What are the risks and possible side effects of each treatment?

- How will I look after treatment?

- How will I speak after treatment? Will I need to work with a speech therapist?

- Will I have problems eating?

- Will I need to change my daily activities?

- When can I return to work?

- What is the treatment likely to cost? Is this treatment covered by my insurance plan?

- Would a clinical trial (research study) be right for me? Can you help me find one?

- How often will I need checkups?

You do not need to ask all your questions or understand all the answers at once. You will have many chances to ask the doctor and the rest of the health care team to explain things that are not clear and to ask for more information.

Methods of Treatment

Cancer of the larynx may be treated with radiation therapy, surgery, or chemotherapy. Some patients have a combination of therapies.

Radiation therapy (also called radiotherapy) uses high-energy x-rays to kill cancer cells. The rays are aimed at the tumor and the tissue around it. Radiation therapy is local therapy. It affects cells only in the treated area. Treatments are usually given five days a week for five to eight weeks.

Laryngeal cancer may be treated with radiation therapy alone or in combination with surgery or chemotherapy:

- **Radiation therapy alone:** Radiation therapy is used alone for small tumors or for patients who cannot have surgery.

- **Radiation therapy combined with surgery:** Radiation therapy may be used to shrink a large tumor before surgery or to destroy cancer cells that may remain in the area after surgery. If a tumor grows back after surgery, it is often treated with radiation.

- **Radiation therapy combined with chemotherapy:** Radiation therapy may be used before, during, or after chemotherapy.

After radiation therapy, some people need feeding tubes placed into the abdomen. The feeding tube is usually temporary.

These are questions you may want to ask your doctor before having radiation therapy:

- Why do I need this treatment?

- What are the risks and side effects of this treatment?

- Are there any long-term effects?

- Should I see my dentist before I start treatment?

- When will the treatments begin? When will they end?

- How will I feel during therapy?

- What can I do to take care of myself during therapy?

- Can I continue my normal activities?

- How will my neck look afterward?

- What is the chance that the tumor will come back?

- How often will I need checkups?

Surgery is an operation in which a doctor removes the cancer using a scalpel or laser while the patient is asleep. When patients need surgery, the type of operation depends mainly on the size and exact location of the tumor.

There are several types of laryngectomy (surgery to remove part or all of the larynx):

- **Total laryngectomy:** The surgeon removes the entire larynx.

- **Partial laryngectomy (hemilaryngectomy):** The surgeon removes part of the larynx.

  - **Supraglottic laryngectomy:** The surgeon takes out the supraglottis, the top part of the larynx.

  - **Cordectomy:** The surgeon removes one or both vocal cords.

Sometimes the surgeon also removes the lymph nodes in the neck. This is called lymph node dissection. The surgeon also may remove the thyroid.

During surgery for cancer of the larynx, the surgeon may need to make a stoma. (This surgery is called a tracheostomy.) The stoma is a new airway through an opening in the front of the neck. Air enters and leaves the windpipe (trachea) and lungs through this opening. A tracheostomy tube, also called a trach ("trake") tube, keeps the new airway open. For many patients, the stoma is temporary. It is needed only until the patient recovers from surgery.

After surgery, some people may need a temporary feeding tube.

Here are some questions to ask the doctor before having surgery:

- How will I feel after the operation?

- Will I need a tracheostomy?

- Will I need to learn how to take care of myself or my incision when I get home?

- Where will the scars be? What will they look like?

- Will surgery affect my ability to speak? If so, who will teach me how to speak in a new way?

- When can I get back to my normal activities?

Chemotherapy is the use of drugs to kill cancer cells. Your doctor may suggest one drug or a combination of drugs. The drugs for cancer of the larynx are usually given by injection into the bloodstream. The drugs enter the bloodstream and travel throughout the body.

Chemotherapy is used to treat laryngeal cancer in several ways:

- **Before surgery or radiation therapy:** In some cases, drugs are given to try to shrink a large tumor before surgery or radiation therapy.

- **After surgery or radiation therapy:** Chemotherapy may be used after surgery or radiation therapy to kill any cancer cells that may be left. It also may be used for cancers that have spread.

- **Instead of surgery:** Chemotherapy may be used with radiation therapy instead of surgery. The larynx is not removed and the voice is spared.

Chemotherapy may be given in an outpatient part of the hospital, at the doctor's office, or at home. Rarely, a hospital stay may be needed.

These are questions you may want to ask your doctor before having chemotherapy:

- Why do I need this treatment?

- What will it do?

- Will I have side effects? What can I do about them?

- How long will I be on this treatment?

- How often will I need checkups?

Side Effects of Cancer Treatment

Cancer treatments are very powerful. Treatments that remove or destroy cancer cells are likely to damage healthy cells, too. That's why treatments often cause side effects. This section describes some of the side effects of each kind of treatment.

Side effects may not be the same for each person, and they may even change from one treatment session to the next. Before treatment starts, your health care team will explain possible side effects and how they can be managed. It may help to know that although some side effects may not go away completely, most of them become less troubling.

It may also help to talk with other patients. A social worker, nurse, or other member of the medical team can set up a visit with someone who has had the same treatment.

Radiation Therapy

People treated with radiation therapy may have some or all of these side effects:

- **Dry mouth:** Drinking lots of fluids can help. Some patients find artificial saliva helpful. It comes in a spray or squeeze bottle.

- **Sore throat or mouth:** Your health care provider may suggest special rinses to numb your throat and mouth and help relieve the soreness.

- **Delayed healing after dental care:** Many doctors recommend having a dental exam and any needed dental work before radiation therapy.

- **Tooth decay:** Good mouth care can help keep your teeth and gums healthy and can help you feel better. If it's hard to floss or brush your teeth in the usual way, you can try using gauze, a soft toothbrush, or a toothbrush that has a spongy tip instead of bristles. A mouthwash made with diluted peroxide, salt water, baking soda, or a combination can keep your mouth fresh and help protect your teeth from decay. It may also be helpful to use fluoride toothpaste or rinse.

- **Changes in sense of taste and smell:** During radiation therapy, food may taste or smell different.

- **Fatigue:** During radiation therapy, you may become very tired, especially in the later weeks of treatment. Resting is important, but doctors usually advise their patients to stay as active as they can.

- **Changes in voice quality:** Your voice may be weak at the end of the day. It may also be affected by changes in the weather. Voice changes and the feeling of a lump in your throat may come from swelling in the larynx caused by the radiation. The doctor may suggest medicine to reduce this swelling.

- **Skin changes in treated area:** The skin in the treated area may become red or dry. Good skin care is important at this time. Try to expose this area to the air but protect it from the sun. Avoid wearing clothes that rub, and do not shave the treated area. You should not put anything on your skin before radiation treatments. Also, you should never use lotion or cream without your doctor's advice.

Surgery

People who have surgery may have any of these side effects:

- **Pain:** You may be uncomfortable for the first few days after surgery. However, medicine can usually control the pain. You should feel free to discuss pain relief with the doctor or nurse.

- **Low energy:** It is common to feel tired or weak after surgery. The length of time it takes to recover from an operation is different for each patient.

- **Swelling in the throat:** For a few days after surgery, you won't be able to eat, drink, or swallow. At first, you will receive fluid through an intravenous (IV) tube placed into your arm. Within a day or two, you will get fluids and nutrition through a feeding tube (put in place during surgery) that goes through your nose and throat into your stomach. When the swelling goes away and the area begins to heal, the feeding tube will be removed. Swallowing may be difficult at first, and you may need the help of a nurse or speech pathologist. Soon you will be eating your regular diet. If you need a feeding tube for longer than one week, you may get a tube that goes directly into the abdomen. Most patients slowly return to eating solid foods by mouth, but for a very few patients, the feeding tube may be permanent.

- **Increased mucus production:** After the operation, the lungs and windpipe produce a lot of mucus, also called sputum. To remove it, the nurse applies gentle suction by placing a small plastic tube in the stoma. You will learn to cough and suction mucus through the stoma without the nurse's help.

- **Numbness, stiffness, or weakness:** After a laryngectomy, parts of the neck and throat may be numb because nerves have been cut. Also, the shoulder, neck, and arm may be weak and stiff. You may need physical therapy to improve your strength and flexibility after surgery.

- **Changes in physical appearance:** Your neck will be somewhat smaller, and it will have scars. Some patients find it helpful to wear clothing that covers the neck area.

- **Tracheostomy:** Patients who have surgery will have a stoma. With most supraglottic and partial laryngectomies, the stoma is temporary. After a short recovery period, the tube can be removed, and the stoma closes up. You should then be able to breathe and talk in the usual way. In some people, however, the voice may be hoarse or weak. After a total laryngectomy, the stoma is permanent. If you have a total laryngectomy, you will need to learn to speak in a new way.

Chemotherapy

The side effects of chemotherapy depend mainly on the specific drugs and the dose. In general, anticancer drugs affect cells that divide rapidly:

- **Blood cells:** These cells fight infection, help your blood to clot, and carry oxygen to all parts of your body. If your blood cells are affected, you are more likely to get infections, may bruise or bleed easily, and may feel very weak and tired.

- **Cells in hair roots:** Chemotherapy can lead to hair loss, but hair will grow back. However, the new hair may be different in color and texture.

- **Cells that line the digestive tract:** Chemotherapy can cause poor appetite, nausea and vomiting, diarrhea, or mouth and lip sores. Many of these side effects can be controlled with new or improved drugs.

Nutrition

Some people who have had treatment for cancer of the larynx may lose their interest in food. Soreness and changes in smell and taste may make eating difficult. Yet good nutrition is important. Eating well means getting enough calories and protein to prevent weight loss, regain strength, and rebuild healthy tissues.

If eating is difficult because your mouth is dry from radiation therapy, you may want to try soft, bland foods moistened with sauces or gravies. Thick soups, puddings, and milkshakes often are easier to swallow. The nurse and the dietitian will help you choose the right foods.

After surgery or radiation therapy, some people need feeding tubes placed into the abdomen. Most people slowly return to a regular diet. Learning to swallow again may take some practice with the help of a nurse or speech pathologist. Some people find liquids easier to swallow; others do better with solid foods. You will find what works best for you.

Living with a Stoma

Learning to live with the changes brought about by cancer of the larynx is a special challenge. The medical team will make every effort to help you return to your normal routine as soon as possible.

If you have a stoma, you will need to learn how to care for it:

- Before leaving the hospital, you will learn to remove and clean the trach tube, suction the trach, and care for the skin around the stoma.

- If the air is too dry, as it may be in heated buildings in the winter, the tissues of the windpipe and lungs may produce extra mucus. Also, the skin around the stoma may get sore. Keeping the skin around the stoma clean and using a humidifier at home or at the office can lessen these problems.

- It is very dangerous for water to get into the windpipe and lungs through the stoma. Wearing a special plastic stoma shield or holding a washcloth over the stoma keeps water out when showering or shaving. Other types of stoma covers—such as scarves, neckties, and specially made covers—help keep moisture in and around the stoma. They help filter smoke and dust from the air before it enters the stoma. They also catch any fluids that come out of the windpipe when you cough or sneeze. Many people choose to wear something over their stoma even after the area heals. Stoma covers can be attractive as well as useful.

- When shaving, men should keep in mind that the neck may be numb for several months after surgery. To avoid nicks and cuts, it may be best to use an electric shaver until the numbness goes away.

People with stomas work in almost every type of business and can do nearly all of the things they did before. However, they cannot hold their breath, so straining and heavy lifting may be difficult. Also, swimming and water skiing are not possible without special instruction and equipment to keep water from entering the stoma.

Some people may feel self-conscious about the way they look and speak. They may be concerned about how other people feel about them. They may be concerned about how their sexual relationships may be affected. Many people find that talking about these concerns helps them. Counseling or support groups may also be helpful.

Learning to Speak Again

Talking is part of nearly everything we do, so it's natural to be scared if your voice box must be removed. Losing the ability to talk—

even for a short time—is hard. Patients and their families and friends need understanding and support during this time.

Within a week or so after a partial laryngectomy, you will be able to talk in the usual way. After a total laryngectomy, however, you must learn to speak in a new way. A speech pathologist usually meets with you before surgery to explain the methods that can be used. In many cases, speech lessons start before you leave the hospital.

Until you begin to talk again, it is important to have other ways to communicate. Here are some ideas that you may find helpful:

- Keep pads of paper and pens or pencils in your pocket or purse.

- Use a typewriter, computer, or other electronic device. Your words can be printed on paper, displayed on a screen, or produced in a male or female voice.

- Carry a small dictionary or a picture book and point to the words you need.

- Write notes on a "magic slate" (a toy with a plastic sheet that covers black wax; lifting the plastic erases the sheet).

The health care team can help patients learn new ways to speak. It takes practice and patience to learn techniques such as esophageal speech or tracheoesophageal puncture speech, and not everyone is successful. How quickly a person learns, how understandable the speech is, and how natural the new voice sounds depend on the extent of the surgery on the larynx.

Esophageal Speech

A speech pathologist can teach you how to force air into the top of your esophagus and then push it out again. The puff of air is like a burp. It vibrates the walls of the throat, making sound for the new voice. The tongue, lips, and teeth form words as the sound passes through the mouth.

This type of speech sounds low pitched and gruff, but it usually sounds more like a natural voice than speech made by a mechanical larynx. There is also no device to carry around, so your hands are free.

Tracheoesophageal Puncture

For tracheoesophageal puncture (TEP), the surgeon makes an opening between the trachea and the esophagus. The opening is made at the time of initial surgery or later. A small plastic or silicone valve fits into this opening. The valve keeps food out of the trachea. After TEP, patients can cover their stoma with a finger and force air into the esophagus through the valve. The air produces sound by making the walls of the throat vibrate. The sound is a lot like natural speech.

Mechanical Speech

You may choose to use a mechanical larynx while you learn esophageal or TEP speech or if you are unable to use these methods. The device may be powered by batteries (electrolarynx) or by air (pneumatic larynx).

Many different mechanical devices are available. The speech pathologist will help you choose the best device for your needs and abilities and will train you to use it.

One kind of electrolarynx looks like a small flashlight. It makes a humming sound. You hold the device against your neck, and the sound travels through your neck to your mouth. Another type of electrolarynx has a flexible plastic tube that carries sound into your mouth from a hand-held device. There are also devices that are built into a denture or retainer and can be worn inside your mouth and operated by a hand-held remote control.

A pneumatic larynx is held over the stoma and uses air from the lungs instead of batteries to make it vibrate. The sound it makes travels to the mouth through a plastic tube.

Follow-up Care

Follow-up care is important after treatment for cancer of the larynx. Regular checkups ensure that any changes in health are noted. Problems can be found and treated as soon as possible. The doctor will check closely to be sure that the cancer has not returned. Checkups include exams of the stoma, neck, and throat. From time to time, the doctor may do a complete physical exam and take x-rays. If you had radiation therapy or a partial laryngectomy, the doctor will also examine you with a laryngoscope.

Treatments for laryngeal cancer can affect the thyroid. A blood test can tell if the thyroid is making enough thyroid hormone. If the level is low, you may need to take thyroid hormone pills.

People who have laryngeal cancer have a chance of developing a new cancer in the mouth, throat, or other areas of the head and neck. This is especially true for those who are smokers or drink alcohol heavily. Most doctors strongly urge their patients to stop smoking and drinking to cut down the risk of a new cancer and other health problems.

Support for People with Cancer of the Larynx

Living with a serious disease such as cancer is not easy. Some people find they need help coping with the emotional and practical aspects of their disease. Support groups can help. In these groups, people living with cancer get together to share what they have learned about coping with the disease and the effects of treatment. People interested in finding a support group may want to talk with their health care provider for suggestions.

People living with cancer may worry about caring for their families, keeping their jobs, or continuing daily activities. Concerns about tests, treatments, hospital stays, and medical bills are also common. Doctors, nurses, and other members of the health care team can answer questions about treatment, working, or other activities. Meeting with a social worker, counselor, or member of the clergy can be helpful for those who want to talk about their feelings or discuss their concerns. Often, a social worker can suggest resources for help with rehabilitation, emotional support, financial aid, transportation, or home care.

The Promise of Cancer Research

Doctors all over the country are conducting many types of clinical trials. These are research studies in which people take part voluntarily. Studies include new ways to treat cancer of the larynx. Research already has led to advances, and researchers continue to search for more effective approaches.

People who join these studies have the first chance to benefit from treatments that have shown promise in earlier research. They also make an important contribution to medical science by helping doctors learn more about the disease. Although clinical trials may pose some risks, researchers take very careful steps to protect their patients.

People with laryngeal cancer are participating in several types of treatment studies:

- **Radiation therapy:** Researchers are studying a new approach to radiation therapy. Patients receive radiation three times a day, five days a week, for just over two weeks, instead of once a day for five to seven weeks.

- **Drugs that reduce side effects:** Researchers are testing therapies that reduce the side effects of radiation therapy. They are testing drugs that may help patients maintain their weight or help lessen damage to the skin during radiation therapy.

- **Chemotherapy:** Scientists are studying drugs that kill cancer cells. These drugs are used alone or in combination with radiation therapy to spare the larynx from surgery.

- **Biological therapy:** Scientists are studying monoclonal antibodies that slow or stop the growth of cancer.

If you are interested in learning more about joining a clinical trial, you may want to talk with your doctor.

Chapter 43

Recent Research in Cancer of the Ear, Nose, and Throat

Cetuximab (Erbitux®) Plus Radiation Boosts Survival for Patients with Head and Neck Cancer

Summary: Adding the drug cetuximab to radiation therapy can nearly double the median survival in patients with head and neck cancer that has not spread to other parts of the body, a large international phase III study has found.

Source: American Society of Clinical Oncology annual meeting, New Orleans, June 5, 2004.

Background: Head and neck cancers account for 3 percent of all cancers in the United States. Most of these cancers begin in squamous cells found in the lining of structures in the head and neck. Initial treatment options for patients with advanced head and neck cancer include

This chapter includes the following publications from the National Cancer Institute: "Cetuximab (Erbitux®) Plus Radiation Boosts Survival for Patients with Head and Neck Cancer," June 5, 2004; "Chemotherapy and Radiation Together May Help Save Voice Box," April 5, 2005; and "Docetaxel (Taxotere®) before Radiation Extends Survival in Patients with Head and Neck Cancer," June 5, 2004. "Chemo Drug Shows Preclinical Promise against Head and Neck Cancer" is reprinted from National Institute of Dental and Craniofacial Research, National Institutes of Health, May 27, 2005. "Zinc Deficiency Linked to Increased Risk of Less-Common Form of Esophageal Cancer," is from a National Institutes of Health press release dated February 15, 2005.

radiation therapy, chemotherapy combined with radiation treatment, or surgery followed by radiation and/or chemotherapy plus radiation for patients whose tumors can be surgically removed.

Many head and neck cancer cells overexpress (make too much of) a protein called the epidermal growth factor receptor (EGFR), which may help cancer cells to grow more aggressively. Cetuximab is a monoclonal antibody that attaches to and blocks EGFRs. Early studies suggested that treatment with cetuximab would boost the effectiveness of radiation therapy in patients with head and neck cancer.

The Study: A total of 424 patients in the United States and Europe were enrolled in this study. All had tumors in their tonsils, tongue, or voice box that may have involved lymph nodes, but had not spread to other parts of the body. Patients were randomly assigned to receive either radiation therapy alone or radiation plus weekly cetuximab. Patients were followed up for a median of just over three years. The study's principal investigator was James A. Bonner, M.D., of the University of Alabama at Birmingham.

Results: Median survival for patients treated with cetuximab was fifty-four months, compared with twenty-eight months for patients who received radiation therapy alone. Fifty-seven percent of the cetuximab-treated patients survived for three years, compared with 44 percent of those in the radiation-only group.

Mucositis (inflammation in the mouth), causing pain and difficulty swallowing, is a common side effect of radiation therapy for head and neck cancer. In this study, patients in both groups suffered from this side effect in roughly equal numbers.

"It is particularly encouraging that the increase in survival achieved with cetuximab was attained with no worsening of radiation-induced adverse effects," said Bonner. Patients treated with cetuximab suffered more frequently from a skin rash on the face and body, but this did not appear to reduce the effectiveness of treatment.

Comments: The addition of chemotherapy to radiation has also previously been shown to improve outcomes in patients with locally advanced head and neck cancer, says Scott Saxman, M.D., of the National Cancer Institute's Cancer Therapy Evaluation Program. Follow-up studies will be necessary to determine the relative benefit of cetuximab compared to chemotherapy, he adds, and to determine whether combining cetuximab with chemotherapy will provide even greater benefit.

Chemotherapy and Radiation Together May Help Save Voice Box

People with cancer of the larynx often face laryngectomy—surgery to remove the voice box—to help stop the spread of the cancer. Now, a new study shows that giving chemotherapy and radiation therapy together can put off the need for a laryngectomy and preserve use of the voice box longer than the currently established practice of giving chemotherapy followed by radiation.

The findings of this large, randomized trial establish a new standard of care for cancer of the larynx, said Arlene Forastiere, M.D., of Johns Hopkins Oncology Center in Baltimore, who reported the finding at the annual meeting of the American Society of Clinical Oncology in San Francisco on May 14, 2002. These data were subsequently published in the November 27, 2003, issue of the *New England Journal of Medicine*.

The trial included 547 patients with locally advanced cancer of the larynx (Stage III and IV) who were randomly assigned to one of three groups. One group received chemotherapy (cisplatin and 5-fluorouracil) followed by radiation therapy, and one received chemotherapy and radiation given concomitantly (over the same time period). The third group received radiation alone.

None of the groups survived any longer than any other. However, the time to laryngectomy was significantly greater in the concomitant-therapy group. At two years, 88 percent of these patients still had their voice box, compared to 74 percent of those who had chemotherapy followed by radiation and 69 percent who had only radiation. The new approach cut the number of laryngectomies needed by 50 percent.

Ten years ago it was standard practice to remove the voice box in all patients with laryngeal cancer, Forastiere said. Over the past decade, the practice of giving chemotherapy followed by radiation therapy evolved, making it possible to save the voice box in about 75 percent of patients. The jump to 88 percent now means that many more patients will have an improved quality of life, she said.

However, one disadvantage to concurrent chemotherapy and radiation therapy is the high number and severity of side effects, said Gregory T. Wolf, M.D., a surgeon from the University of Michigan. Appointed to discuss the study following its presentation, Wolf pointed out that 80 percent of the patients who received radiation and chemotherapy together experienced moderate to severe side effects. He also emphasized that there was no survival benefit to using the more toxic therapy.

Wolf recommended continued study to find the optimum ways to improve survival, larynx preservation, and quality of life in patients with laryngeal cancer.

Chemo Drug Shows Preclinical Promise against Head and Neck Cancer

A hallmark of cancer cells is that their internal wiring has been modified to prompt their abnormal growth. This has led some cancer researchers to suspect the most effective chemotherapeutic drugs might be those that target proteins influencing not one but multiple wires within the tumor cells. One such protein is called heat shock protein 90, or Hsp90, a so-called molecular chaperone that helps to fold various cancer-causing proteins into their proper three-dimensional configurations. Studies indicate Hsp90 is present at two- to tenfold higher levels in tumor cells than in normal cells. They also show Hsp90 is found in tumor cells in a distinct molecular form that has a one-hundred-fold higher affinity for ansamycin antibiotics, natural compounds that microbes produce to protect themselves from disease-causing substances, than the Hsp90 present in normal cells. The challenge has been to synthesize an ansamycin-derived compound that kills tumor cells but that also is relatively straightforward to formulate. In the May 15, 2005, issue of the journal *Clinical Cancer Research*, National Institute of Dental and Craniofacial Research (NIDCR) grantees report promising early results with such a compound called EC5 [E-cadherin-5]. It is a novel dimerized, or two-headed, form of geldanamycin, an ansamycin-derived compound. As reported in their paper, EC5 proved more effective at inhibiting the growth of eight head and neck cancer cell lines than the related compound 17-AAG [17-(Allylamino)-17-demethoxy-geldanamycin], which is already in clinical trials. In addition, EC5 shrunk a type of head and neck tumor in mice that 17-AAG proved ineffective against. As the scientists noted, "EC5 is one of the most active of a series of divalent Hsp90 inhibitors and the length and flexibility of the linker between the two geldanamycin pharmacores is critical to potency of EC5 and other highly active dimers."

Docetaxel (Taxotere®) Before Radiation Extends Survival in Patients with Head and Neck Cancer

Summary: In a phase III study of patients with inoperable head and neck cancer, a multidrug chemotherapy regimen including the drug docetaxel (Taxotere®) that was given before radiation extended patients' survival by about four months, with fewer side effects, compared to standard therapy.

Source: American Society of Clinical Oncology annual meeting, New Orleans, June 5, 2004.

Background: Head and neck cancers account for 3 percent of all cancers in the United States. Most of these cancers begin in squamous cells found in the lining of structures in the head and neck. Initial treatment options for most patients with head and neck cancer include surgery and/or radiation or, for patients with advanced tumors, chemotherapy combined with radiation.

Patients are sometimes given chemotherapy before other treatment, when it is thought that giving the drugs first may improve the effectiveness of the treatment that follows. This strategy is known as neoadjuvant chemotherapy. For patients with inoperable head and neck cancer, however, previous studies have not identified a neoadjuvant chemotherapy regimen that extended patients' lives.

The Study: This study involved 358 patients with inoperable head and neck cancer whose tumors had spread to lymph nodes in the neck. Patients were randomly assigned to receive standard chemotherapy with the drugs cisplatin and 5-fluorouracil or the same chemotherapy plus docetaxel. After chemotherapy, both groups of patients also received standard radiation therapy.

The European Organization for Research and Treatment of Cancer conducted the study. The principal investigator was Jan B. Vermorken, M.D., Ph.D., of the University of Antwerp in Belgium.

Results: After a median follow-up period of 32 months, patients treated with docetaxel survived for a median of 18.6 months, compared with 14.5 months for patients who received the standard platinum-based chemotherapy. In addition, patients in the docetaxel group lived for a median of 12.7 months before their disease progressed, compared with 8.4 months for standard-therapy patients. More patients in the docetaxel group than in the standard therapy group (67.8 percent vs. 53.6 percent) responded to treatment.

Fewer patients treated with docetaxel suffered side effects such as nausea, vomiting, and stomatitis (mouth sores). In addition, fewer patients in the docetaxel group died from adverse reactions to chemotherapy.

Comments: Previous randomized trials involving patients with advanced head and neck cancer have suggested that chemotherapy is most effective when administered concurrently with (at the same time as) radiation, notes Scott Saxman, M.D., of the National Cancer Institute's Cancer Therapy Evaluation Program. Further study will be necessary, he says, to determine whether adding docetaxel concurrently with platinum-based chemotherapy and radiation is feasible and, perhaps, even more beneficial.

Zinc Deficiency Linked to Increased Risk of Less–Common Form of Esophageal Cancer

Researchers at the National Cancer Institute (NCI), part of the National Institutes of Health, have found that zinc deficiency in humans is associated with an increased risk of developing esophageal squamous cell carcinoma, an often-fatal form of esophageal cancer that has about seven thousand cases a year. NCI researchers used a novel approach to measure the concentration of zinc and other elements directly in the esophageal tissue. Their results, appearing in the February 15, 2005, *Journal of the National Cancer Institute*, showed an inverse relationship between tissue zinc concentration and subsequent risk of esophageal squamous cell carcinoma.

Dietary deficiency of zinc, an essential mineral, has been associated with esophageal cancer in rodents. So far, though, examining this association in humans has been hampered by the difficulty of measuring zinc levels in the body through traditional methods. "Measuring zinc levels in the blood is not very sensitive," noted lead author Christian Abnet, Ph.D., of NCI's Cancer Prevention Studies Branch. "Because zinc is maintained in a state of equilibrium, just like body temperature, the readings will tend to be similar. Calculating zinc from intake of meat and other dietary sources isn't very sensitive either since other compounds, like phytates in whole grains, will inhibit zinc absorption."

Abnet turned to a different technique: x-ray fluorescence spectroscopy, which involves bombarding a sample with high-intensity x-rays, causing the elements in the sample to fluoresce, or glow, with a characteristic energy signature. "This allowed us to measure element concentrations directly in the tissue of interest," said Abnet, "so it should be the best indicator of the effects of zinc or other metals."

Esophageal tissue samples were obtained from a population in Linzhou, China, that was followed from 1985 through 2001. People in this region are at high risk for squamous esophageal cancer and tend to consume little meat and a lot of whole grain, and therefore are more likely to be zinc deficient. An earlier publication estimated that residents of this region get only 62 to 72 percent of the U.S. dietary recommendations for zinc, whereas most Americans meet current dietary recommendation levels.

A subset of the population underwent endoscopy with biopsy in 1985, and the NCI team, with the aid of Barry Lai, Ph.D., at Argonne National Laboratories, in Argonne, Illinois, examined these specimens. They measured zinc, copper, iron, nickel, and sulfur levels in samples from sixty subjects who developed esophageal squamous cell carcinoma during the sixteen-year follow-up and from seventy-two histology-matched subjects at the start of the study who did not develop the disease.

The average tissue zinc concentration was significantly lower in subjects who developed esophageal cancer than in control subjects (44 ng/cm2 compared to 57 ng/cm2). When the researchers ranked the study participants by quartiles based on zinc concentration, they found that those in the highest quartile had a fivefold lower risk of developing esophageal cancer than those in the lowest quartile. Overall, 90 percent of subjects in the highest quartile were alive and cancer-free after sixteen years, while only 65 percent of the subjects in the lowest quartile were alive and cancer-free. There were no consistent associations with cancer risk for any of the other elements studied.

These findings establish an initial connection between zinc and esophageal squamous cell carcinoma in humans, although further research is needed to ensure this association is more than a local phenomenon in an area of extreme zinc deficiency. However, Abnet believes the technique itself holds great promise for future element studies. "X-ray fluorescence spectroscopy has many advantages," said Abnet. "You can apply it to most elements and you only need a tiny tissue sample. Also, it doesn't damage the tissue, so you can make multiple measurements on one sample." Abnet also noted that they successfully measured samples collected and embedded in paraffin in 1985, demonstrating that other researchers could apply this technique to archived tissue samples.

Reference

Christian C. Abnet, Barry Lai, You-Lin Qiao, Stefan Vogt, Xian-Mao Luo, Philip R. Taylor, Zhi-Wei Dong, Steven D. Mark, Sanford M. Dawsey. Zinc concentration in esophageal biopsy specimens measured by x-ray fluorescence and esophageal cancer risk. *Journal of the National Cancer Institute*, 2005; February 16, 2005, 97(4).

Part Seven

Additional Help
and Information

Chapter 44

Glossary of Terms Related to the Ears, Nose, and Throat

acoustic neurinoma: tumor, usually benign, which may develop on the hearing and balance nerves and can cause gradual hearing loss, tinnitus, and/or dizziness (sometimes called vestibular schwannoma). Also see neurofibromatosis type 2.

acquired deafness: loss of hearing that occurs or develops some time during the lifespan but is not present at birth.

ageusia: loss of the sense of taste.

Alport syndrome: hereditary condition characterized by kidney disease, sensorineural hearing loss, and sometimes eye defects.

American Sign Language (ASL): manual language with its own syntax and grammar, used primarily by people who are deaf.

anosmia: absence of the sense of smell.

aphonia: complete loss of voice.

articulation disorder: inability to correctly produce speech sounds (phonemes) because of imprecise placement, timing, pressure, speed, or flow of movement of the lips, tongue, or throat.

assistive devices: technical tools and devices such as alphabet boards, text telephones, or text-to-speech conversion software used to

Reprinted from National Institute on Deafness and Other Communication Disorders, National Institutes of Health, September 9, 2005.

aid individuals who have communication disorders perform actions, tasks, and activities.

audiologist: health care professional who is trained to evaluate hearing loss and related disorders, including balance (vestibular) disorders and tinnitus, and to rehabilitate individuals with hearing loss and related disorders. An audiologist uses a variety of tests and procedures to assess hearing and balance function and to fit and dispense hearing aids and other assistive devices for hearing.

auditory brainstem response (ABR) test: a test for brain functioning in comatose, unresponsive, etc., patients, and for hearing in infants and young children; involves attaching electrodes to the head to record electrical activity from the hearing nerve and other parts of the brain.

auditory nerve: eighth cranial nerve that connects the inner ear to the brainstem and is responsible for hearing and balance.

auditory perception: ability to identify, interpret, and attach meaning to sound.

auditory prosthesis: device that substitutes or enhances the ability to hear.

augmentative devices: tools that help individuals with limited or absent speech to communicate, such as communication boards, pictographs (symbols that look like the things they represent), or ideographs (symbols representing ideas).

aural rehabilitation: techniques used with people who are hearing impaired to improve their ability to speak and communicate.

autoimmune deafness: individual's immune system produces abnormal antibodies that react against the body's healthy tissues.

balance: biological system that enables individuals to know where their bodies are in the environment and to maintain a desired position. Normal balance depends on information from the labyrinth in the inner ear, from other senses such as sight and touch, and from muscle movement.

balance disorder: disruption in the labyrinth, the inner ear organ that controls the balance system, which allows individuals to know where their bodies are in the environment. The labyrinth works with other systems in the body, such as the visual and skeletal systems, to maintain posture.

barotrauma: injury to the middle ear caused by a reduction of air pressure.

benign paroxysmal positional vertigo (BPPV): balance disorder that results in sudden onset of dizziness, spinning, or vertigo when moving the head.

brainstem implant: auditory prosthesis that bypasses the cochlea and auditory nerve. This type of implant helps individuals who cannot benefit from a cochlear implant because the auditory nerves are not working.

captioning: text display of spoken words, presented on a television or a movie screen, that allows a deaf or hard-of-hearing viewer to follow the dialogue and the action of a program simultaneously.

central auditory processing disorder: inability to differentiate, recognize, or understand sounds; hearing and intelligence are normal.

chemosensory disorders: diseases or problems associated with the sense of smell or the sense of taste.

cholesteatoma: accumulation of dead cells in the middle ear, caused by repeated middle ear infections.

cochlea: snail-shaped structure in the inner ear that contains the organ of hearing.

cochlear implant: medical device that bypasses damaged structures in the inner ear and directly stimulates the auditory nerve, allowing some deaf individuals to learn to hear and interpret sounds and speech.

conductive hearing impairment: hearing loss caused by dysfunction of the outer or middle ear.

cued speech: method of communication that combines speech reading with a system of handshapes placed near the mouth to help deaf or hard-of-hearing individuals differentiate words that look similar on the lips (e.g., bunch vs. punch) or are hidden (e.g., gag).

cytomegalovirus (congenital): one group of herpes viruses that infects humans and can cause a variety of clinical symptoms, including deafness or hearing impairment; infection with the virus may be either before or after birth.

decibel: unit that measures the intensity or loudness of sound.

dizziness: physical unsteadiness, imbalance, and lightheadedness associated with balance disorders.

dysarthria: group of speech disorders caused by disturbances in the strength or coordination of the muscles of the speech mechanism as a result of damage to the brain or nerves.

dysequilibrium: any disturbance of balance.

dysfluency: disruption in the smooth flow or expression of speech.

dysgeusia: distortion or absence of the sense of taste.

dysosmia: distortion or absence of the sense of smell.

dysphagia: difficulty swallowing.

dysphonia: any impairment of the voice or speaking ability.

dyspraxia of speech: in individuals with normal muscle tone and speech muscle coordination, partial loss of the ability to consistently pronounce words.

ear infection: presence and growth of bacteria or viruses in the ear.

ear wax: yellow secretion from glands in the outer ear (cerumen) that keeps the skin of the ear dry and protected from infection.

endolymph: fluid in the labyrinth (the organ of balance located in the inner ear that consists of three semicircular canals and the vestibule).

gustation: act or sensation of tasting.

hair cells: sensory cells of the inner ear, which are topped with hair-like structures, the stereocilia, and which transform the mechanical energy of sound waves into nerve impulses.

haptic sense: sense of physical contact or touch.

haptometer: instrument for measuring sensitivity to touch.

hearing: series of events in which sound waves in the air are converted to electrical signals, which are sent as nerve impulses to the brain, where they are interpreted.

hearing aid: electronic device that brings amplified sound to the ear. A hearing aid usually consists of a microphone, amplifier, and receiver.

hearing disorder: disruption in the normal hearing process that may occur in outer, middle, or inner ear, whereby sound waves are not converted to electrical signals and nerve impulses are not transmitted to the brain to be interpreted.

hereditary hearing impairment: hearing loss passed down through generations of a family.

hoarseness: abnormally rough or harsh-sounding voice caused by vocal abuse and other disorders such as gastroesophageal reflux, thyroid problems, or trauma to the larynx (voice box).

hypogeusia: diminished sensitivity to taste.

hyposmia: diminished sensitivity to smell.

inner ear: part of the ear that contains both the organ of hearing (the cochlea) and the organ of balance (the labyrinth).

Kallmann syndrome: disorder that can include several characteristics such as absence of the sense of smell and decreased functional activity of the gonads (organs that produce sex cells), affecting growth and sexual development.

labyrinth: organ of balance located in the inner ear. The labyrinth consists of three semicircular canals and the vestibule.

labyrinthine hydrops: excessive fluid in the organ of balance (labyrinth); can cause pressure or fullness in the ears, hearing loss, dizziness, and loss of balance.

labyrinthitis: viral or bacterial infection or inflammation of the inner ear that can cause dizziness, loss of balance, and temporary hearing loss.

Landau-Kleffner syndrome: childhood disorder of unknown origin that often extends into adulthood and can be identified by gradual or sudden loss of the ability to understand and use spoken language.

language disorders: any of a number of problems with verbal communication and the ability to use or understand a symbol system for communication.

laryngeal neoplasms: abnormal growths in the larynx (voice box) that can be cancerous or noncancerous.

laryngeal nodules: noncancerous, callous-like growths on the inner parts of the vocal folds (vocal cords); usually caused by vocal abuse or misuse.

laryngeal paralysis: loss of function or feeling of one or both of the vocal folds caused by injury or disease to the nerves of the larynx.

laryngectomy: surgery to remove part or all of the larynx (voice box).

laryngitis: hoarse voice or the complete loss of the voice because of irritation to the vocal folds (vocal cords).

larynx: valve structure between the trachea (windpipe) and the pharynx (the upper throat) that is the primary organ of voice production.

mastoid: back portion of the temporal bone that contains the inner ear.

mastoid surgery: surgical procedure to remove infection from the mastoid bone.

Ménière disease: inner ear disorder that can affect both hearing and balance. It can cause episodes of vertigo, hearing loss, tinnitus, and the sensation of fullness in the ear.

meningitis: inflammation of the meninges, the membranes that envelop the brain and the spinal cord; may cause hearing loss or deafness.

middle ear: part of the ear that includes the eardrum and three tiny bones of the middle ear, ending at the round window that leads to the inner ear.

motion sickness: dizziness, sweating, nausea, vomiting, and generalized discomfort experienced when an individual is in motion.

motor speech disorders: group of disorders caused by the inability to accurately produce speech sounds (phonemes) because of muscle weakness or incoordination or difficulty performing voluntary muscle movements.

neural prostheses: devices that substitute for an injured or diseased part of the nervous system, such as the cochlear implant.

neural stimulation: to activate or energize a nerve through an external source.

neurofibromatosis type 1 (NF-1 von Recklinghausen): group of inherited disorders in which noncancerous tumors grow on several nerves that may include the hearing nerve. The symptoms of NF-1 include coffee-colored spots on the skin, enlargement, deformation of bones, and neurofibromas.

neurofibromatosis type 2 (NF-2): group of inherited disorders in which noncancerous tumors grow on several nerves that usually include the hearing nerve. The symptoms of NF-2 include tumors on the hearing nerve that can affect hearing and balance. NF-2 may occur in the teenage years with hearing loss. Also see acoustic neurinoma.

neurogenic communication disorder: inability to exchange information with others because of hearing, speech, and/or language problems caused by impairment of the nervous system (brain or nerves).

noise-induced hearing loss: hearing loss caused by exposure to harmful sounds, either very loud impulse sound(s) or repeated exposure to sounds over 90-decibel level over an extended period of time that damage the sensitive structures of the inner ear.

nonsyndromic hereditary hearing impairment: hearing loss or deafness that is inherited and is not associated with other inherited clinical characteristics.

odorant: substance that stimulates the sense of smell.

olfaction: the act of smelling.

olfactometer: device for estimating the intensity of the sense of smell.

open-set speech recognition: understanding speech without visual clues (speech reading).

otitis externa: inflammation of the outer part of the ear extending to the auditory canal.

otitis media: inflammation of the middle ear caused by infection.

otoacoustic emissions: low-intensity sounds produced by the inner ear that can be quickly measured with a sensitive microphone placed in the ear canal.

otolaryngologist: physician/surgeon who specializes in diseases of the ears, nose, throat, and head and neck.

otologist: physician/surgeon who specializes in diseases of the ear.

otosclerosis: abnormal growth of bone of the inner ear. This bone prevents structures within the ear from working properly and causes hearing loss. For some people with otosclerosis, the hearing loss may become severe.

ototoxic drugs: drugs such as a special class of antibiotics, aminoglycoside antibiotics, that can damage the hearing and balance organs located in the inner ear for some individuals.

outer ear: external portion of the ear, consisting of the pinna, or auricle, and the ear canal.

papillomavirus: group of viruses that can cause noncancerous wartlike tumors to grow on the surface of skin and internal organs such as the respiratory tract; can be life-threatening.

parosmia: any disease or perversion of the sense of smell, especially the subjective perception of odors that do not exist.

perilymph fistula: leakage of inner ear fluid to the middle ear that occurs without apparent cause or that is associated with head trauma, physical exertion, or barotrauma.

phonology: study of speech sounds.

postlingually deafened: individual who becomes deaf after having acquired language.

prelingually deafened: individual who is either born deaf or who lost his or her hearing early in childhood, before acquiring language.

presbycusis: loss of hearing that gradually occurs because of changes in the inner or middle ear in individuals as they grow older.

round window: membrane separating the middle ear and inner ear.

sensorineural hearing loss: hearing loss caused by damage to the sensory cells and/or nerve fibers of the inner ear.

sign language: method of communication for people who are deaf or hard-of-hearing in which hand movements, gestures, and facial expressions convey thoughts and feelings.

smell: to perceive odor or scent through stimuli affecting the olfactory nerves.

smell disorder: inability to perceive odors. It may be temporary, caused by a head cold or swelling or blockage of the nasal passages. It can be permanent when any part of the olfactory region is damaged by factors such as brain injury, tumor, disease, or chronic rhinitis.

sound vocalization: ability to produce voice.

spasmodic dysphonia: momentary disruption of voice caused by involuntary movements of one or more muscles of the larynx or voice box.

specific language impairment (SLI): difficulty with language or the organized-symbol system used for communication in the absence of problems such as mental retardation, hearing loss, or emotional disorders.

speech disorder: any defect or abnormality that prevents an individual from communicating by means of spoken words. Speech disorders may develop from nerve injury to the brain, muscular paralysis, structural defects, hysteria, or mental retardation.

speech processor: part of a cochlear implant that converts speech sounds into electrical impulses to stimulate the auditory nerve, allowing an individual to understand sound and speech.

speech-language pathologist: health professional trained to evaluate and treat people who have voice, speech, language, or swallowing disorders (including hearing impairment) that affect their ability to communicate.

stuttering: frequent repetition of words or parts of words that disrupts the smooth flow of speech.

sudden deafness: loss of hearing that occurs quickly due to such causes as explosion, a viral infection, or the use of some drugs.

swallowing disorders: any of a group of problems that interferes with the transfer of food from the mouth to the stomach.

syndromic hearing impairment: hearing loss or deafness that, along with other characteristics, is inherited or passed down through generations of a family.

tactile devices: mechanical instruments that make use of touch to help individuals who have certain disabilities, such as deaf-blindness, to communicate.

taste: sensation produced by a stimulus applied to the gustatory nerve endings in the tongue. The four tastes are salt, sour, sweet, and bitter. Some scientists indicate the existence of a fifth taste, described as savory.

taste buds: groups of cells located on the tongue that enable one to recognize different tastes.

taste disorder: inability to perceive different flavors. Taste disorders may result from poor oral hygiene, gum disease, hepatitis, or medicines and chemotherapeutic drugs. Taste disorders may also be neurological.

throat disorders: disorders or diseases of the larynx (voice box), pharynx, or esophagus.

thyroplasty: surgical technique to improve voice by altering the cartilages of the larynx, which houses the vocal folds (vocal cords), in order to change the position or length of the vocal folds. Also known as laryngeal framework surgery.

tinnitus: sensation of a ringing, roaring, or buzzing sound in the ears or head. It is often associated with many forms of hearing impairment and noise exposure.

tongue: large muscle on the floor of the mouth that manipulates food for chewing and swallowing. It is the main organ of taste, and assists in forming speech sounds.

tracheostomy: surgical opening into the trachea (windpipe) to help someone breathe who has an obstruction or swelling in the larynx (voice box) or upper throat or who has had the larynx surgically removed.

tympanoplasty: surgical repair of the eardrum (tympanic membrane) or bones of the middle ear.

Usher syndrome: hereditary disease that affects hearing and vision and sometimes balance.

velocardiofacial syndrome: inherited disorder characterized by cleft palate (opening in the roof of the mouth), heart defects, characteristic facial appearance, minor learning problems, and speech and feeding problems.

vertigo: illusion of movement; a sensation as if the external world were revolving around an individual (objective vertigo) or as if the individual were revolving in space (subjective vertigo).

vestibular neuronitis: infection at the vestibular nerve.

vestibular system: system in the body that is responsible for maintaining balance, posture, and the body's orientation in space. This system also regulates locomotion and other movements and keeps objects in visual focus as the body moves.

vestibule: bony cavity of the inner ear.

vibrotactile aids: mechanical instruments that help individuals who are deaf to detect and interpret sound through the sense of touch.

vocal cord paralysis: inability of one or both vocal folds (vocal cords) to move because of damage to the brain or nerves.

vocal cords (vocal folds): muscularized folds of mucous membrane that extend from the larynx (voice box) wall. The folds are enclosed in elastic vocal ligament and muscle that control the tension and rate of vibration of the cords as air passes through them.

vocal folds: see vocal cords.

vocal tremor: trembling or shaking of one or more of the muscles of the larynx, resulting in an unsteady-sounding voice.

voice: sound produced by air passing out through the larynx and upper respiratory tract.

voice disorders: group of problems involving abnormal pitch, loudness, or quality of the sound produced by the larynx (voice box).

Waardenburg syndrome: hereditary disorder that is characterized by hearing impairment, a white shock of hair and/or distinctive blue color to one or both eyes, and wide-set inner corners of the eyes. Balance problems are also associated with some types of Waardenburg syndrome.

Chapter 45

Ear, Nose, and Throat Disorders: Resources for Information and Support

General Information

American Academy of Otolaryngology-Head and Neck Surgery (AAO-HNS)
One Prince Street
Alexandria, VA 22314-3357
Phone: 703-836-4444
TTY: 703-519-1585
Website: http://www.entnet.org
E-mail: webmaster@entnet.org

American Head and Neck Society
11300 W. Olympic Blvd.
Suite 600
Los Angeles, CA 90064
Phone: 310-437-0559
Fax: 310-437-0585
Website: http://www.ahns.info
E-mail: admin@ahns.info

Massachusetts Eye and Ear Infirmary
243 Charles Street
Boston, MA 02114
Phone: 617-523-7900
TDD: 617-523-5498
Website: http://www.meei.harvard.edu

National Organization for Rare Disorders (NORD)
55 Kenosia Ave., P.O. Box 1968
Danbury, CT 06813-1968
Toll-Free: 800-999-6673
TDD 203-797-9590
Phone: 203-744-0100
Fax: 203-798-2291
Website: http://www.rarediseases.org
E-mail: orphan@rarediseases.org

The information in this chapter was compiled from various sources deemed accurate. All contact information was verified and updated in February 2006. Inclusion does not imply endorsement. This list is intended to serve as a starting point for information gathering; it is not comprehensive.

New York Eye and Ear Infirmary
310 East 14th Street
New York, NY 10003
Phone: 212-979-4000
Website: http://www.nyee.edu

Government Sources

Agency for Healthcare Research and Quality (AHRQ)
540 Gaither Road
Rockville, MD 20850
Clearinghouse Toll-Free:
800-358-9295
Clearinghouse TTY: 888-586-6340
Phone: 301-427-1364
Website: http://www.ahrq.gov
E-mail: info@ahrq.gov

Centers for Disease Control and Prevention (CDC)
1600 Clifton Road, MS D31
Atlanta, GA 30333
Toll-Free: (800) 311-3435
TTY: 800-243-7889
Phone: (404) 639-3311
Website: http://www.cdc.gov
E-mail: cdcinfo@cdc.gov

National Cancer Institute
NCI Public Inquiries Office
6116 Executive Boulevard
Room 3036A
Bethesda, MD 20892-8322
Toll-Free: 800-4-CANCER
800-422-6237
TTY Toll-Free: (800) 332-8615
Website: http://www.cancer.gov
E-mail: cancergovstaff@mail
.nih.gov

National Center on Sleep Disorders Research
Rockledge Two Centre
6701 Rockledge Drive
Suite 10181
Bethesda, MD 20892-7921
Phone: 301-435-0199
Fax: 301-480-3451
Website: http://www.nhlbi
.nih.gov/about/ncsdr

National Heart, Lung, and Blood Institute (NHLBI)
NHLBI Information Center
P.O. Box 30105
Bethesda, MD 20824-0105
Phone: (301) 592-8573
TTY: (240) 629-3255
Fax: (240) 629-3246
Website: http://www
.nhlbi.nih.gov
E-mail: nhlbiinfo@nhlbi.nih.gov

National Institute on Aging Information Center
Building 31C, Room 5C27
31 Center Drive, MSC 2292
Bethesda, MD 20892
Publications Toll-Free:
800-222-2225
Phone: (301) 496-1752
TTY: (800) 222-4225
Fax: (301) 496-1072
Website: http://www.nia.nih.gov
Publications Website: http://
www.niapublications.org
E-mail: niainfo@nia.nih.gov

National Institute of Dental and Craniofacial Research (NIDCR)

National Oral Health
Information Clearinghouse
One NOHIC Way
Bethesda, MD 20892–3500
Phone: 301-402–7364
Fax: 301-480-4098
Website: http://www.nidr.nih.gov
E-mail: nidcrinfo@mail.nih.gov

National Institute of Diabetes and Digestive and Kidney Diseases (NIDDK)

National Institutes of Health
Building 31, Room 9A04
31 Center Drive, MSC 2560
Bethesda, MD 20892-2560
NIDDK Information Clearing-
house Toll-Free: 800-891-5390
Website: http://www.niddk.nih.gov
E-mail: dkwebmaster@extra
.niddk.nih.gov

National Institute on Deafness and Other Communication Disorders NIDCD Clearinghouse

1 Communication Avenue
Bethesda, MD 20892-3456
Toll-Free: 800-241-1044
TTY: 800-241-1055
Fax: 301-770-8977
Website: http://www.nidcd.nih.gov
Website for WISE EARS! A Public
Education Campaign to Prevent
Noise-Induced Hearing Loss:
http://www.nidcd.nih.gov/health/
wise
E-mail: nidcdinfo@nidcd.nih.gov

National Organization for Rare Disorders (NORD)

55 Kenosia Ave., P.O. Box 1968
Danbury, CT 06813-1968
Toll-Free: 800-999-6673
Phone: 203-744-0100
TTY: 203-797-9590
Fax: 203-798-2291
Website: http://www
.rarediseases.org
E-mail: orphan@rarediseases.org

Acoustic Neuroma

Acoustic Neuroma Association (ANA)

600 Peachtree Parkway, Suite 108
Cumming, GA 30041
Phone: 770-205-8211
Fax: 770-205-0239
Website: http://www.anausa.org
E-mail: info@anausa.org

American Hearing Research Foundation

8 South Michigan Avenue
Suite #814
Chicago, IL 60603-4539
Phone: 312-726-9670
Fax: 312-726-9695
Website: http://www
.american-hearing.org
E-mail:
lkoch@american-hearing.org

Neurofibromatosis, Inc. (NF, Inc.)

P.O. Box 18246
Minneapolis, MN 55418
Toll-Free: 800-942-6825
Phone: 301-918-4600
Website: http://www.nfinc.org

Hearing Loss

Alexander Graham Bell Association for the Deaf and Hard of Hearing (AG Bell)
3417 Volta Place, NW
Washington, DC 20007-2778
Toll-Free: 866-337-5220
Phone: 202-337-5220
TTY: 202-337-5221
Fax: 202-337-8314
Website: http://www.agbell.org
E-mail: info@agbell.org

American Academy of Audiology
11730 Plaza America Drive,
Suite 300
Reston, VA 20190
Toll-Free: 800-AAA-2336
Phone: 703-790-8466
Fax: 703-790-8631
Website: http://
www.audiology.org

American Association of the Deaf-Blind (AADB)
8630 Fenton Street
Suite 121
Silver Spring, MD 20910-3803
Phone: 301-495-4403
TTY: 301-495-4402
Fax: 301-495-4404
Website: http://www.aadb.org
E-mail: AADB-info@aadb.org

American Hearing Research Foundation
8 South Michigan Avenue
Suite #814
Chicago, IL 60603-4539
Phone: 312-726-9670
Fax: 312-726-9695
Website:
http://www.american-hearing.org
E-mail:
lkoch@american-hearing.org

American Society for Deaf Children (ASDC)
3820 Hartzdale Drive
Camp Hill, PA 17011
Toll-Free: 866-895-4206 (V/TTY)
Parent Hotline:
800-942-ASDC (2732)
Phone: 717-703-0073
Fax: 717-909-5599
Website: http://www
.deafchildren.org
E-mail: ASDC4U@aol.com

American Speech-Language-Hearing Association
10801 Rockville Pike
Rockville, MA 20852
Toll-Free: 800-638-8255
Phone: 301-897-8682
Fax: 301-571-0457
Website: http://www.asha.org
E-mail: actioncenter@asha.org

Association of Late-Deafened Adults

ALDA Inc.
8038 Macintosh Lane
Rockford, IL 61107
Toll-Free:
866-402-ALDA (2532) (V/TTY)
Phone: 815-332-1515
Website: http://www.alda.org

Beginnings for Parents of Hearing Impaired Children, Inc.

P.O. Box 17646
Raleigh, NC 27619
Phone: 919-850-2746 (V/TTY)
Website: http://www.ncbegin.com
E-mail: ncbegin.org

Better Hearing Institute (BHI)

515 King Street
Suite 420
Alexandria, VA 22314
Toll-Free: 888-432-7435
Helpline:
800-EAR-WELL (327-9355)
Phone: 703-684-3391
Fax: 703-684-6048
Website: http://www
.betterhearing.org
E-mail: mail@betterhearing.org

Clerc National Deaf Education Center

Office of Publications and
Information Dissemination
800 Florida Avenue, NE
Washington, DC 20002
Phone: 202-651-5051 (V/TTY)
Fax: 202-651-5708
Website: http://clerccenter
.gallaudet.edu
E-mail: clearinghouse.infotogo
@gallaudet.edu

Boys Town National Research Hospital (BTNRH)

555 North 30th Street
Omaha, NE 68131
Phone: 402-498-6511
TTY: 402-498-6543
Websites:
http://www.boystownhospital.org
http://www.babyhearing.org

Deafness and Family Communication Center

Children's Hospital of
Philadelphia
3440 Market St., 4th floor
Philadelphia, PA 19104
Phone: 215-590-7440
TTY: 215-590-6817
Fax: 215-590-1335
Website: http://www
.raisingdeafkids.org
E-mail: bainl@email.chop.edu

Deafness Research Foundation (DRF) and the World Council on Hearing Health (WCHH)
2801 M Street, NW
Washington, DC 20007
Toll-Free: 866-454-3924
Phone: 202-719-8088
TTY: 888-435-6104
Fax: 202-338-8182
Websites:
http://www.drf.org
http://www.wchh.com
http://www.hearinghealthmag.com
E-mail: info@drf.org

EAR Foundation
955 Woodland Street
Nashville, TN 37206
Toll-Free: 800-545-4327 (V/TDD)
Phone: 615-627-2724 (V/TDD)
Fax: 615-627-2728
Websites:
http://www.earfoundation.org
http://www.seniorears.org
E-mail: info@earfoundation.org

Harvard Medical School Center for Hereditary Deafness
Laboratory for Molecular Medicine
65 Landsdowne Street
Cambridge, MA 02139
Phone: 617-768-8291
Fax: 617-768-8513
Website:
http://hearing.harvard.edu
E-mail:
hearing@hms.harvard.edu

HealthyHearing.com
5282 Medical Drive
Suite 150
San Antonio, TX 78229
Toll-Free: 800-567-1692
Fax: 210-615-6832
Website:
http://www.healthyhearing.com

HEAR NOW
6700 Washington Avenue S.
Eden Prairie, MN 55344
Toll-Free: 800-769-2799
Fax: 952-828-6946
Website: http://www
.sotheworldmayhear.org
E-mail: joanita
@sotheworldmayhear.org

House Ear Institute
2100 W. Third Street, 5th Floor
Los Angeles, CA 90057
Toll-Free: 800-388-8612
Phone: 213-483-4431
TDD: 213-483-2642
Fax: 213-483-8789
Website: http://www.hei.org
E-mail: webmaster@hei.org

League for the Hard of Hearing
50 Broadway, 6th Floor
New York, NY 10004
Phone: 917-305-7700
TTY: 917-305-7999
Fax: 917-305-7888
Website: http://www.lhh.org
E-mail: info@lhh.org

National Association of the Deaf (NAD)
814 Thayer Avenue
Suite 250
Silver Spring, MD 20910-4500
Phone: 301-587-1788
TTY: 301-587-1789
Fax: 301-587-1791
Website: http://www.nad.org
E-mail: nadinfo@nad.org

National Black Association for Speech-Language and Hearing (NBASLH)
800 Perry Hwy., Suite 3
Pittsburgh, PA 15229
Phone: 412-366-1177
Fax: 412-366-8804
Website: http://www.nbaslh.org
E-mail: NBASLH@nbaslh.org

National Cued Speech Association (NCSA), Deaf Children's Literacy Project
23970 Hermitage Road
Cleveland, OH 44122-4008
Toll-Free: 800-459-3529 (V/TTY)
Phone: 216-292-6213 (V/TTY)
Website: http://www
.cuedspeech.org
E-mail: info@cuedspeech.com

National Family Association for Deaf-Blind (NFADB)
141 Middle Neck Road
Sands Point, NY 11050
Toll-Free: 800-255-0411
Fax: 516-767-1738
Website: http://www.nfadb.org
E-mail: NFADB@aol.com

National Information Clearinghouse on Children Who Are Deaf-Blind (DB-LINK)
345 N. Monmouth Avenue
Monmouth, OR 97361
Toll-Free: 800-438-9376
TTY: 800-854-7013
Fax: 503-838-8150
Website: http://www.dblink.org
E-mail: dblink@tr.wou.edu

SEE Center for the Advancement of Deaf Children
P.O. Box 1181
Los Alamitos, CA 90720
Phone/TTY: 562-430-1467
Fax: 562-795-6614
Website: http://www.seecenter.org
E-mail: seecenter@seecenter.org

Self Help for Hard of Hearing People
7910 Woodmont Ave, Suite 1200
Bethesda, MD 20814
Phone: 301-657-2248
TTY: 301-657-2249
Fax: 301-913-9413
Website: http://
www.hearingloss.org
E-mail: info@hearingloss.org

Tracy (John) Clinic
806 W. Adams Blvd.
Los Angeles, CA 90007-2505
Toll-Free: 800-522-4582
Phone: 213-748-5481
TTY: 213-747-2924
Fax: 213-749-1651
Website: http://www.jtc.org
E-mail: bhecht@jtc.org

Laryngeal Papillomatosis

International Recurrent Respiratory Papillomatosis (RRP) Information, Service, and Advocacy Center
International RRP ISA Center
P.O. Box 4330
Bellingham, WA 98227
Phone: 360-756-8185
Website: http://www
.rrpwebsite.org
E-mail:
webmaster@rrpwebsite.org

Recurrent Respiratory Papillomatosis Foundation (RRPF)
Phone: 609-530-1443
Website: http://www.rrpf.org

Nasal and Sinus Disorders

American Academy of Allergy, Asthma and Immunology
555 E. Wells Street, Suite 1100
Milwaukee, WI 53202-3823
Toll-Free: 800-822-2762
Phone: 414-272-6071
Fax: 414-272-6070
Website: http://www.aaaai.org
E-mail: info@aaaai.org

American College of Allergy, Asthma and Immunology
85 West Algonquin Road
Suite 550
Arlington Heights, IL 60005
Phone: 847-427-1200
Website: http://www.acaai.org
E-mail: mail@acaai.org

American Rhinologic Society
9 Sunset Terrace
Warwick, NY 10990
Phone: 845-988-1631
Fax: 845-986-1527
Website: http://www
.american-rhinologic.org
E-mail: arsinfo@
american-rhinologic.org

Joint Council of Allergy, Asthma, and Immunology
50 N. Brockway
Suite 3-3
Palatine, IL 60067
Phone: 847-934-1918
Website: http://www.jcaai.org
E-mail: info@jcaai.org

Sleep Apnea

American Sleep Apnea Association
1424 K Street NW
Suite 302
Washington, DC 20005
Phone: 202-293-3650
Fax: 202-293-3656
Website: http://
www.sleepapnea.org
E-mail: asaa@sleepapnea.org

Apnea Patients' News, Education and Awareness Network
Website: http://
www.apneanet.org
E-mail:
webmaster@apneanet.org

National Center on Sleep Disorders Research

Rockledge Two Centre
6701 Rockledge Drive
Suite 10181
Bethesda, MD 20892-7921
Phone: 301-435-0199
Fax: 301-480-3451
Website: http://www
.nhlbi.nih.gov/about/ncsdr

National Sleep Foundation

1522 K Street NW
Suite 500
Washington, DC 20005
Phone: 202-347-3471
Website: http://
www.sleepfoundation.org
E-mail: nsf@sleepfoundation.org

Smell and Taste Disorders

Monell Chemical Senses Center

3500 Market Street
Philadelphia, PA 19104-3308
Phone: 215-898-6666
Fax: 215-898-2084
Website: http://www.monell.org
E-mail: mcsc@monell.org

Rocky Mountain Taste and Smell Center (RMTSC)

University of Colorado Health
Sciences Center
4200 East Ninth Avenue
Box B205
Denver, CO 80262
Phone: 303-315-6600
Fax: 303-315-8787

State University of New York (SUNY) Smell and Taste Disorders Clinic

750 East Adams Street
Syracuse, NY 13210
Phone: 315-464-5588
Fax: 315-464-7712
Website: http://www.upstate
.edu/ent/smelltaste.shtml
E-mail:
kurtzd@mail.upstate.edu

University of Pennsylvania Smell and Taste Center

3400 Spruce Street
Ravdin Bldg., 5th Floor
Philadelphia, PA 19104
Phone: 215-662-6580
Fax: 215-349-5266
Website: http://www.med
.upenn.edu/stc

Spasmodic Dysphonia

National Spasmodic Dysphonia Association, Inc. (NSDA)

300 Park Blvd.
Suite 350
Itasca, IL 60143
Toll-Free: 800-795-NSDA (6732)
Fax: 630-250-4505
Website: http://www
.dysphonia.org
E-mail: NSDA@dysphonia.org

Tinnitus

American Tinnitus Association National Headquarters
P.O. Box 5
Portland, OR 97207-0005
Toll-Free: 800-634-8978
Phone: 503-248-9985
Fax: 503-248-0024
Website: http://www.ata.org
E-mail: tinnitus@ata.org

Vestibular Disorders

Vestibular Disorders Association
P.O. Box 13305
Portland, OR 97213-0305
Toll-Free: 800-837-8428
Phone: 503-229-7705
Fax: 503-229-8064
Website: http://www
.vestibular.org
E-mail: veda@vestibular.org

Vocal Disorders

American Academy of Otolaryngic Allergy
1990 M Street, NW, Suite 680
Washington, DC 20036
Phone: 202-955-5010
Fax: 202-955-5016
Website: http://www.aaoaf.org
E-mail: info@aaoaf.org

American Laryngological Association (ALA)
OtoRhinoLaryngology-Head and Neck Surgery
3400 Bainbridge Ave., 3rd Floor
Bronx, NY 10467-2490
Phone: 718-920-2991
Fax: 718-405-9014
Website: http://www.alahns.org

National Center for Voice and Speech (NCVS)
NCVS, The Denver Center for the Performing Arts
1101 13th Street
Denver, CO 80204
Phone: 303-446-4834
Fax: 303-893-6487
Website: http://www.ncvs.org
E-mail:
NCVSWebmaster@dcpa.org

Voice Foundation
1721 Pine Street
Philadelphia, PA 19103
Phone: 215-735-7999
Fax: 215-735-9293
Website: http://
www.voicefoundation.org
E-mail:
office@voicefoundation.org

Index

Index

Page numbers followed by 'n' indicate a footnote. Page numbers in *italics* indicate a table or illustration.

601

hyposmia
  defined 581
  described 397
HZ *see* hertz

I

ibuprofen 257, 412
ideographs, described 578
IEDCS *see* inner ear
  decompression sickness
IgE *see* immunoglobulin E
immune system
  deafness 578
  otitis media 23
  sudden deafness 147
immunoglobulin E (IgE),
  allergic reactions 342–43, 351
immunotherapy
  allergies 356
  rhinitis 337
implants, brainstem 579
implosive mechanism theory 55
IMRT *see* intensity-modulated
  radiation therapy
incus (anvil)
  described 5–6, 22, 71, 136
  noise-induced hearing loss 158
infants
  air travel 57, 59
  hearing tests 96–98
infections
  adenoids 427–28
  alternative treatments 38–46
  balance 287
  balance disorders 227–28
  bone-anchored hearing aids 183
  chronic middle ear 29–32
  cochlear implants 188, 199–204
  ear examinations 7–8
  ear plugs 162–63
  ear tubes 26, 34–37
  labyrinthitis 164
  mastoiditis 33–34
  middle ear 29–32, 48
  otitis media 22–28, 583
  post-nasal drip 339
  sore throat 410–12

infections, continued
  strep throat 413–16
  swimmer's ear 18–21
  see also sinusitis
infectious rhinitis, described 333
inner ear
  air pressure 58
  balance disorder 226
  barotrauma 55
  defined 581
  described 6, 123, 136
  dizziness 286
  see also cochlea; labyrinth
inner ear decompression sickness
  (IEDCS), described 53–54
insects, ear emergencies 62
insurance coverage
  botulinum toxin 462
  cochlear implants 192–94
  hearing aids 139
  nasal endoscopy 322
  otoplasty 16
  rhinoplasty 372
intensity-modulated radiation
  therapy (IMRT), nasopharyngeal
  cancer 510
International Recurrent Respiratory
  Papillomatosis (RRP) Information,
  Service, and Advocacy Center,
  contact information 596
in-the-ear hearing aids,
  described 178
intonation, described 207
inverting papilloma, described 514
ipratropium bromide 337
irritants
  laryngitis 433
  rhinitis 335
Isordil 453

J

JCAAI *see* Joint Council of Allergy,
  Asthma, and Immunology
"Jervell and Lange-Nielsen
  Syndrome" (NIH) 115n
Jervell and Lange-Nielsen syndrome,
  described 104, 116–17

622

Health Reference Series
COMPLETE CATALOG

List price $87 per volume. **School and library price $78 per volume.**

Adolescent Health Sourcebook, 2nd Edition

Basic Consumer Health Information about the Physical, Mental, and Emotional Growth and Development of Adolescents, Including Medical Care, Nutritional and Physical Activity Requirements, Puberty, Sexual Activity, Acne, Tanning, Body Piercing, Common Physical Illnesses and Disorders, Eating Disorders, Attention Deficit Hyperactivity Disorder, Depression, Bullying, Hazing, and Adolescent Injuries Related to Sports, Driving, and Work

Along with Substance Abuse Information about Nicotine, Alcohol, and Drug Use, a Glossary, and Directory of Additional Resources

Edited by Joyce Brennfleck Shannon. 650 pages. 2006. 0-7808-0943-2.

"It is written in clear, nontechnical language aimed at general readers. . . . Recommended for public libraries, community colleges, and other agencies serving health care consumers."
— *American Reference Books Annual, 2003*

"Recommended for school and public libraries. Parents and professionals dealing with teens will appreciate the easy-to-follow format and the clearly written text. This could become a 'must have' for every high school teacher." — *E-Streams, Jan '03*

"A good starting point for information related to common medical, mental, and emotional concerns of adolescents." — *School Library Journal, Nov '02*

"This book provides accurate information in an easy to access format. It addresses topics that parents and caregivers might not be aware of and provides practical, useable information."
— *Doody's Health Sciences Book Review Journal, Sep-Oct '02*

"Recommended reference source."
— *Booklist, American Library Association, Sep '02*

AIDS Sourcebook, 3rd Edition

Basic Consumer Health Information about Acquired Immune Deficiency Syndrome (AIDS) and Human Immunodeficiency Virus (HIV) Infection, Including Facts about Transmission, Prevention, Diagnosis, Treatment, Opportunistic Infections, and Other Complications, with a Section for Women and Children, Including Details about Associated Gynecological Concerns, Pregnancy, and Pediatric Care

Along with Updated Statistical Information, Reports on Current Research Initiatives, a Glossary, and Directories of Internet, Hotline, and Other Resources

Edited by Dawn D. Matthews. 664 pages. 2003. 0-7808-0631-X.

"The 3rd edition of the *AIDS Sourcebook*, part of Omnigraphics' *Health Reference Series*, is a welcome update. . . . This resource is highly recommended for academic and public libraries."
— *American Reference Books Annual, 2004*

"Excellent sourcebook. This continues to be a highly recommended book. There is no other book that provides as much information as this book provides."
— *AIDS Book Review Journal, Dec-Jan '00*

"Recommended reference source."
— *Booklist, American Library Association, Dec '99*

Alcoholism Sourcebook, 2nd Edition

Basic Consumer Health Information about Alcohol Use, Abuse, and Dependence, Featuring Facts about the Physical, Mental, and Social Health Effects of Alcohol Addiction, Including Alcoholic Liver Disease, Pancreatic Disease, Cardiovascular Disease, Neurological Disorders, and the Effects of Drinking during Pregnancy

Along with Information about Alcohol Treatment, Medications, and Recovery Programs, in Addition to Tips for Reducing the Prevalence of Underage Drinking, Statistics about Alcohol Use, a Glossary of Related Terms, and Directories of Resources for More Help and Information

Edited by Amy L. Sutton. 625 pages. 2006. 0-7808-0942-4.

"This title is one of the few reference works on alcoholism for general readers. For some readers this will be a welcome complement to the many self-help books on the market. Recommended for collections serving general readers and consumer health collections."
— *E-Streams, Mar '01*

"This book is an excellent choice for public and academic libraries."
— *American Reference Books Annual, 2001*

"Recommended reference source."
— *Booklist, American Library Association, Dec '00*

"Presents a wealth of information on alcohol use and abuse and its effects on the body and mind, treatment, and prevention." — *SciTech Book News, Dec '00*

"Important new health guide which packs in the latest consumer information about the problems of alcoholism." — *Reviewer's Bookwatch, Nov '00*

SEE ALSO *Drug Abuse Sourcebook, Substance Abuse Sourcebook*

633

Allergies Sourcebook, 2nd Edition

Basic Consumer Health Information about Allergic Disorders, Triggers, Reactions, and Related Symptoms, Including Anaphylaxis, Rhinitis, Sinusitis, Asthma, Dermatitis, Conjunctivitis, and Multiple Chemical Sensitivity

Along with Tips on Diagnosis, Prevention, and Treatment, Statistical Data, a Glossary, and a Directory of Sources for Further Help and Information

Edited by Annemarie S. Muth. 598 pages. 2002. 0-7808-0376-0.

"This book brings a great deal of useful material together. . . . This is an excellent addition to public and consumer health library collections."
— *American Reference Books Annual, 2003*

"This second edition would be useful to laypersons with little or advanced knowledge of the subject matter. This book would also serve as a resource for nursing and other health care professions students. It would be useful in public, academic, and hospital libraries with consumer health collections." — *E-Streams, Jul '02*

Alternative Medicine Sourcebook

SEE Complementary & Alternative Medicine Sourcebook, 3rd Edition

Alzheimer's Disease Sourcebook, 3rd Edition

Basic Consumer Health Information about Alzheimer's Disease, Other Dementias, and Related Disorders, Including Multi-Infarct Dementia, AIDS Dementia Complex, Dementia with Lewy Bodies, Huntington's Disease, Wernicke-Korsakoff Syndrome (Alcohol-Reated Dementia), Delirium, and Confusional States

Along with Information for People Newly Diagnosed with Alzheimer's Disease and Caregivers, Reports Detailing Current Research Efforts in Prevention, Diagnosis, and Treatment, Facts about Long-Term Care Issues, and Listings of Sources for Additional Information

Edited by Karen Bellenir. 645 pages. 2003. 0-7808-0666-2.

"This very informative and valuable tool will be a great addition to any library serving consumers, students and health care workers."
— *American Reference Books Annual, 2004*

"This is a valuable resource for people affected by dementias such as Alzheimer's. It is easy to navigate and includes important information and resources."
— *Doody's Review Service, Feb '04*

"Recommended reference source."
— *Booklist, American Library Association, Oct '99*

SEE ALSO Brain Disorders Sourcebook

Arthritis Sourcebook, 2nd Edition

Basic Consumer Health Information about Osteoarthritis, Rheumatoid Arthritis, Other Rheumatic Disorders, Infectious Forms of Arthritis, and Diseases with Symptoms Linked to Arthritis, Featuring Facts about Diagnosis, Pain Management, and Surgical Therapies

Along with Coping Strategies, Research Updates, a Glossary, and Resources for Additional Help and Information

Edited by Amy L. Sutton. 593 pages. 2004. 0-7808-0667-0.

"This easy-to-read volume is recommended for consumer health collections within public or academic libraries." —*E-Streams, May '05*

"As expected, this updated edition continues the excellent reputation of this series in providing sound, usable health information. . . . Highly recommended."
— *American Reference Books Annual, 2005*

"Excellent reference." — *The Bookwatch, Jan '05*

Asthma Sourcebook, 2nd Edition

Basic Consumer Health Information about the Causes, Symptoms, Diagnosis, and Treatment of Asthma in Infants, Children, Teenagers, and Adults, Including Facts about Different Types of Asthma, Common Co-Occurring Conditions, Asthma Management Plans, Triggers, Medications, and Medication Delivery Devices

Along with Asthma Statistics, Research Updates, a Glossary, a Directory of Asthma-Related Resources, and More

Edited by Karen Bellenir. 609 pages. 2006. 0-7808-0866-5.

"A worthwhile reference acquisition for public libraries and academic medical libraries whose readers desire a quick introduction to the wide range of asthma information." — *Choice, Association of College & Research Libraries, Jun '01*

"Recommended reference source."
— *Booklist, American Library Association, Feb '01*

"Highly recommended." — *The Bookwatch, Jan '01*

"There is much good information for patients and their families who deal with asthma daily."
— *American Medical Writers Association Journal, Winter '01*

"This informative text is recommended for consumer health collections in public, secondary school, and community college libraries and the libraries of universities with a large undergraduate population."
— *American Reference Books Annual, 2001*

Attention Deficit Disorder Sourcebook

Basic Consumer Health Information about Attention Deficit/Hyperactivity Disorder in Children and Adults, Including Facts about Causes, Symptoms, Diagnostic Criteria, and Treatment Options Such as Medications, Behavior Therapy, Coaching, and Homeopathy

Along with Reports on Current Research Initiatives, Legal Issues, and Government Regulations, and Featuring a Glossary of Related Terms, Internet Resources, and a List of Additional Reading Material

Edited by Dawn D. Matthews. 470 pages. 2002. 0-7808-0624-7.

"Recommended reference source."
— Booklist, American Library Association, Jan '03

"This book is recommended for all school libraries and the reference or consumer health sections of public libraries." — American Reference Books Annual, 2003

■

Back & Neck Sourcebook, 2nd Edition

Basic Consumer Health Information about Spinal Pain, Spinal Cord Injuries, and Related Disorders, Such as Degenerative Disk Disease, Osteoarthritis, Scoliosis, Sciatica, Spina Bifida, and Spinal Stenosis, and Featuring Facts about Maintaining Spinal Health, Self-Care, Pain Management, Rehabilitative Care, Chiropractic Care, Spinal Surgeries, and Complementary Therapies

Along with Suggestions for Preventing Back and Neck Pain, a Glossary of Related Terms, and a Directory of Resources

Edited by Amy L. Sutton. 633 pages. 2004. 0-7808-0738-3.

"Recommended . . . an easy to use, comprehensive medical reference book." — E-Streams, Sep '05

"The strength of this work is its basic, easy-to-read format. Recommended." — Reference and User Services Quarterly, American Library Association, Winter '97

■

Blood & Circulatory Disorders Sourcebook, 2nd Edition

Basic Consumer Health Information about the Blood and Circulatory System and Related Disorders, Such as Anemia and Other Hemoglobin Diseases, Cancer of the Blood and Associated Bone Marrow Disorders, Clotting and Bleeding Problems, and Conditions That Affect the Veins, Blood Vessels, and Arteries, Including Facts about the Donation and Transplantation of Bone Marrow, Stem Cells, and Blood and Tips for Keeping the Blood and Circulatory System Healthy

Along with a Glossary of Related Terms and Resources for Additional Help and Information

Edited by Amy L. Sutton. 659 pages. 2005. 0-7808-0746-4.

"Highly recommended pick for basic consumer health reference holdings at all levels."
— The Bookwatch, Aug '05

"Recommended reference source."
—Booklist, American Library Association, Feb '99

"An important reference sourcebook written in simple language for everyday, non-technical users. "
— Reviewer's Bookwatch, Jan '99

Brain Disorders Sourcebook, 2nd Edition

Basic Consumer Health Information about Acquired and Traumatic Brain Injuries, Infections of the Brain, Epilepsy and Seizure Disorders, Cerebral Palsy, and Degenerative Neurological Disorders, Including Amyotrophic Lateral Sclerosis (ALS), Dementias, Multiple Sclerosis, and More

Along with Information on the Brain's Structure and Function, Treatment and Rehabilitation Options, Reports on Current Research Initiatives, a Glossary of Terms Related to Brain Disorders and Injuries, and a Directory of Sources for Further Help and Information

Edited by Sandra J. Judd. 625 pages. 2005. 0-7808-0744-8.

"Highly recommended pick for basic consumer health reference holdings at all levels."
—The Bookwatch, Aug '05

"Belongs on the shelves of any library with a consumer health collection." — E-Streams, Mar '00

"Recommended reference source."
— Booklist, American Library Association, Oct '99

SEE ALSO Alzheimer's Disease Sourcebook

■

Breast Cancer Sourcebook, 2nd Edition

Basic Consumer Health Information about Breast Cancer, Including Facts about Risk Factors, Prevention, Screening and Diagnostic Methods, Treatment Options, Complementary and Alternative Therapies, Post-Treatment Concerns, Clinical Trials, Special Risk Populations, and New Developments in Breast Cancer Research

Along with Breast Cancer Statistics, a Glossary of Related Terms, and a Directory of Resources for Additional Help and Information

Edited by Sandra J. Judd. 595 pages. 2004. 0-7808-0668-9.

"This book will be an excellent addition to public, community college, medical, and academic libraries."
— American Reference Books Annual, 2006

"It would be a useful reference book in a library or on loan to women in a support group."
— Cancer Forum, Mar '03

"Recommended reference source."
— Booklist, American Library Association, Jan '02

"This reference source is highly recommended. It is quite informative, comprehensive and detailed in nature, and yet it offers practical advice in easy-to-read language. It could be thought of as the 'bible' of breast cancer for the consumer." — E-Streams, Jan '02

"From the pros and cons of different screening methods and results to treatment options, Breast Cancer Sourcebook provides the latest information on the subject."
— Library Bookwatch, Dec '01

"This thoroughgoing, very readable reference covers all aspects of breast health and cancer. . . . Readers will find

635

much to consider here. Recommended for all public and patient health collections."

— *Library Journal, Sep '01*

SEE ALSO *Cancer Sourcebook for Women, Women's Health Concerns Sourcebook*

■

Breastfeeding Sourcebook

Basic Consumer Health Information about the Benefits of Breastmilk, Preparing to Breastfeed, Breastfeeding as a Baby Grows, Nutrition, and More, Including Information on Special Situations and Concerns Such as Mastitis, Illness, Medications, Allergies, Multiple Births, Prematurity, Special Needs, and Adoption

Along with a Glossary and Resources for Additional Help and Information

Edited by Jenni Lynn Colson. 388 pages. 2002. 0-7808-0332-9.

"Particularly useful is the information about professional lactation services and chapters on breastfeeding when returning to work. . . . *Breastfeeding Sourcebook* will be useful for public libraries, consumer health libraries, and technical schools offering nurse assistant training, especially in areas where Internet access is problematic."

— *American Reference Books Annual, 2003*

SEE ALSO *Pregnancy & Birth Sourcebook*

■

Burns Sourcebook

Basic Consumer Health Information about Various Types of Burns and Scalds, Including Flame, Heat, Cold, Electrical, Chemical, and Sun Burns

Along with Information on Short-Term and Long-Term Treatments, Tissue Reconstruction, Plastic Surgery, Prevention Suggestions, and First Aid

Edited by Allan R. Cook. 604 pages. 1999. 0-7808-0204-7.

"This is an exceptional addition to the series and is highly recommended for all consumer health collections, hospital libraries, and academic medical centers."

— *E-Streams, Mar '00*

"This key reference guide is an invaluable addition to all health care and public libraries in confronting this ongoing health issue."

— *American Reference Books Annual, 2000*

"Recommended reference source."

— *Booklist, American Library Association, Dec '99*

SEE ALSO *Dermatological Disorders Sourcebook*

■

Cancer Sourcebook, 4th Edition

Basic Consumer Health Information about Major Forms and Stages of Cancer, Featuring Facts about Head and Neck Cancers, Lung Cancers, Gastrointestinal Cancers, Genitourinary Cancers, Lymphomas, Blood Cell Cancers, Endocrine Cancers, Skin Cancers, Bone Cancers, Sarcomas, and Others, and Including Information about Cancer Treatments and Therapies,

Identifying and Reducing Cancer Risks, and Strategies for Coping with Cancer and the Side Effects of Treatment

Along with a Cancer Glossary, Statistical and Demographic Data, and a Directory of Sources for Additional Help and Information

Edited by Karen Bellenir. 1,119 pages. 2003. 0-7808-0633-6.

"With cancer being the second leading cause of death for Americans, a prodigious work such as this one, which locates centrally so much cancer-related information, is clearly an asset to this nation's citizens and others."

— *Journal of the National Medical Association, 2004*

"This title is recommended for health sciences and public libraries with consumer health collections."

— *E-Streams, Feb '01*

". . . can be effectively used by cancer patients and their families who are looking for answers in a language they can understand. Public and hospital libraries should have it on their shelves."

— *American Reference Books Annual, 2001*

"Recommended reference source."

— *Booklist, American Library Association, Dec '00*

SEE ALSO *Breast Cancer Sourcebook, Cancer Sourcebook for Women, Pediatric Cancer Sourcebook, Prostate Cancer Sourcebook*

■

Cancer Sourcebook for Women, 3rd Edition

Basic Consumer Health Information about Leading Causes of Cancer in Women, Featuring Facts about Gynecologic Cancers and Related Concerns, Such as Breast Cancer, Cervical Cancer, Endometrial Cancer, Uterine Sarcoma, Vaginal Cancer, Vulvar Cancer, and Common Non-Cancerous Gynecologic Conditions, in Addition to Facts about Lung Cancer, Colorectal Cancer, and Thyroid Cancer in Women

Along with Information about Cancer Risk Factors, Screening and Prevention, Treatment Options, and Tips on Coping with Life after Cancer Treatment, a Glossary of Cancer Terms, and a Directory of Resources for Additional Help and Information

Edited by Amy L. Sutton. 715 pages. 2006. 0-7808-0867-3.

"An excellent addition to collections in public, consumer health, and women's health libraries."

— *American Reference Books Annual, 2003*

"Overall, the information is excellent, and complex topics are clearly explained. As a reference book for the consumer it is a valuable resource to assist them to make informed decisions about cancer and its treatments." — *Cancer Forum, Nov '02*

"Highly recommended for academic and medical reference collections." — *Library Bookwatch, Sep '02*

"This is a highly recommended book for any public or consumer library, being reader friendly and containing accurate and helpful information."

— *E-Streams, Aug '02*

"Recommended reference source."
—*Booklist, American Library Association, Jul '02*

SEE ALSO *Breast Cancer Sourcebook, Women's Health Concerns Sourcebook*

Cardiovascular Diseases & Disorders Sourcebook, 3rd Edition

Basic Consumer Health Information about Heart and Vascular Diseases and Disorders, Such as Angina, Heart Attacks, Arrhythmias, Cardiomyopathy, Valve Disease, Atherosclerosis, and Aneurysms, with Information about Managing Cardiovascular Risk Factors and Maintaining Heart Health, Medications and Procedures Used to Treat Cardiovascular Disorders, and Concerns of Special Significance to Women

Along with Reports on Current Research Initiatives, a Glossary of Related Medical Terms, and a Directory of Sources for Further Help and Information

Edited by Sandra J. Judd. 713 pages. 2005. 0-7808-0739-1.

"This updated sourcebook is still the best first stop for comprehensive introductory information on cardiovascular diseases."
—*American Reference Books Annual, 2006*

"Recommended for public libraries and libraries supporting health care professionals."
—*E-Streams, Sep '05*

"This should be a standard health library reference."
—*The Bookwatch, Jun '05*

"Recommended reference source."
—*Booklist, American Library Association, Dec '00*

". . . comprehensive format provides an extensive overview on this subject."
—*Choice, Association of College & Research Libraries*

Caregiving Sourcebook

Basic Consumer Health Information for Caregivers, Including a Profile of Caregivers, Caregiving Responsibilities and Concerns, Tips for Specific Conditions, Care Environments, and the Effects of Caregiving

Along with Facts about Legal Issues, Financial Information, and Future Planning, a Glossary, and a Listing of Additional Resources

Edited by Joyce Brennfleck Shannon. 600 pages. 2001. 0-7808-0331-0.

"Essential for most collections."
—*Library Journal, Apr 1, 2002*

"An ideal addition to the reference collection of any public library. Health sciences information professionals may also want to acquire the *Caregiving Sourcebook* for their hospital or academic library for use as a ready reference tool by health care workers interested in aging and caregiving."
—*E-Streams, Jan '02*

"Recommended reference source."
—*Booklist, American Library Association, Oct '01*

Child Abuse Sourcebook

Basic Consumer Health Information about the Physical, Sexual, and Emotional Abuse of Children, with Additional Facts about Neglect, Munchausen Syndrome by Proxy (MSBP), Shaken Baby Syndrome, and Controversial Issues Related to Child Abuse, Such as Withholding Medical Care, Corporal Punishment, and Child Maltreatment in Youth Sports, and Featuring Facts about Child Protective Services, Foster Care, Adoption, Parenting Challenges, and Other Abuse Prevention Efforts

Along with a Glossary of Related Terms and Resources for Additional Help and Information

Edited by Dawn D. Matthews. 620 pages. 2004. 0-7808-0705-7.

"A valuable and highly recommended resource for school, academic and public libraries whether used on its own or as a starting point for more in-depth research."
—*E-Streams, Apr '05*

"Every week the news brings cases of child abuse or neglect, so it is useful to have a source that supplies so much helpful information. . . . Recommended. Public and academic libraries, and child welfare offices."
—*Choice, Association of College & Research Libraries, Mar '05*

"Packed with insights on all kinds of issues, from foster care and adoption to parenting and abuse prevention."
—*The Bookwatch, Nov '04*

SEE ALSO: *Domestic Violence Sourcebook, 2nd Edition*

Childhood Diseases & Disorders Sourcebook

Basic Consumer Health Information about Medical Problems Often Encountered in Pre-Adolescent Children, Including Respiratory Tract Ailments, Ear Infections, Sore Throats, Disorders of the Skin and Scalp, Digestive and Genitourinary Diseases, Infectious Diseases, Inflammatory Disorders, Chronic Physical and Developmental Disorders, Allergies, and More

Along with Information about Diagnostic Tests, Common Childhood Surgeries, and Frequently Used Medications, with a Glossary of Important Terms and Resource Directory

Edited by Chad T. Kimball. 662 pages. 2003. 0-7808-0458-9.

"This is an excellent book for new parents and should be included in all health care and public libraries."
—*American Reference Books Annual, 2004*

SEE ALSO: *Healthy Children Sourcebook*

Colds, Flu & Other Common Ailments Sourcebook

Basic Consumer Health Information about Common Ailments and Injuries, Including Colds, Coughs, the Flu, Sinus Problems, Headaches, Fever, Nausea and

Vomiting, Menstrual Cramps, Diarrhea, Constipation, Hemorrhoids, Back Pain, Dandruff, Dry and Itchy Skin, Cuts, Scrapes, Sprains, Bruises, and More

Along with Information about Prevention, Self-Care, Choosing a Doctor, Over-the-Counter Medications, Folk Remedies, and Alternative Therapies, and Including a Glossary of Important Terms and a Directory of Resources for Further Help and Information

Edited by Chad T. Kimball. 638 pages. 2001. 0-7808-0435-X.

"A good starting point for research on common illnesses. It will be a useful addition to public and consumer health library collections."
— *American Reference Books Annual, 2002*

"Will prove valuable to any library seeking to maintain a current, comprehensive reference collection of health resources. . . . Excellent reference."
— *The Bookwatch, Aug '01*

"Recommended reference source."
— *Booklist, American Library Association, Jul '01*

■

Communication Disorders Sourcebook

Basic Information about Deafness and Hearing Loss, Speech and Language Disorders, Voice Disorders, Balance and Vestibular Disorders, and Disorders of Smell, Taste, and Touch

Edited by Linda M. Ross. 533 pages. 1996. 0-7808-0077-X.

"This is skillfully edited and is a welcome resource for the layperson. It should be found in every public and medical library." — *Booklist Health Sciences Supplement, American Library Association, Oct '97*

■

Complementary & Alternative Medicine Sourcebook, 3rd Edition

Basic Consumer Health Information about Complementary and Alternative Medical Therapies, Including Acupuncture, Ayurveda, Traditional Chinese Medicine, Herbal Medicine, Homeopathy, Naturopathy, Biofeedback, Hypnotherapy, Yoga, Art Therapy, Aromatherapy, Clinical Nutrition, Vitamin and Mineral Supplements, Chiropractic, Massage, Reflexology, Crystal Therapy, Therapeutic Touch, and More

Along with Facts about Alternative and Complementary Treatments for Specific Conditions Such as Cancer, Diabetes, Osteoarthritis, Chronic Pain, Menopause, Gastrointestinal Disorders, Headaches, and Mental Illness, a Glossary, and a Resource List for Additional Help and Information

Edited by Sandra J. Judd. 657 pages. 2006. 0-7808-0864-9.

"Recommended for public, high school, and academic libraries that have consumer health collections. Hospital libraries that also serve the public will find this to be a useful resource." — *E-Streams, Feb '03*

"Recommended reference source."
— *Booklist, American Library Association, Jan '03*

"An important alternate health reference."
— *MBR Bookwatch, Oct '02*

"A great addition to the reference collection of every type of library." — *American Reference Books Annual, 2000*

■

Congenital Disorders Sourcebook

Basic Information about Disorders Acquired during Gestation, Including Spina Bifida, Hydrocephalus, Cerebral Palsy, Heart Defects, Craniofacial Abnormalities, Fetal Alcohol Syndrome, and More

Along with Current Treatment Options and Statistical Data

Edited by Karen Bellenir. 607 pages. 1997. 0-7808-0205-5.

"Recommended reference source."
— *Booklist, American Library Association, Oct '97*

SEE ALSO Pregnancy & Birth Sourcebook

■

Consumer Issues in Health Care Sourcebook

Basic Information about Health Care Fundamentals and Related Consumer Issues, Including Exams and Screening Tests, Physician Specialties, Choosing a Doctor, Using Prescription and Over-the-Counter Medications Safely, Avoiding Health Scams, Managing Common Health Risks in the Home, Care Options for Chronically or Terminally Ill Patients, and a List of Resources for Obtaining Help and Further Information

Edited by Karen Bellenir. 618 pages. 1998. 0-7808-0221-7.

"Both public and academic libraries will want to have a copy in their collection for readers who are interested in self-education on health issues."
— *American Reference Books Annual, 2000*

"The editor has researched the literature from government agencies and others, saving readers the time and effort of having to do the research themselves. Recommended for public libraries."
— *Reference and User Services Quarterly, American Library Association, Spring '99*

"Recommended reference source."
— *Booklist, American Library Association, Dec '98*

■

Contagious Diseases Sourcebook

Basic Consumer Health Information about Infectious Diseases Spread by Person-to-Person Contact through Direct Touch, Airborne Transmission, Sexual Contact, or Contact with Blood or Other Body Fluids, Including Hepatitis, Herpes, Influenza, Lice, Measles, Mumps, Pinworm, Ringworm, Severe Acute Respiratory Syndrome (SARS), Streptococcal Infections, Tuberculosis, and Others

Along with Facts about Disease Transmission, Antimicrobial Resistance, and Vaccines, with a Glossary and Directories of Resources for More Information

Edited by Karen Bellenir. 643 pages. 2004. 0-7808-0736-7.

Contagious & Non-Contagious Infectious Diseases Sourcebook

Basic Information about Contagious Diseases like Measles, Polio, Hepatitis B, and Infectious Mononucleosis, and Non-Contagious Infectious Diseases like Tetanus and Toxic Shock Syndrome, and Diseases Occurring as Secondary Infections Such as Shingles and Reye Syndrome

Along with Vaccination, Prevention, and Treatment Information, and a Section Describing Emerging Infectious Disease Threats

Edited by Karen Bellenir and Peter D. Dresser. 566 pages. 1996. 0-7808-0075-3.

SEE ALSO *Infectious Diseases Sourcebook*

Death & Dying Sourcebook, 2nd Edition

Basic Consumer Health Information about End-of-Life Care and Related Perspectives and Ethical Issues, Including End-of-Life Symptoms and Treatments, Pain Management, Quality-of-Life Concerns, the Use of Life Support, Patients' Rights and Privacy Issues, Advance Directives, Physician-Assisted Suicide, Caregiving, Organ and Tissue Donation, Autopsies, Funeral Arrangements, and Grief

Along with Statistical Data, Information about the Leading Causes of Death, a Glossary, and Directories of Support Groups and Other Resources

Edited by Joyce Brennfleck Shannon. 653 pages. 2006. 0-7808-0871-1.

Dental Care & Oral Health Sourcebook, 2nd Edition

Basic Consumer Health Information about Dental Care, Including Oral Hygiene, Dental Visits, Pain Management, Cavities, Crowns, Bridges, Dental Implants, and Fillings, and Other Oral Health Concerns, Such as Gum Disease, Bad Breath, Dry Mouth, Genetic and Developmental Abnormalities, Oral Cancers, Orthodontics, and Temporomandibular Disorders

Along with Updates on Current Research in Oral Health, a Glossary, a Directory of Dental and Oral Health Organizations, and Resources for People with Dental and Oral Health Disorders

Edited by Amy L. Sutton. 609 pages. 2003. 0-7808-0634-4.

Depression Sourcebook

Basic Consumer Health Information about Unipolar Depression, Bipolar Disorder, Postpartum Depression, Seasonal Affective Disorder, and Other Types of Depression in Children, Adolescents, Women, Men, the Elderly, and Other Selected Populations

Along with Facts about Causes, Risk Factors, Diagnostic Criteria, Treatment Options, Coping Strategies, Suicide Prevention, a Glossary, and a Directory of Sources for Additional Help and Information

Edited by Karen Belleni. 602 pages. 2002. 0-7808-0611-5.

Dermatological Disorders Sourcebook, 2nd Edition

Basic Consumer Health Information about Conditions and Disorders Affecting the Skin, Hair, and Nails, Such as Acne, Rosacea, Rashes, Dermatitis, Pigmentation Disorders, Birthmarks, Skin Cancer, Skin Injuries, Psoriasis, Scleroderma, and Hair Loss, Including Facts about Medications and Treatments for Dermatological

Disorders and Tips for Maintaining Healthy Skin, Hair, and Nails

Along with Information about How Aging Affects the Skin, a Glossary of Related Terms, and a Directory of Resources for Additional Help and Information

Edited by Amy L. Sutton. 645 pages. 2005. 0-7808-0795-2.

"... comprehensive, easily read reference book."
—Doody's Health Sciences Book Reviews, Oct '97

SEE ALSO Burns Sourcebook

Diabetes Sourcebook, 3rd Edition

Basic Consumer Health Information about Type 1 Diabetes (Insulin-Dependent or Juvenile-Onset Diabetes), Type 2 Diabetes (Noninsulin-Dependent or Adult-Onset Diabetes), Gestational Diabetes, Impaired Glucose Tolerance (IGT), and Related Complications, Such as Amputation, Eye Disease, Gum Disease, Nerve Damage, and End-Stage Renal Disease, Including Facts about Insulin, Oral Diabetes Medications, Blood Sugar Testing, and the Role of Exercise and Nutrition in the Control of Diabetes

Along with a Glossary and Resources for Further Help and Information

Edited by Dawn D. Matthews. 622 pages. 2003. 0-7808-0629-8.

"This edition is even more helpful than earlier versions. . . . It is a truly valuable tool for anyone seeking readable and authoritative information on diabetes."
— American Reference Books Annual, 2004

"An invaluable reference." — Library Journal, May '00

Selected as one of the 250 "Best Health Sciences Books of 1999." — Doody's Rating Service, Mar-Apr '00

"Provides useful information for the general public."
— Healthlines, University of Michigan Health Management Research Center, Sep/Oct '99

"... provides reliable mainstream medical information . . . belongs on the shelves of any library with a consumer health collection." — E-Streams, Sep '99

"Recommended reference source."
— Booklist, American Library Association, Feb '99

Diet & Nutrition Sourcebook, 3rd Edition

Basic Consumer Health Information about Dietary Guidelines and the Food Guidance System, Recommended Daily Nutrient Intakes, Serving Proportions, Weight Control, Vitamins and Supplements, Nutrition Issues for Different Life Stages and Lifestyles, and the Needs of People with Specific Medical Concerns, Including Cancer, Celiac Disease, Diabetes, Eating Disorders, Food Allergies, and Cardiovascular Disease

Along with Facts about Federal Nutrition Support Programs, a Glossary of Nutrition and Dietary Terms, and Directories of Additional Resources for More Information about Nutrition

Edited by Joyce Brennfleck Shannon. 633 pages. 2006. 0-7808-0800-2.

"This book is an excellent source of basic diet and nutrition information." — Booklist Health Sciences Supplement, American Library Association, Dec '00

"This reference document should be in any public library, but it would be a very good guide for beginning students in the health sciences. If the other books in this publisher's series are as good as this, they should all be in the health sciences collections."
—American Reference Books Annual, 2000

"This book is an excellent general nutrition reference for consumers who desire to take an active role in their health care for prevention. Consumers of all ages who select this book can feel confident they are receiving current and accurate information." — Journal of Nutrition for the Elderly, Vol. 19, No. 4, 2000

SEE ALSO Digestive Diseases & Disorders Sourcebook, Eating Disorders Sourcebook, Gastrointestinal Diseases & Disorders Sourcebook, Vegetarian Sourcebook

---

Digestive Diseases & Disorders Sourcebook

Basic Consumer Health Information about Diseases and Disorders that Impact the Upper and Lower Digestive System, Including Celiac Disease, Constipation, Crohn's Disease, Cyclic Vomiting Syndrome, Diarrhea, Diverticulosis and Diverticulitis, Gallstones, Heartburn, Hemorrhoids, Hernias, Indigestion (Dyspepsia), Irritable Bowel Syndrome, Lactose Intolerance, Ulcers, and More

Along with Information about Medications and Other Treatments, Tips for Maintaining a Healthy Digestive Tract, a Glossary, and Directory of Digestive Diseases Organizations

Edited by Karen Bellenir. 335 pages. 2000. 0-7808-0327-2.

"This title would be an excellent addition to all public or patient-research libraries."
— American Reference Books Annual, 2001

"This title is recommended for public, hospital, and health sciences libraries with consumer health collections." - — E-Streams, Jul-Aug '00

"Recommended reference source."
— Booklist, American Library Association, May '00

SEE ALSO Eating Disorders Sourcebook, Gastrointestinal Diseases & Disorders Sourcebook

---

Disabilities Sourcebook

Basic Consumer Health Information about Physical and Psychiatric Disabilities, Including Descriptions of Major Causes of Disability, Assistive and Adaptive Aids, Workplace Issues, and Accessibility Concerns

Along with Information about the Americans with Disabilities Act, a Glossary, and Resources for Additional Help and Information

Edited by Dawn D. Matthews. 616 pages. 2000. 0-7808-0389-2.

"It is a must for libraries with a consumer health section." — *American Reference Books Annual, 2002*

"A much needed addition to the Omnigraphics Health Reference Series. A current reference work to provide people with disabilities, their families, caregivers or those who work with them, a broad range of information in one volume, has not been available until now. . . . It is recommended for all public and academic library reference collections." — *E-Streams, May '01*

"An excellent source book in easy-to-read format covering many current topics; highly recommended for all libraries." — *Choice, Association of College & Research Libraries, Jan '01*

"Recommended reference source." *Booklist, American Library Association, Jul '00*

Domestic Violence Sourcebook, 2nd Edition

Basic Consumer Health Information about the Causes and Consequences of Abusive Relationships, Including Physical Violence, Sexual Assault, Battery, Stalking, and Emotional Abuse, and Facts about the Effects of Violence on Women, Men, Young Adults, and the Elderly, with Reports about Domestic Violence in Selected Populations, and Featuring Facts about Medical Care, Victim Assistance and Protection, Prevention Strategies, Mental Health Services, and Legal Issues

Along with a Glossary of Related Terms and Resources for Additional Help and Information

Edited by Dawn D. Matthews. 628 pages. 2004. 0-7808-0669-7.

"Educators, clergy, medical professionals, police, and victims and their families will benefit from this realistic and easy-to-understand resource." — *American Reference Books Annual, 2005*

"Recommended for all collections supporting consumer health information. It should also be considered for any collection needing general, readable information on domestic violence." — *E-Streams, Jan '05*

"This sourcebook complements other books in its field, providing a one-stop resource . . . Recommended." — *Choice, Association of College & Research Libraries, Jan '05*

"Interested lay persons should find the book extremely beneficial. . . . A copy of *Domestic Violence and Child Abuse Sourcebook* should be in every public library in the United States." — *Social Science & Medicine, No. 56, 2003*

"This is important information. The Web has many resources but this sourcebook fills an important societal need. I am not aware of any other resources of this type." — *Doody's Review Service, Sep '01*

"Recommended reference source." — *Booklist, American Library Association, Apr '01*

"Important pick for college-level health reference libraries." — *The Bookwatch, Mar '01*

"Because this problem is so widespread and because this book includes a lot of issues within one volume, this work is recommended for all public libraries." — *American Reference Books Annual, 2001*

SEE ALSO *Child Abuse Sourcebook*

Drug Abuse Sourcebook, 2nd Edition

Basic Consumer Health Information about Illicit Substances of Abuse and the Misuse of Prescription and Over-the-Counter Medications, Including Depressants, Hallucinogens, Inhalants, Marijuana, Stimulants, and Anabolic Steroids

Along with Facts about Related Health Risks, Treatment Programs, Prevention Programs, a Glossary of Abuse and Addiction Terms, a Glossary of Drug-Related Street Terms, and a Directory of Resources for More Information

Edited by Catherine Ginther. 607 pages. 2004. 0-7808-0740-5.

"Commendable for organizing useful, normally scattered government and association-produced data into a logical sequence." — *American Reference Books Annual, 2006*

"This easy-to-read volume is recommended for consumer health collections within public or academic libraries." — *E-Streams, Sep '05*

"An excellent library reference." — *The Bookwatch, May '05*

"Containing a wealth of information, this book will be useful to the college student just beginning to explore the topic of substance abuse. This resource belongs in libraries that serve a lower-division undergraduate or community college clientele as well as the general public." — *Choice, Association of College & Research Libraries, Jun '01*

"Recommended reference source." — *Booklist, American Library Association, Feb '01*

SEE ALSO *Alcoholism Sourcebook, Substance Abuse Sourcebook*

Ear, Nose & Throat Disorders Sourcebook, 2nd Edition

Basic Consumer Health Information about Disorders of the Ears, Hearing Loss, Vestibular Disorders, Nasal and Sinus Problems, Throat and Vocal Cord Disorders, and Otolaryngologic Cancers, Including Facts about Ear Infections and Injuries, Genetic and Congenital Deafness, Sensorineural Hearing Disorders, Tinnitus, Vertigo, Ménière Disease, Rhinitis, Sinusitis, Snoring, Sore Throats, Hoarseness, and More

Along with Reports on Current Research Initiatives, a Glossary of Related Medical Terms, and a Directory of Sources for Further Help and Information

Edited by Sandra J. Judd. 659 pages. 2006. 0-7808-0872-X.

"Overall, this sourcebook is helpful for the consumer seeking information on ENT issues. It is recommended for public libraries."
—*American Reference Books Annual, 1999*

"Recommended reference source."
—*Booklist, American Library Association, Dec '98*

■

Eating Disorders Sourcebook

Basic Consumer Health Information about Eating Disorders, Including Information about Anorexia Nervosa, Bulimia Nervosa, Binge Eating, Body Dysmorphic Disorder, Pica, Laxative Abuse, and Night Eating Syndrome

Along with Information about Causes, Adverse Effects, and Treatment and Prevention Issues, and Featuring a Section on Concerns Specific to Children and Adolescents, a Glossary, and Resources for Further Help and Information

Edited by Dawn D. Matthews. 322 pages. 2001. 0-7808-0335-3.

"Recommended for health science libraries that are open to the public, as well as hospital libraries. This book is a good resource for the consumer who is concerned about eating disorders." —*E-Streams, Mar '02*

"This volume is another convenient collection of excerpted articles. Recommended for school and public library patrons; lower-division undergraduates; and two-year technical program students."
—*Choice, Association of College & Research Libraries, Jan '02*

"Recommended reference source."
—*Booklist, American Library Association, Oct '01*

SEE ALSO *Diet & Nutrition Sourcebook, Digestive Diseases & Disorders Sourcebook, Gastrointestinal Diseases & Disorders Sourcebook*

■

Emergency Medical Services Sourcebook

Basic Consumer Health Information about Preventing, Preparing for, and Managing Emergency Situations, When and Who to Call for Help, What to Expect in the Emergency Room, the Emergency Medical Team, Patient Issues, and Current Topics in Emergency Medicine

Along with Statistical Data, a Glossary, and Sources of Additional Help and Information

Edited by Jenni Lynn Colson. 494 pages. 2002. 0-7808-0420-1.

"Handy and convenient for home, public, school, and college libraries. Recommended."
— *Choice, Association of College & Research Libraries, Apr '03*

"This reference can provide the consumer with answers to most questions about emergency care in the United States, or it will direct them to a resource where the answer can be found."
—*American Reference Books Annual, 2003*

"Recommended reference source."
— *Booklist, American Library Association, Feb '03*

■

Endocrine & Metabolic Disorders Sourcebook

Basic Information for the Layperson about Pancreatic and Insulin-Related Disorders Such as Pancreatitis, Diabetes, and Hypoglycemia; Adrenal Gland Disorders Such as Cushing's Syndrome, Addison's Disease, and Congenital Adrenal Hyperplasia; Pituitary Gland Disorders Such as Growth Hormone Deficiency, Acromegaly, and Pituitary Tumors; Thyroid Disorders Such as Hypothyroidism, Graves' Disease, Hashimoto's Disease, and Goiter; Hyperparathyroidism; and Other Diseases and Syndromes of Hormone Imbalance or Metabolic Dysfunction

Along with Reports on Current Research Initiatives

Edited by Linda M. Shin. 574 pages. 1998. 0-7808-0207-1.

"Omnigraphics has produced another needed resource for health information consumers."
—*American Reference Books Annual, 2000*

"Recommended reference source."
— *Booklist, American Library Association, Dec '98*

■

Environmental Health Sourcebook, 2nd Edition

Basic Consumer Health Information about the Environment and Its Effect on Human Health, Including the Effects of Air Pollution, Water Pollution, Hazardous Chemicals, Food Hazards, Radiation Hazards, Biological Agents, Household Hazards, Such as Radon, Asbestos, Carbon Monoxide, and Mold, and Information about Associated Diseases and Disorders, Including Cancer, Allergies, Respiratory Problems, and Skin Disorders

Along with Information about Environmental Concerns for Specific Populations, a Glossary of Related Terms, and Resources for Further Help and Information

Edited by Dawn D. Matthews. 673 pages. 2003. 0-7808-0632-8.

"This recently updated edition continues the level of quality and the reputation of the numerous other volumes in Omnigraphics' Health Reference Series."
—*American Reference Books Annual, 2004*

"An excellent updated edition."
— *The Bookwatch, Oct '03*

"Recommended reference source."
—*Booklist, American Library Association, Sep '98*

"This book will be a useful addition to anyone's library." — *Choice Health Sciences Supplement, Association of College & Research Libraries, May '98*

"... a good survey of numerous environmentally induced physical disorders ... a useful addition to anyone's library."

— *Doody's Health Sciences Book Reviews, Jan '98*

Environmentally Induced Disorders Sourcebook

SEE *Environmental Health Sourcebook, 2nd Edition*

Ethnic Diseases Sourcebook

Basic Consumer Health Information for Ethnic and Racial Minority Groups in the United States, Including General Health Indicators and Behaviors, Ethnic Diseases, Genetic Testing, the Impact of Chronic Diseases, Women's Health, Mental Health Issues, and Preventive Health Care Services

Along with a Glossary and a Listing of Additional Resources

Edited by Joyce Brennfleck Shannon. 664 pages. 2001. 0-7808-0336-1.

"Recommended for health sciences libraries where public health programs are a priority."

— *E-Streams, Jan '02*

"Not many books have been written on this topic to date, and the *Ethnic Diseases Sourcebook* is a strong addition to the list. It will be an important introductory resource for health consumers, students, health care personnel, and social scientists. It is recommended for public, academic, and large hospital libraries."

— *American Reference Books Annual, 2002*

"Recommended reference source."

— *Booklist, American Library Association, Oct '01*

"Will prove valuable to any library seeking to maintain a current, comprehensive reference collection of health resources.... An excellent source of health information about genetic disorders which affect particular ethnic and racial minorities in the U.S."

— *The Bookwatch, Aug '01*

Eye Care Sourcebook, 2nd Edition

Basic Consumer Health Information about Eye Care and Eye Disorders, Including Facts about the Diagnosis, Prevention, and Treatment of Common Refractive Problems Such as Myopia, Hyperopia, Astigmatism, and Presbyopia, and Eye Diseases, Including Glaucoma, Cataract, Age-Related Macular Degeneration, and Diabetic Retinopathy

Along with a Section on Vision Correction and Refractive Surgeries, Including LASIK and LASEK, a Glossary, and Directories of Resources for Additional Help and Information

Edited by Amy L. Sutton. 543 pages. 2003. 0-7808-0635-2.

"... a solid reference tool for eye care and a valuable addition to a collection."

— *American Reference Books Annual, 2004*

Family Planning Sourcebook

Basic Consumer Health Information about Planning for Pregnancy and Contraception, Including Traditional Methods, Barrier Methods, Hormonal Methods, Permanent Methods, Future Methods, Emergency Contraception, and Birth Control Choices for Women at Each Stage of Life

Along with Statistics, a Glossary, and Sources of Additional Information

Edited by Amy Marcaccio Keyzer. 520 pages. 2001. 0-7808-0379-5.

"Recommended for public, health, and undergraduate libraries as part of the circulating collection."

— *E-Streams, Mar '02*

"Information is presented in an unbiased, readable manner, and the sourcebook will certainly be a necessary addition to those public and high school libraries where Internet access is restricted or otherwise problematic."   — *American Reference Books Annual, 2002*

"Recommended reference source."

— *Booklist, American Library Association, Oct '01*

"Will prove valuable to any library seeking to maintain a current, comprehensive reference collection of health resources. ... Excellent reference."

— *The Bookwatch, Aug '01*

SEE ALSO *Pregnancy & Birth Sourcebook*

Fitness & Exercise Sourcebook, 2nd Edition

Basic Consumer Health Information about the Fundamentals of Fitness and Exercise, Including How to Begin and Maintain a Fitness Program, Fitness as a Lifestyle, the Link between Fitness and Diet, Advice for Specific Groups of People, Exercise as It Relates to Specific Medical Conditions, and Recent Research in Fitness and Exercise

Along with a Glossary of Important Terms and Resources for Additional Help and Information

Edited by Kristen M. Gledhill. 646 pages. 2001. 0-7808-0334-5.

"This work is recommended for all general reference collections."

— *American Reference Books Annual, 2002*

"Highly recommended for public, consumer, and school grades fourth through college."   — *E-Streams, Nov '01*

"Recommended reference source."

— *Booklist, American Library Association, Oct '01*

"The information appears quite comprehensive and is considered reliable. ... This second edition is a welcomed addition to the series."

— *Doody's Review Service, Sep '01*

Food & Animal Borne Diseases Sourcebook

Basic Information about Diseases That Can Be Spread to Humans through the Ingestion of Contaminated Food or Water or by Contact with Infected Animals and Insects, Such as Botulism, E. Coli, Hepatitis A, Trichinosis, Lyme Disease, and Rabies

Along with Information Regarding Prevention and Treatment Methods, and Including a Special Section for International Travelers Describing Diseases Such as Cholera, Malaria, Travelers' Diarrhea, and Yellow Fever, and Offering Recommendations for Avoiding Illness

Edited by Karen Bellenir and Peter D. Dresser. 535 pages. 1995. 0-7808-0033-8.

"Targeting general readers and providing them with a single, comprehensive source of information on selected topics, this book continues, with the excellent caliber of its predecessors, to catalog topical information on health matters of general interest. Readable and thorough, this valuable resource is highly recommended for all libraries."
— *Academic Library Book Review, Summer '96*

"A comprehensive collection of authoritative information."   — *Emergency Medical Services, Oct '95*

Food Safety Sourcebook

Basic Consumer Health Information about the Safe Handling of Meat, Poultry, Seafood, Eggs, Fruit Juices, and Other Food Items, and Facts about Pesticides, Drinking Water, Food Safety Overseas, and the Onset, Duration, and Symptoms of Foodborne Illnesses, Including Types of Pathogenic Bacteria, Parasitic Protozoa, Worms, Viruses, and Natural Toxins

Along with the Role of the Consumer, the Food Handler, and the Government in Food Safety; a Glossary, and Resources for Additional Help and Information

Edited by Dawn D. Matthews. 339 pages. 1999. 0-7808-0326-4.

"This book is recommended for public libraries and universities with home economic and food science programs."   — *E-Streams, Nov '00*

"Recommended reference source."
— *Booklist, American Library Association, May '00*

"This book takes the complex issues of food safety and foodborne pathogens and presents them in an easily understood manner. [It does] an excellent job of covering a large and often confusing topic."
— *American Reference Books Annual, 2000*

Forensic Medicine Sourcebook

Basic Consumer Information for the Layperson about Forensic Medicine, Including Crime Scene Investigation, Evidence Collection and Analysis, Expert Testimony, Computer-Aided Criminal Identification, Digital Imaging in the Courtroom, DNA Profiling, Accident Reconstruction, Autopsies, Ballistics, Drugs and

Explosives Detection, Latent Fingerprints, Product Tampering, and Questioned Document Examination

Along with Statistical Data, a Glossary of Forensics Terminology, and Listings of Sources for Further Help and Information

Edited by Annemarie S. Muth. 574 pages. 1999. 0-7808-0232-2.

"Given the expected widespread interest in its content and its easy to read style, this book is recommended for most public and all college and university libraries."
— *E-Streams, Feb '01*

"Recommended for public libraries."
— *Reference & User Services Quarterly, American Library Association, Spring 2000*

"Recommended reference source."
— *Booklist, American Library Association, Feb '00*

"A wealth of information, useful statistics, references are up-to-date and extremely complete. This wonderful collection of data will help students who are interested in a career in any type of forensic field. It is a great resource for attorneys who need information about types of expert witnesses needed in a particular case. It also offers useful information for fiction and nonfiction writers whose work involves a crime. A fascinating compilation. All levels."
— *Choice, Association of College & Research Libraries, Jan '00*

"There are several items that make this book attractive to consumers who are seeking certain forensic data. . . . This is a useful current source for those seeking general forensic medical answers."
— *American Reference Books Annual, 2000*

Gastrointestinal Diseases & Disorders Sourcebook, 2nd Edition

Basic Consumer Health Information about the Upper and Lower Gastrointestinal (GI) Tract, Including the Esophagus, Stomach, Intestines, Rectum, Liver, and Pancreas, with Facts about Gastroesophageal Reflux Disease, Gastritis, Hernias, Ulcers, Celiac Disease, Diverticulitis, Irritable Bowel Syndrome, Hemorrhoids, Gastrointestinal Cancers, and Other Diseases and Disorders Related to the Digestive Process

Along with Information about Commonly Used Diagnostic and Surgical Procedures, Statistics, Reports on Current Research Initiatives and Clinical Trials, a Glossary, and Resources for Additional Help and Information

Edited by Sandra J. Judd. 681 pages. 2006. 0-7808-0798-7.

". . . very readable form. The successful editorial work that brought this material together into a useful and understandable reference makes accessible to all readers information that can help them more effectively understand and obtain help for digestive tract problems."
— *Choice, Association of College & Research Libraries, Feb '97*

Genetic Disorders Sourcebook, 3rd Edition

Basic Consumer Health Information about Hereditary Diseases and Disorders, Including Facts about the Human Genome, Genetic Inheritance Patterns, Disorders Associated with Specific Genes, Such as Sickle Cell Disease, Hemophilia, and Cystic Fibrosis, Chromosome Disorders, Such as Down Syndrome, Fragile X Syndrome, and Turner Syndrome, and Complex Diseases and Disorders Resulting from the Interaction of Environmental and Genetic Factors, Such as Allergies, Cancer, and Obesity

Along with Facts about Genetic Testing, Suggestions for Parents of Children with Special Needs, Reports on Current Research Initiatives, a Glossary of Genetic Terminology, and Resources for Additional Help and Information

Edited by Karen Bellenir. 777 pages. 2004. 0-7808-0742-1.

"This text is recommended for any library with an interest in providing consumer health resources."
— *E-Streams, Aug '05*

"This is a valuable resource for anyone wishing to have an understandable description of any of the topics or disorders included. The editor succeeds in making complex genetic issues understandable."
— *Doody's Book Review Service, May '05*

"A good acquisition for public libraries."
— *American Reference Books Annual, 2005*

"Excellent reference." — *The Bookwatch, Jan '05*

"Recommended reference source."
— *Booklist, American Library Association, Apr '01*

"Important pick for college-level health reference libraries." — *The Bookwatch, Mar '01*

Head Trauma Sourcebook

Basic Information for the Layperson about Open-Head and Closed-Head Injuries, Treatment Advances, Recovery, and Rehabilitation

Along with Reports on Current Research Initiatives

Edited by Karen Bellenir. 414 pages. 1997. 0-7808-0208-X.

Headache Sourcebook

Basic Consumer Health Information about Migraine, Tension, Cluster, Rebound and Other Types of Headaches, with Facts about the Cause and Prevention of Headaches, the Effects of Stress and the Environment, Headaches during Pregnancy and Menopause, and Childhood Headaches

Along with a Glossary and Other Resources for Additional Help and Information

Edited by Dawn D. Matthews. 362 pages. 2002. 0-7808-0337-X.

"Highly recommended for academic and medical reference collections." — *Library Bookwatch, Sep '02*

Health Insurance Sourcebook

Basic Information about Managed Care Organizations, Traditional Fee-for-Service Insurance, Insurance Portability and Pre-Existing Conditions Clauses, Medicare, Medicaid, Social Security, and Military Health Care

Along with Information about Insurance Fraud

Edited by Wendy Wilcox. 530 pages. 1997. 0-7808-0222-5.

"Particularly useful because it brings much of this information together in one volume. This book will be a handy reference source in the health sciences library, hospital library, college and university library, and medium to large public library."
— *Medical Reference Services Quarterly, Fall '98*

Awarded "Books of the Year Award"
— *American Journal of Nursing, 1997*

"The layout of the book is particularly helpful as it provides easy access to reference material. A most useful addition to the vast amount of information about health insurance. The use of data from U.S. government agencies is most commendable. Useful in a library or learning center for healthcare professional students."
— *Doody's Health Sciences Book Reviews, Nov '97*

Healthy Aging Sourcebook

Basic Consumer Health Information about Maintaining Health through the Aging Process, Including Advice on Nutrition, Exercise, and Sleep, Help in Making Decisions about Midlife Issues and Retirement, and Guidance Concerning Practical and Informed Choices in Health Consumerism

Along with Data Concerning the Theories of Aging, Different Experiences in Aging by Minority Groups, and Facts about Aging Now and Aging in the Future; and Featuring a Glossary, a Guide to Consumer Help, Additional Suggested Reading, and Practical Resource Directory

Edited by Jenifer Swanson. 536 pages. 1999. 0-7808-0390-6.

"Recommended reference source."
— *Booklist, American Library Association, Feb '00*

SEE ALSO *Physical & Mental Issues in Aging Sourcebook*

Healthy Children Sourcebook

Basic Consumer Health Information about the Physical and Mental Development of Children between the Ages of 3 and 12, Including Routine Health Care, Preventative Health Services, Safety and First Aid, Healthy Sleep, Dental Care, Nutrition, and Fitness, and Featuring Parenting Tips on Such Topics as Bed-

wetting, Choosing Day Care, Monitoring TV and Other Media, and Establishing a Foundation for Substance Abuse Prevention

Along with a Glossary of Commonly Used Pediatric Terms and Resources for Additional Help and Information.

Edited by Chad T. Kimball. 647 pages. 2003. 0-7808-0247-0.

"It is hard to imagine that any other single resource exists that would provide such a comprehensive guide of timely information on health promotion and disease prevention for children aged 3 to 12."
—American Reference Books Annual, 2004

"The strengths of this book are many. It is clearly written, presented and structured."
—Journal of the National Medical Association, 2004

SEE ALSO Childhood Diseases & Disorders Sourcebook

Healthy Heart Sourcebook for Women

Basic Consumer Health Information about Cardiac Issues Specific to Women, Including Facts about Major Risk Factors and Prevention, Treatment and Control Strategies, and Important Dietary Issues

Along with a Special Section Regarding the Pros and Cons of Hormone Replacement Therapy and Its Impact on Heart Health, and Additional Help, Including Recipes, a Glossary, and a Directory of Resources

Edited by Dawn D. Matthews. 336 pages. 2000. 0-7808-0329-9.

"A good reference source and recommended for all public, academic, medical, and hospital libraries."
—Medical Reference Services Quarterly, Summer '01

"Because of the lack of information specific to women on this topic, this book is recommended for public libraries and consumer libraries."
—American Reference Books Annual, 2001

"Contains very important information about coronary artery disease that all women should know. The information is current and presented in an easy-to-read format. The book will make a good addition to any library."
—American Medical Writers Association Journal, Summer '00

"Important, basic reference."
—Reviewer's Bookwatch, Jul '00

SEE ALSO Cardiovascular Diseases & Disorders Sourcebook, Women's Health Concerns Sourcebook

Heart Diseases & Disorders Sourcebook

SEE Cardiovascular Diseases & Disorders Sourcebook, 3rd Edition

Hepatitis Sourcebook

Basic Consumer Health Information about Hepatitis A, Hepatitis B, Hepatitis C, and Other Forms of Hepatitis, Including Autoimmune Hepatitis, Alcoholic Hepatitis, Nonalcoholic Steatohepatitis, and Toxic Hepatitis, with Facts about Risk Factors, Screening Methods, Diagnostic Tests, and Treatment Options

Along with Information on Liver Health, Tips for People Living with Chronic Hepatitis, Reports on Current Research Initiatives, a Glossary of Terms Related to Hepatitis, and a Directory of Sources for Further Help and Information

Edited by Sandra J. Judd. 597 pages. 2005. 0-7808-0749-9.

"Highly recommended."
—American Reference Books Annual, 2006

Household Safety Sourcebook

Basic Consumer Health Information about Household Safety, Including Information about Poisons, Chemicals, Fire, and Water Hazards in the Home

Along with Advice about the Safe Use of Home Maintenance Equipment, Choosing Toys and Nursery Furniture, Holiday and Recreation Safety, a Glossary, and Resources for Further Help and Information

Edited by Dawn D. Matthews. 606 pages. 2002. 0-7808-0338-8.

"This work will be useful in public libraries with large consumer health and wellness departments."
—American Reference Books Annual, 2003

"As a sourcebook on household safety this book meets its mark. It is encyclopedic in scope and covers a wide range of safety issues that are commonly seen in the home."
—E-Streams, Jul '02

Hypertension Sourcebook

Basic Consumer Health Information about the Causes, Diagnosis, and Treatment of High Blood Pressure, with Facts about Consequences, Complications, and Co-Occurring Disorders, Such as Coronary Heart Disease, Diabetes, Stroke, Kidney Disease, and Hypertensive Retinopathy, and Issues in Blood Pressure Control, Including Dietary Choices, Stress Management, and Medications

Along with Reports on Current Research Initiatives and Clinical Trials, a Glossary, and Resources for Additional Help and Information

Edited by Dawn D. Matthews and Karen Bellenir. 613 pages. 2004. 0-7808-0674-3.

"Academic, public, and medical libraries will want to add the *Hypertension Sourcebook* to their collections."
—E-Streams, Aug '05

"The strength of this source is the wide range of information given about hypertension."
—American Reference Books Annual, 2005

Immune System Disorders Sourcebook, 2nd Edition

Basic Consumer Health Information about Disorders of the Immune System, Including Immune System Function and Response, Diagnosis of Immune Disorders, Information about Inherited Immune Disease, Acquired Immune Disease, and Autoimmune Diseases, Including Primary Immune Deficiency, Acquired Immunodeficiency Syndrome (AIDS), Lupus, Multiple Sclerosis, Type 1 Diabetes, Rheumatoid Arthritis, and Graves' Disease

Along with Treatments, Tips for Coping with Immune Disorders, a Glossary, and a Directory of Additional Resources.

Edited by Joyce Brennfleck Shannon. 671 pages. 2005. 0-7808-0748-0

"Highly recommended for academic and public libraries." — *American Reference Books Annual, 2006*

"The updated second edition is a 'must' for any consumer health library seeking a solid resource covering the treatments, symptoms, and options for immune disorder sufferers. . . . An excellent guide."
— *MBR Bookwatch, Jan '06*

■

Infant & Toddler Health Sourcebook

Basic Consumer Health Information about the Physical and Mental Development of Newborns, Infants, and Toddlers, Including Neonatal Concerns, Nutrition Recommendations, Immunization Schedules, Common Pediatric Disorders, Assessments and Milestones, Safety Tips, and Advice for Parents and Other Caregivers

Along with a Glossary of Terms and Resource Listings for Additional Help

Edited by Jenifer Swanson. 585 pages. 2000. 0-7808-0246-2.

"As a reference for the general public, this would be useful in any library." — *E-Streams, May '01*

"Recommended reference source."
— *Booklist, American Library Association, Feb '01*

"This is a good source for general use."
— *American Reference Books Annual, 2001*

■

Infectious Diseases Sourcebook

Basic Consumer Health Information about Non-Contagious Bacterial, Viral, Prion, Fungal, and Parasitic Diseases Spread by Food and Water, Insects and Animals, or Environmental Contact, Including Botulism, E. Coli, Encephalitis, Legionnaires' Disease, Lyme Disease, Malaria, Plague, Rabies, Salmonella, Tetanus, and Others, and Facts about Newly Emerging Diseases, Such as Hantavirus, Mad Cow Disease, Monkeypox, and West Nile Virus

Along with Information about Preventing Disease Transmission, the Threat of Bioterrorism, and Current

Research Initiatives, with a Glossary and Directory of Resources for More Information

Edited by Karen Bellenir. 634 pages. 2004. 0-7808-0675-1.

"This reference continues the excellent tradition of the *Health Reference Series* in consolidating a wealth of information on a selected topic into a format that is easy to use and accessible to the general public."
— *American Reference Books Annual, 2005*

"Recommended for public and academic libraries."
— *E-Streams, Jan '05*

■

Injury & Trauma Sourcebook

Basic Consumer Health Information about the Impact of Injury, the Diagnosis and Treatment of Common and Traumatic Injuries, Emergency Care, and Specific Injuries Related to Home, Community, Workplace, Transportation, and Recreation

Along with Guidelines for Injury Prevention, a Glossary, and a Directory of Additional Resources

Edited by Joyce Brennfleck Shannon. 696 pages. 2002. 0-7808-0421-X.

"This publication is the most comprehensive work of its kind about injury and trauma."
— *American Reference Books Annual, 2003*

"This sourcebook provides concise, easily readable, basic health information about injuries. . . . This book is well organized and an easy to use reference resource suitable for hospital, health sciences and public libraries with consumer health collections."
— *E-Streams, Nov '02*

"Practitioners should be aware of guides such as this in order to facilitate their use by patients and their families." — *Doody's Health Sciences Book Review Journal, Sep-Oct '02*

"Recommended reference source."
— *Booklist, American Library Association, Sep '02*

"Highly recommended for academic and medical reference collections." — *Library Bookwatch, Sep '02*

■

Kidney & Urinary Tract Diseases & Disorders Sourcebook

SEE *Urinary Tract & Kidney Diseases & Disorders Sourcebook, 2nd Edition*

■

Learning Disabilities Sourcebook, 2nd Edition

Basic Consumer Health Information about Learning Disabilities, Including Dyslexia, Developmental Speech and Language Disabilities, Non-Verbal Learning Disorders, Developmental Arithmetic Disorder, Developmental Writing Disorder, and Other Conditions That Impede Learning Such as Attention Deficit/ Hyperac-

tivity Disorder, Brain Injury, Hearing Impairment, Kline-
felter Syndrome, Dyspraxia, and Tourette's Syndrome

Along with Facts about Educational Issues and Assistive Technology, Coping Strategies, a Glossary of Related Terms, and Resources for Further Help and
Information

Edited by Dawn D. Matthews. 621 pages. 2003. 0-7808-
0626-3.

"The second edition of Learning Disabilities Sourcebook far surpasses the earlier edition in that it is more
focused on information that will be useful as a consumer health resource."
— American Reference Books Annual, 2004

"Teachers as well as consumers will find this an essential guide to understanding various syndromes and their
latest treatments. [An] invaluable reference for public
and school library collections alike."
— Library Bookwatch, Apr '03

Named "Outstanding Reference Book of 1999."
— New York Public Library, Feb 2000

"An excellent candidate for inclusion in a public library
reference section. It's a great source of information.
Teachers will also find the book useful. Definitely
worth reading."
— Journal of Adolescent & Adult Literacy, Feb 2000

"Readable . . . provides a solid base of information
regarding successful techniques used with individuals
who have learning disabilities, as well as practical suggestions for educators and family members. Clear language, concise descriptions, and pertinent information
for contacting multiple resources add to the strength of
this book as a useful tool." — Choice,
Association of College & Research Libraries, Feb '99

"Recommended reference source."
— Booklist, American Library Association, Sep '98

"A useful resource for libraries and for those who don't
have the time to identify and locate the individual publications." — Disability Resources Monthly, Sep '98

Leukemia Sourcebook

Basic Consumer Health Information about Adult and
Childhood Leukemias, Including Acute Lymphocytic
Leukemia (ALL), Chronic Lymphocytic Leukemia
(CLL), Acute Myelogenous Leukemia (AML), Chronic
Myelogenous Leukemia (CML), and Hairy Cell Leuke-
mia, and Treatments Such as Chemotherapy, Radia-
tion Therapy, Peripheral Blood Stem Cell and Marrow
Transplantation, and Immunotherapy

Along with Tips for Life During and After Treatment, a
Glossary, and Directories of Additional Resources

Edited by Joyce Brennfleck Shannon. 587 pages. 2003.
0-7808-0627-1.

"Unlike other medical books for the layperson, . . . the
language does not talk down to the reader. . . . This volume is highly recommended for all libraries."
— American Reference Books Annual, 2004

"... a fine title which ranges from diagnosis to alternative treatments, staging, and tips for life during and
after diagnosis." — The Bookwatch, Dec '03

Liver Disorders Sourcebook

Basic Consumer Health Information about the Liver
and How It Works; Liver Diseases, Including Cancer,
Cirrhosis, Hepatitis, and Toxic and Drug Related Diseases; Tips for Maintaining a Healthy Liver; Laboratory
Tests, Radiology Tests, and Facts about Liver Transplantation

Along with a Section on Support Groups, a Glossary,
and Resource Listings

Edited by Joyce Brennfleck Shannon. 591 pages. 2000.
0-7808-0383-3.

"A valuable resource."
— American Reference Books Annual, 2001

"This title is recommended for health sciences and
public libraries with consumer health collections."
— E-Streams, Oct '00

"Recommended reference source."
— Booklist, American Library Association, Jun '00

Lung Disorders Sourcebook

Basic Consumer Health Information about Emphyse-
ma, Pneumonia, Tuberculosis, Asthma, Cystic Fibro-
sis, and Other Lung Disorders, Including Facts about
Diagnostic Procedures, Treatment Strategies, Disease
Prevention Efforts, and Such Risk Factors as Smoking,
Air Pollution, and Exposure to Asbestos, Radon, and
Other Agents

Along with a Glossary and Resources for Additional
Help and Information

Edited by Dawn D. Matthews. 678 pages. 2002. 0-7808-
0339-6.

"This title is a great addition for public and school
libraries because it provides concise health information
on the lungs."
— American Reference Books Annual, 2003

"Highly recommended for academic and medical reference collections." — Library Bookwatch, Sep '02

SEE ALSO Respiratory Diseases & Disorders
Sourcebook

Medical Tests Sourcebook,
2nd Edition

Basic Consumer Health Information about Medical
Tests, Including Age-Specific Health Tests, Important
Health Screenings and Exams, Home-Use Tests, Blood
and Specimen Tests, Electrical Tests, Scope Tests,
Genetic Testing, and Imaging Tests, Such as X-Rays,
Ultrasound, Computed Tomography, Magnetic Reso-
nance Imaging, Angiography, and Nuclear Medicine

Along with a Glossary and Directory of Additional Resources

Edited by Joyce Brennfleck Shannon. 654 pages. 2004. 0-7808-0670-0.

"Recommended for hospital and health sciences libraries with consumer health collections."
— E-Streams, Mar '00

"This is an overall excellent reference with a wealth of general knowledge that may aid those who are reluctant to get vital tests performed."
— Today's Librarian, Jan '00

"A valuable reference guide."
— American Reference Books Annual, 2000

■

Men's Health Concerns Sourcebook, 2nd Edition

Basic Consumer Health Information about the Medical and Mental Concerns of Men, Including Theories about the Shorter Male Lifespan, the Leading Causes of Death and Disability, Physical Concerns of Special Significance to Men, Reproductive and Sexual Concerns, Sexually Transmitted Diseases, Men's Mental and Emotional Health, and Lifestyle Choices That Affect Wellness, Such as Nutrition, Fitness, and Substance Use

Along with a Glossary of Related Terms and a Directory of Organizational Resources in Men's Health

Edited by Robert Aquinas McNally. 644 pages. 2004. 0-7808-0671-9.

"A very accessible reference for non-specialist general readers and consumers." *— The Bookwatch, Jun '04*

"This comprehensive resource and the series are highly recommended."
—American Reference Books Annual, 2000

"Recommended reference source."
— Booklist, American Library Association, Dec '98

■

Mental Health Disorders Sourcebook, 3rd Edition

Basic Consumer Health Information about Mental and Emotional Health and Mental Illness, Including Facts about Depression, Bipolar Disorder, and Other Mood Disorders, Phobias, Post-Traumatic Stress Disorder (PTSD), Obsessive-Compulsive Disorder, and Other Anxiety Disorders, Impulse Control Disorders, Eating Disorders, Personality Disorders, and Psychotic Disorders, Including Schizophrenia and Dissociative Disorders

Along with Statistical Information, a Special Section Concerning Mental Health Issues in Children and Adolescents, a Glossary, and Directories of Resources for Additional Help and Information

Edited by Karen Bellenir. 661 pages. 2005. 0-7808-0747-2.

"Recommended for public libraries and academic libraries with an undergraduate program in psychology."
— American Reference Books Annual, 2006

"Recommended reference source."
—Booklist, American Library Association, Jun '00

■

Mental Retardation Sourcebook

Basic Consumer Health Information about Mental Retardation and Its Causes, Including Down Syndrome, Fetal Alcohol Syndrome, Fragile X Syndrome, Genetic Conditions, Injury, and Environmental Sources

Along with Preventive Strategies, Parenting Issues, Educational Implications, Health Care Needs, Employment and Economic Matters, Legal Issues, a Glossary, and a Resource Listing for Additional Help and Information

Edited by Joyce Brennfleck Shannon. 642 pages. 2000. 0-7808-0377-9.

"Public libraries will find the book useful for reference and as a beginning research point for students, parents, and caregivers."
— American Reference Books Annual, 2001

"The strength of this work is that it compiles many basic fact sheets and addresses for further information in one volume. It is intended and suitable for the general public. This sourcebook is relevant to any collection providing health information to the general public."
— E-Streams, Nov '00

"From preventing retardation to parenting and family challenges, this covers health, social and legal issues and will prove an invaluable overview."
— Reviewer's Bookwatch, Jul '00

■

Movement Disorders Sourcebook

Basic Consumer Health Information about Neurological Movement Disorders, Including Essential Tremor, Parkinson's Disease, Dystonia, Cerebral Palsy, Huntington's Disease, Myasthenia Gravis, Multiple Sclerosis, and Other Early-Onset and Adult-Onset Movement Disorders, Their Symptoms and Causes, Diagnostic Tests, and Treatments

Along with Mobility and Assistive Technology Information, a Glossary, and a Directory of Additional Resources

Edited by Joyce Brennfleck Shannon. 655 pages. 2003. 0-7808-0628-X.

". . . a good resource for consumers and recommended for public, community college and undergraduate libraries." *— American Reference Books Annual, 2004*

■

Muscular Dystrophy Sourcebook

Basic Consumer Health Information about Congenital, Childhood-Onset, and Adult-Onset Forms of Muscular Dystrophy, Such as Duchenne, Becker, Emery-Dreifuss, Distal, Limb-Girdle, Facioscapulohumeral (FSHD), Myotonic, and Ophthalmoplegic Muscular Dystro-

phies, Including Facts about Diagnostic Tests, Medical and Physical Therapies, Management of Co-Occurring Conditions, and Parenting Guidelines

Along with Practical Tips for Home Care, a Glossary, and Directories of Additional Resources

Edited by Joyce Brennfleck Shannon. 577 pages. 2004. 0-7808-0676-X.

"This book is highly recommended for public and academic libraries as well as health care offices that support the information needs of patients and their families."
— E-Streams, Apr '05

"Excellent reference." — The Bookwatch, Jan '05

Obesity Sourcebook

Basic Consumer Health Information about Diseases and Other Problems Associated with Obesity, and Including Facts about Risk Factors, Prevention Issues, and Management Approaches

Along with Statistical and Demographic Data, Information about Special Populations, Research Updates, a Glossary, and Source Listings for Further Help and Information

Edited by Wilma Caldwell and Chad T. Kimball. 376 pages. 2001. 0-7808-0333-7.

"The book synthesizes the reliable medical literature on obesity into one easy-to-read and useful resource for the general public."
— American Reference Books Annual, 2002

"This is a very useful resource book for the lay public."
— Doody's Review Service, Nov '01

"Well suited for the health reference collection of a public library or an academic health science library that serves the general population." — E-Streams, Sep '01

"Recommended reference source."
— Booklist, American Library Association, Apr '01

"Recommended pick both for specialty health library collections and any general consumer health reference collection." — The Bookwatch, Apr '01

Ophthalmic Disorders Sourcebook

SEE Eye Care Sourcebook, 2nd Edition

Oral Health Sourcebook

SEE Dental Care & Oral Health Sourcebook, 2nd Edition

Osteoporosis Sourcebook

Basic Consumer Health Information about Primary and Secondary Osteoporosis and Juvenile Osteoporosis and Related Conditions, Including Fibrous Dysplasia,

Gaucher Disease, Hyperthyroidism, Hypophosphatasia, Myeloma, Osteopetrosis, Osteogenesis Imperfecta, and Paget's Disease

Along with Information about Risk Factors, Treatments, Traditional and Non-Traditional Pain Management, a Glossary of Related Terms, and a Directory of Resources

Edited by Allan R. Cook. 584 pages. 2001. 0-7808-0239-X.

"This would be a book to be kept in a staff or patient library. The targeted audience is the layperson, but the therapist who needs a quick bit of information on a particular topic will also find the book useful."
— Physical Therapy, Jan '02

"This resource is recommended as a great reference source for public, health, and academic libraries, and is another triumph for the editors of Omnigraphics."
— American Reference Books Annual, 2002

"Recommended for all public libraries and general health collections, especially those supporting patient education or consumer health programs."
— E-Streams, Nov '01

"Will prove valuable to any library seeking to maintain a current, comprehensive reference collection of health resources. . . . From prevention to treatment and associated conditions, this provides an excellent survey."
— The Bookwatch, Aug '01

"Recommended reference source."
— Booklist, American Library Association, Jul '01

SEE ALSO Healthy Aging Sourcebook, Physical & Mental Issues in Aging Sourcebook, Women's Health Concerns Sourcebook

Pain Sourcebook, 2nd Edition

Basic Consumer Health Information about Specific Forms of Acute and Chronic Pain, Including Muscle and Skeletal Pain, Nerve Pain, Cancer Pain, and Disorders Characterized by Pain, Such as Fibromyalgia, Shingles, Angina, Arthritis, and Headaches

Along with Information about Pain Medications and Management Techniques, Complementary and Alternative Pain Relief Options, Tips for People Living with Chronic Pain, a Glossary, and a Directory of Sources for Further Information

Edited by Karen Bellenir. 670 pages. 2002. 0-7808-0612-3.

"A source of valuable information. . . . This book offers help to nonmedical people who need information about pain and pain management. It is also an excellent reference for those who participate in patient education."
— Doody's Review Service, Sep '02

"Highly recommended for academic and medical reference collections." — Library Bookwatch, Sep '02

"The text is readable, easily understood, and well indexed. This excellent volume belongs in all patient education libraries, consumer health sections of public libraries, and many personal collections."
— American Reference Books Annual, 1999

"The information is basic in terms of scholarship and is appropriate for general readers. Written in journalistic style . . . intended for non-professionals. Quite thorough in its coverage of different pain conditions and summarizes the latest clinical information regarding pain treatment."
— *Choice, Association of College and Research Libraries, Jun '98*

"Recommended reference source."
— *Booklist, American Library Association, Mar '98*

Pediatric Cancer Sourcebook

Basic Consumer Health Information about Leukemias, Brain Tumors, Sarcomas, Lymphomas, and Other Cancers in Infants, Children, and Adolescents, Including Descriptions of Cancers, Treatments, and Coping Strategies

Along with Suggestions for Parents, Caregivers, and Concerned Relatives, a Glossary of Cancer Terms, and Resource Listings

Edited by Edward J. Prucha. 587 pages. 1999. 0-7808-0245-4.

"An excellent source of information. Recommended for public, hospital, and health science libraries with consumer health collections." — *E-Streams, Jun '00*

"Recommended reference source."
— *Booklist, American Library Association, Feb '00*

"A valuable addition to all libraries specializing in health services and many public libraries."
— *American Reference Books Annual, 2000*

SEE ALSO Childhood Diseases & Disorders Sourcebook, Healthy Children Sourcebook

Physical & Mental Issues in Aging Sourcebook

Basic Consumer Health Information on Physical and Mental Disorders Associated with the Aging Process, Including Concerns about Cardiovascular Disease, Pulmonary Disease, Oral Health, Digestive Disorders, Musculoskeletal and Skin Disorders, Metabolic Changes, Sexual and Reproductive Issues, and Changes in Vision, Hearing, and Other Senses

Along with Data about Longevity and Causes of Death, Information on Acute and Chronic Pain, Descriptions of Mental Concerns, a Glossary of Terms, and Resource Listings for Additional Help

Edited by Jenifer Swanson. 660 pages. 1999. 0-7808-0233-0.

"This is a treasure of health information for the layperson." — *Choice Health Sciences Supplement, Association of College & Research Libraries, May '00*

"Recommended for public libraries."
— *American Reference Books Annual, 2000*

"Recommended reference source."
— *Booklist, American Library Association, Oct '99*

SEE ALSO Healthy Aging Sourcebook

Podiatry Sourcebook

Basic Consumer Health Information about Foot Conditions, Diseases, and Injuries, Including Bunions, Corns, Calluses, Athlete's Foot, Plantar Warts, Hammertoes and Clawtoes, Clubfoot, Heel Pain, Gout, and More

Along with Facts about Foot Care, Disease Prevention, Foot Safety, Choosing a Foot Care Specialist, a Glossary of Terms, and Resource Listings for Additional Information

Edited by M. Lisa Weatherford. 380 pages. 2001. 0-7808-0215-2.

"Recommended reference source."
— *Booklist, American Library Association, Feb '02*

"There is a lot of information presented here on a topic that is usually only covered sparingly in most larger comprehensive medical encyclopedias."
— *American Reference Books Annual, 2002*

Pregnancy & Birth Sourcebook, 2nd Edition

Basic Consumer Health Information about Conception and Pregnancy, Including Facts about Fertility, Infertility, Pregnancy Symptoms and Complications, Fetal Growth and Development, Labor, Delivery, and the Postpartum Period, as Well as Information about Maintaining Health and Wellness during Pregnancy and Caring for a Newborn

Along with Information about Public Health Assistance for Low-Income Pregnant Women, a Glossary, and Directories of Agencies and Organizations Providing Help and Support

Edited by Amy L. Sutton. 626 pages. 2004. 0-7808-0672-7.

"Will appeal to public and school reference collections strong in medicine and women's health. . . . Deserves a spot on any medical reference shelf."
— *The Bookwatch, Jul '04*

"A well-organized handbook. Recommended."
— *Choice, Association of College & Research Libraries, Apr '98*

"Recommended reference source."
— *Booklist, American Library Association, Mar '98*

"Recommended for public libraries."
— *American Reference Books Annual, 1998*

SEE ALSO Breastfeeding Sourcebook, Congenital Disorders Sourcebook, Family Planning Sourcebook

Prostate Cancer Sourcebook

Basic Consumer Health Information about Prostate Cancer, Including Information about the Associated Risk Factors, Detection, Diagnosis, and Treatment of Prostate Cancer

Along with Information on Non-Malignant Prostate Conditions, and Featuring a Section Listing Support and Treatment Centers and a Glossary of Related Terms

Edited by Dawn D. Matthews. 358 pages. 2001. 0-7808-0324-8.

"Recommended reference source."
— *Booklist, American Library Association, Jan '02*

"A valuable resource for health care consumers seeking information on the subject.... All text is written in a clear, easy-to-understand language that avoids technical jargon. Any library that collects consumer health resources would strengthen their collection with the addition of the Prostate Cancer Sourcebook."
— *American Reference Books Annual, 2002*

SEE ALSO Men's Health Concerns Sourcebook

Prostate & Urological Disorders Sourcebook

Basic Consumer Health Information about Urogenital and Sexual Disorders in Men, Including Prostate and Other Andrological Cancers, Prostatitis, Benign Prostatic Hyperplasia, Testicular and Penile Trauma, Cryptorchidism, Peyronie Disease, Erectile Dysfunction, and Male Factor Infertility, and Facts about Commonly Used Tests and Procedures, Such as Prostatectomy, Vasectomy, Vasectomy Reversal, Penile Implants, and Semen Analysis

Along with a Glossary of Andrological Terms and a Directory of Resources for Additional Information

Edited by Karen Bellenir. 631 pages. 2005. 0-7808-0797-9.

Public Health Sourcebook

Basic Information about Government Health Agencies, Including National Health Statistics and Trends, Healthy People 2000 Program Goals and Objectives, the Centers for Disease Control and Prevention, the Food and Drug Administration, and the National Institutes of Health

Along with Full Contact Information for Each Agency

Edited by Wendy Wilcox. 698 pages. 1998. 0-7808-0220-9.

"Recommended reference source."
— *Booklist, American Library Association, Sep '98*

"This consumer guide provides welcome assistance in navigating the maze of federal health agencies and their data on public health concerns."
— *SciTech Book News, Sep '98*

Reconstructive & Cosmetic Surgery Sourcebook

Basic Consumer Health Information on Cosmetic and Reconstructive Plastic Surgery, Including Statistical Information about Different Surgical Procedures, Things to Consider Prior to Surgery, Plastic Surgery Techniques and Tools, Emotional and Psychological Considerations, and Procedure-Specific Information

Along with a Glossary of Terms and a Listing of Resources for Additional Help and Information

Edited by M. Lisa Weatherford. 374 pages. 2001. 0-7808-0214-4.

"An excellent reference that addresses cosmetic and medically necessary reconstructive surgeries.... The style of the prose is calm and reassuring, discussing the many positive outcomes now available due to advances in surgical techniques."
— *American Reference Books Annual, 2002*

"Recommended for health science libraries that are open to the public, as well as hospital libraries that are open to the patients. This book is a good resource for the consumer interested in plastic surgery."
— *E-Streams, Dec '01*

"Recommended reference source."
— *Booklist, American Library Association, Jul '01*

Rehabilitation Sourcebook

Basic Consumer Health Information about Rehabilitation for People Recovering from Heart Surgery, Spinal Cord Injury, Stroke, Orthopedic Impairments, Amputation, Pulmonary Impairments, Traumatic Injury, and More, Including Physical Therapy, Occupational Therapy, Speech/Language Therapy, Massage Therapy, Dance Therapy, Art Therapy, and Recreational Therapy

Along with Information on Assistive and Adaptive Devices, a Glossary, and Resources for Additional Help and Information

Edited by Dawn D. Matthews. 531 pages. 1999. 0-7808-0236-5.

"This is an excellent resource for public library reference and health collections."
— *American Reference Books Annual, 2001*

"Recommended reference source."
— *Booklist, American Library Association, May '00*

Respiratory Diseases & Disorders Sourcebook

Basic Information about Respiratory Diseases and Disorders, Including Asthma, Cystic Fibrosis, Pneumonia, the Common Cold, Influenza, and Others, Featuring Facts about the Respiratory System, Statistical and Demographic Data, Treatments, Self-Help Management Suggestions, and Current Research Initiatives

Edited by Allan R. Cook and Peter D. Dresser. 771 pages. 1995. 0-7808-0037-0.

"Designed for the layperson and for patients and their families coping with respiratory illness.... an extensive array of information on diagnosis, treatment, management, and prevention of respiratory illnesses for the general reader." — *Choice, Association of College & Research Libraries, Jun '96*

"A highly recommended text for all collections. It is a comforting reminder of the power of knowledge that good books carry between their covers."
— *Academic Library Book Review, Spring '96*

"A comprehensive collection of authoritative information presented in a nontechnical, humanitarian style for patients, families, and caregivers."
—*Association of Operating Room Nurses, Sep/Oct '95*

SEE ALSO Lung Disorders Sourcebook

Sexually Transmitted Diseases Sourcebook, 3rd Edition

Basic Consumer Health Information about Chlamydial Infections, Gonorrhea, Hepatitis, Herpes, HIV/AIDS, Human Papillomavirus, Pubic Lice, Scabies, Syphilis, Trichomoniasis, Vaginal Infections, and Other Sexually Transmitted Diseases, Including Facts about Risk Factors, Symptoms, Diagnosis, Treatment, and the Prevention of Sexually Transmitted Infections

Along with Updates on Current Research Initiatives, a Glossary of Related Terms, and Resources for Additional Help and Information

Edited by Amy L. Sutton. 629 pages. 2006. 0-7808-0824-X.

"Recommended for consumer health collections in public libraries, and secondary school and community college libraries."
—*American Reference Books Annual, 2002*

"Every school and public library should have a copy of this comprehensive and user-friendly reference book."
—*Choice, Association of College & Research Libraries, Sep '01*

"This is a highly recommended book. This is an especially important book for all school and public libraries."
—*AIDS Book Review Journal, Jul-Aug '01*

"Recommended reference source."
—*Booklist, American Library Association, Apr '01*

Skin Disorders Sourcebook

SEE Dermatological Disorders Sourcebook, 2nd Edition

Sleep Disorders Sourcebook, 2nd Edition

Basic Consumer Health Information about Sleep and Sleep Disorders, Including Insomnia, Sleep Apnea, Restless Legs Syndrome, Narcolepsy, Parasomnias, and Other Health Problems That Affect Sleep, Plus Facts about Diagnostic Procedures, Treatment Strategies, Sleep Medications, and Tips for Improving Sleep Quality

Along with a Glossary of Related Terms and Resources for Additional Help and Information

Edited by Amy L. Sutton. 567 pages. 2005. 0-7808-0743-X.

"This book will be useful for just about everybody, especially the 40 million Americans with sleep disorders."
—*American Reference Books Annual, 2006*

"Recommended for public libraries and libraries supporting health care professionals." —*E-Streams, Sep '05*

". . . key medical library acquisition."
—*The Bookwatch, Jun '05*

Smoking Concerns Sourcebook

Basic Consumer Health Information about Nicotine Addiction and Smoking Cessation, Featuring Facts about the Health Effects of Tobacco Use, Including Lung and Other Cancers, Heart Disease, Stroke, and Respiratory Disorders, Such as Emphysema and Chronic Bronchitis

Along with Information about Smoking Prevention Programs, Suggestions for Achieving and Maintaining a Smoke-Free Lifestyle, Statistics about Tobacco Use, Reports on Current Research Initiatives, a Glossary of Related Terms, and Directories of Resources for Additional Help and Information

Edited by Karen Bellenir. 621 pages. 2004. 0-7808-0323-X.

"Provides everything needed for the student or general reader seeking practical details on the effects of tobacco use." —*The Bookwatch, Mar '05*

"Public libraries and consumer health care libraries will find this work useful."
—*American Reference Books Annual, 2005*

Sports Injuries Sourcebook, 2nd Edition

Basic Consumer Health Information about the Diagnosis, Treatment, and Rehabilitation of Common Sports-Related Injuries in Children and Adults

Along with Suggestions for Conditioning and Training, Information and Prevention Tips for Injuries Frequently Associated with Specific Sports and Special Populations, a Glossary, and a Directory of Additional Resources

Edited by Joyce Brennfleck Shannon. 614 pages. 2002. 0-7808-0604-2.

"This is an excellent reference for consumers and it is recommended for public, community college, and undergraduate libraries."
—*American Reference Books Annual, 2003*

"Recommended reference source."
—*Booklist, American Library Association, Feb '03*

Stress-Related Disorders Sourcebook

Basic Consumer Health Information about Stress and Stress-Related Disorders, Including Stress Origins and Signals, Environmental Stress at Work and Home, Mental and Emotional Stress Associated with Depression, Post-Traumatic Stress Disorder, Panic Disorder, Suicide, and the Physical Effects of Stress on the Cardiovascular, Immune, and Nervous Systems

Along with Stress Management Techniques, a Glossary, and a Listing of Additional Resources

Edited by Joyce Brennfleck Shannon. 610 pages. 2002. 0-7808-0560-7.

"Well written for a general readership, the *Stress-Related Disorders Sourcebook* is a useful addition to the health reference literature."
— *American Reference Books Annual, 2003*

"I am impressed by the amount of information. It offers a thorough overview of the causes and consequences of stress for the layperson. . . . A well-done and thorough reference guide for professionals and nonprofessionals alike."
— *Doody's Review Service, Dec '02*

Stroke Sourcebook

Basic Consumer Health Information about Stroke, Including Ischemic, Hemorrhagic, Transient Ischemic Attack (TIA), and Pediatric Stroke, Stroke Triggers and Risks, Diagnostic Tests, Treatments, and Rehabilitation Information

Along with Stroke Prevention Guidelines, Legal and Financial Information, a Glossary, and a Directory of Additional Resources

Edited by Joyce Brennfleck Shannon. 606 pages. 2003. 0-7808-0630-1.

"This volume is highly recommended and should be in every medical, hospital, and public library."
— *American Reference Books Annual, 2004*

"Highly recommended for the amount and variety of topics and information covered." — *Choice, Nov '03*

Substance Abuse Sourcebook

Basic Health-Related Information about the Abuse of Legal and Illegal Substances Such as Alcohol, Tobacco, Prescription Drugs, Marijuana, Cocaine, and Heroin; and Including Facts about Substance Abuse Prevention Strategies, Intervention Methods, Treatment and Recovery Programs, and a Section Addressing the Special Problems Related to Substance Abuse during Pregnancy

Edited by Karen Bellenir. 573 pages. 1996. 0-7808-0038-9.

"A valuable addition to any health reference section. Highly recommended."
— *The Book Report, Mar/Apr '97*

". . . a comprehensive collection of substance abuse information that's both highly readable and compact. Families and caregivers of substance abusers will find the information enlightening and helpful, while teachers, social workers and journalists should benefit from the concise format. Recommended."
— *Drug Abuse Update, Winter '96/'97*

SEE ALSO Alcoholism Sourcebook, Drug Abuse Sourcebook

Surgery Sourcebook

Basic Consumer Health Information about Inpatient and Outpatient Surgeries, Including Cardiac, Vascular, Orthopedic, Ocular, Reconstructive, Cosmetic, Gynecologic, and Ear, Nose, and Throat Procedures and More

Along with Information about Operating Room Policies and Instruments, Laser Surgery Techniques, Hospital Errors, Statistical Data, a Glossary, and Listings of Sources for Further Help and Information

Edited by Annemarie S. Muth and Karen Bellenir. 596 pages. 2002. 0-7808-0380-9.

"Large public libraries and medical libraries would benefit from this material in their reference collections."
— *American Reference Books Annual, 2004*

"Invaluable reference for public and school library collections alike." — *Library Bookwatch, Apr '03*

Thyroid Disorders Sourcebook

Basic Consumer Health Information about Disorders of the Thyroid and Parathyroid Glands, Including Hypothyroidism, Hyperthyroidism, Graves Disease, Hashimoto Thyroiditis, Thyroid Cancer, and Parathyroid Disorders, Featuring Facts about Symptoms, Risk Factors, Tests, and Treatments

Along with Information about the Effects of Thyroid Imbalance on Other Body Systems, Environmental Factors That Affect the Thyroid Gland, a Glossary, and a Directory of Additional Resources

Edited by Joyce Brennfleck Shannon. 599 pages. 2005. 0-7808-0745-6.

"Recommended for consumer health collections."
— *American Reference Books Annual, 2006*

"Highly recommended pick for basic consumer health reference holdings at all levels."
— *The Bookwatch, Aug '05*

Transplantation Sourcebook

Basic Consumer Health Information about Organ and Tissue Transplantation, Including Physical and Financial Preparations, Procedures and Issues Relating to Specific Solid Organ and Tissue Transplants, Rehabilitation, Pediatric Transplant Information, the Future of Transplantation, and Organ and Tissue Donation

Along with a Glossary and Listings of Additional Resources

Edited by Joyce Brennfleck Shannon. 628 pages. 2002. 0-7808-0322-1.

"Along with these advances [in transplantation technology] have come a number of daunting questions for potential transplant patients, their families, and their health care providers. This reference text is the best single tool to address many of these questions. . . . It will be a much-needed addition to the reference collections in health care, academic, and large public libraries."
— *American Reference Books Annual, 2003*

654

"Recommended for libraries with an interest in offering consumer health information." — *E-Streams, Jul '02*

"This is a unique and valuable resource for patients facing transplantation and their families." — *Doody's Review Service, Jun '02*

Traveler's Health Sourcebook

Basic Consumer Health Information for Travelers, Including Physical and Medical Preparations, Transportation Health and Safety, Essential Information about Food and Water, Sun Exposure, Insect and Snake Bites, Camping and Wilderness Medicine, and Travel with Physical or Medical Disabilities

Along with International Travel Tips, Vaccination Recommendations, Geographical Health Issues, Disease Risks, a Glossary, and a Listing of Additional Resources

Edited by Joyce Brennfleck Shannon. 613 pages. 2000. 0-7808-0384-1.

"Recommended reference source." — *Booklist, American Library Association, Feb '01*

"This book is recommended for any public library, any travel collection, and especially any collection for the physically disabled." — *American Reference Books Annual, 2001*

SEE ALSO *Worldwide Health Sourcebook*

Urinary Tract & Kidney Diseases & Disorders Sourcebook, 2nd Edition

Basic Consumer Health Information about the Urinary System, Including the Bladder, Urethra, Ureters, and Kidneys, with Facts about Urinary Tract Infections, Incontinence, Congenital Disorders, Kidney Stones, Cancers of the Urinary Tract and Kidneys, Kidney Failure, Dialysis, and Kidney Transplantation

Along with Statistical and Demographic Information, Reports on Current Research in Kidney and Urologic Health, a Summary of Commonly Used Diagnostic Tests, a Glossary of Related Terms, and a Directory of Resources for Additional Help and Information

Edited by Ivy L. Alexander. 649 pages. 2005. 0-7808-0750-2.

"A good choice for a consumer health information library or for a medical library needing information to refer to their patients." — *American Reference Books Annual, 2006*

Vegetarian Sourcebook

Basic Consumer Health Information about Vegetarian Diets, Lifestyle, and Philosophy, Including Definitions of Vegetarianism and Veganism, Tips about Adopting Vegetarianism, Creating a Vegetarian Pantry, and Meeting Nutritional Needs of Vegetarians, with Facts Regarding Vegetarianism's Effect on Pregnant and Lactating Women, Children, Athletes, and Senior Citizens

Along with a Glossary of Commonly Used Vegetarian Terms and Resources for Additional Help and Information

Edited by Chad T. Kimball. 360 pages. 2002. 0-7808-0439-2.

"Organizes into one concise volume the answers to the most common questions concerning vegetarian diets and lifestyles. This title is recommended for public and secondary school libraries." — *E-Streams, Apr '03*

"Invaluable reference for public and school library collections alike." — *Library Bookwatch, Apr '03*

"The articles in this volume are easy to read and come from authoritative sources. The book does not necessarily support the vegetarian diet but instead provides the pros and cons of this important decision. The Vegetarian Sourcebook is recommended for public libraries and consumer health libraries." — *American Reference Books Annual, 2003*

SEE ALSO *Diet & Nutrition Sourcebook*

Women's Health Concerns Sourcebook, 2nd Edition

Basic Consumer Health Information about the Medical and Mental Concerns of Women, Including Maintaining Health and Wellness, Gynecological Concerns, Breast Health, Sexuality and Reproductive Issues, Menopause, Cancer in Women, Leading Causes of Death and Disability among Women, Physical Concerns of Special Significance to Women, and Women's Mental and Emotional Health

Along with a Glossary of Related Terms and Directories of Resources for Additional Help and Information

Edited by Amy L. Sutton. 746 pages. 2004. 0-7808-0673-5.

"This is a useful reference book, which makes the reader knowledgeable about several issues that concern women's health. It is recommended for public libraries and home library collections." — *E-Streams, May '05*

"A useful addition to public and consumer health library collections." — *American Reference Books Annual, 2005*

"A highly recommended title." — *The Bookwatch, May '04*

"Handy compilation. There is an impressive range of diseases, devices, disorders, procedures, and other physical and emotional issues covered . . . well organized, illustrated, and indexed." — *Choice, Association of College & Research Libraries, Jan '98*

SEE ALSO *Breast Cancer Sourcebook, Cancer Sourcebook for Women, Healthy Heart Sourcebook for Women, Osteoporosis Sourcebook*

Workplace Health & Safety Sourcebook

Basic Consumer Health Information about Workplace Health and Safety, Including the Effect of Workplace Hazards on the Lungs, Skin, Heart, Ears, Eyes, Brain, Reproductive Organs, Musculoskeletal System, and Other Organs and Body Parts

Along with Information about Occupational Cancer, Personal Protective Equipment, Toxic and Hazardous Chemicals, Child Labor, Stress, and Workplace Violence

Edited by Chad T. Kimball. 626 pages. 2000. 0-7808-0231-4.

"As a reference for the general public, this would be useful in any library." *— E-Streams, Jun '01*

"Provides helpful information for primary care physicians and other caregivers interested in occupational medicine. . . . General readers; professionals."
— Choice, Association of College & Research Libraries, May '01

"Recommended reference source."
— Booklist, American Library Association, Feb '01

"Highly recommended." *— The Bookwatch, Jan '01*

Worldwide Health Sourcebook

Basic Information about Global Health Issues, Including Malnutrition, Reproductive Health, Disease Dispersion and Prevention, Emerging Diseases, Risky Health Behaviors, and the Leading Causes of Death

Along with Global Health Concerns for Children, Women, and the Elderly, Mental Health Issues, Research and Technology Advancements, and Economic, Environmental, and Political Health Implications, a Glossary, and a Resource Listing for Additional Help and Information

Edited by Joyce Brennfleck Shannon. 614 pages. 2001. 0-7808-0330-2.

"Named an Outstanding Academic Title."
— Choice, Association of College & Research Libraries, Jan '02

"Yet another handy but also unique compilation in the extensive Health Reference Series, this is a useful work because many of the international publications reprinted or excerpted are not readily available. Highly recommended." *— Choice, Association of College & Research Libraries, Nov '01*

"Recommended reference source."
— Booklist, American Library Association, Oct '01

SEE ALSO *Traveler's Health Sourcebook*

Teen Health Series

Helping Young Adults Understand, Manage, and Avoid Serious Illness

List price $65 per volume. **School and library price $58 per volume.**

Alcohol Information for Teens

Health Tips about Alcohol and Alcoholism

Including Facts about Underage Drinking, Preventing Teen Alcohol Use, Alcohol's Effects on the Brain and the Body, Alcohol Abuse Treatment, Help for Children of Alcoholics, and More

Edited by Joyce Brennfleck Shannon. 370 pages. 2005. 0-7808-0741-3.

"Boxed facts and tips add visual interest to the well-researched and clearly written text."
— *Curriculum Connection, Apr '06*

Allergy Information for Teens

Health Tips about Allergic Reactions Such as Anaphylaxis, Respiratory Problems, and Rashes

Including Facts about Identifying and Managing Allergies to Food, Pollen, Mold, Animals, Chemicals, Drugs, and Other Substances

Edited by Karen Bellenir. 410 pages. 2006. 0-7808-0799-5.

Asthma Information for Teens

Health Tips about Managing Asthma and Related Concerns

Including Facts about Asthma Causes, Triggers, Symptoms, Diagnosis, and Treatment

Edited by Karen Bellenir. 386 pages. 2005. 0-7808-0770-7.

"**Highly recommended for medical libraries, public school libraries, and public libraries.**"
— *American Reference Books Annual, 2006*

"**It is so clearly written and well organized that even hesitant readers will be able to find the facts they need, whether for reports or personal information. . . . A succinct but complete resource.**"
— *School Library Journal, Sep '05*

Cancer Information for Teens

Health Tips about Cancer Awareness, Prevention, Diagnosis, and Treatment

Including Facts about Frequently Occurring Cancers, Cancer Risk Factors, and Coping Strategies for Teens Fighting Cancer or Dealing with Cancer in Friends or Family Members

Edited by Wilma R. Caldwell. 428 pages. 2004. 0-7808-0678-6.

"**Recommended for school libraries, or consumer libraries that see a lot of use by teens.**"
— *E-Streams, May 2005*

"**A valuable educational tool.**"
— *American Reference Books Annual, 2005*

"**Young adults and their parents alike will find this new addition to the** *Teen Health Series* **an important reference to cancer in teens.**"
— *Children's Bookwatch, Feb '05*

Diabetes Information for Teens

Health Tips about Managing Diabetes and Preventing Related Complications

Including Information about Insulin, Glucose Control, Healthy Eating, Physical Activity, and Learning to Live with Diabetes

Edited by Sandra Augustyn Lawton. 410 pages. 2006. 0-7808-0811-8.

Diet Information for Teens, 2nd Edition

Health Tips about Diet and Nutrition

Including Facts about Dietary Guidelines, Food Groups, Nutrients, Healthy Meals, Snacks, Weight Control, Medical Concerns Related to Diet, and More

Edited by Karen Bellenir. 432 pages. 2006. 0-7808-0820-7.

"**Full of helpful insights and facts throughout the book. . . . An excellent resource to be placed in public libraries or even in personal collections.**"
— *American Reference Books Annual, 2002*

"**Recommended for middle and high school libraries and media centers as well as academic libraries that educate future teachers of teenagers. It is also a suitable addition to health science libraries that serve patrons who are interested in teen health promotion and education.**"
— *E-Streams, Oct '01*

"**This comprehensive book would be beneficial to collections that need information about nutrition, dietary guidelines, meal planning, and weight control. . . . This reference is so easy to use that its purchase is recommended.**"
— *The Book Report, Sep-Oct '01*

"This book is written in an easy to understand format describing issues that many teens face every day, and then provides thoughtful explanations so that teens can make informed decisions. This is an interesting book that provides important facts and information for today's teens." —*Doody's Health Sciences Book Review Journal, Jul-Aug '01*

"A comprehensive compendium of diet and nutrition. The information is presented in a straightforward, plain-spoken manner. This title will be useful to those working on reports on a variety of topics, as well as to general readers concerned about their dietary health." —*School Library Journal, Jun '01*

■

Drug Information for Teens, 2nd Edition

Health Tips about the Physical and Mental Effects of Substance Abuse

Including Information about Marijuana, Inhalants, Club Drugs, Stimulants, Hallucinogens, Opiates, Prescription and Over-the-Counter Drugs, Herbal Products, Tobacco, Alcohol, and More

Edited by Sandra Augustyn Lawton. 468 pages. 2006. 0-7808-0862-2.

"A clearly written resource for general readers and researchers alike." —*School Library Journal*

"This book is well-balanced. . . . a must for public and school libraries." —*VOYA: Voice of Youth Advocates, Dec '03*

"The chapters are quick to make a connection to their teenage reading audience. The prose is straightforward and the book lends itself to spot reading. It should be useful both for practical information and for research, and it is suitable for public and school libraries." —*American Reference Books Annual, 2003*

"Recommended reference source." —*Booklist, American Library Association, Feb '03*

"This is an excellent resource for teens and their parents. Education about drugs and substances is key to discouraging teen drug abuse and this book provides this much needed information in a way that is interesting and factual." —*Doody's Review Service, Dec '02*

■

Eating Disorders Information for Teens

Health Tips about Anorexia, Bulimia, Binge Eating, and Other Eating Disorders

Including Information on the Causes, Prevention, and Treatment of Eating Disorders, and Such Other Issues as Maintaining Healthy Eating and Exercise Habits

Edited by Sandra Augustyn Lawton. 337 pages. 2005. 0-7808-0783-9.

"An excellent resource for teens and those who work with them." —*VOYA: Voice of Youth Advocates, Apr '06*

"A welcome addition to high school and undergraduate libraries." —*American Reference Books Annual, 2006*

"This book covers the topic in a lucid manner but delves deeper into every aspect of an eating disorder. A solid addition for any nonfiction or reference collection." —*School Library Journal, Dec '05*

■

Fitness Information for Teens

Health Tips about Exercise, Physical Well-Being, and Health Maintenance

Including Facts about Aerobic and Anaerobic Conditioning, Stretching, Body Shape and Body Image, Sports Training, Nutrition, and Activities for Non-Athletes

Edited by Karen Bellenir. 425 pages. 2004. 0-7808-0679-4.

"Another excellent offering from Omnigraphics in their *Teen Health Series*. . . . This book will be a great addition to any public, junior high, senior high, or secondary school library." —*American Reference Books Annual, 2005*

■

Learning Disabilities Information for Teens

Health Tips about Academic Skills Disorders and Other Disabilities That Affect Learning

Including Information about Common Signs of Learning Disabilities, School Issues, Learning to Live with a Learning Disability, and Other Related Issues

Edited by Sandra Augustyn Lawton. 337 pages. 2005. 0-7808-0796-0.

"This book provides a wealth of information for any reader interested in the signs, causes, and consequences of learning disabilities, as well as related legal rights and educational interventions. . . . Public and academic libraries should want this title for both students and general readers." —*American Reference Books Annual, 2006*

■

Mental Health Information for Teens, 2nd Edition

Health Tips about Mental Wellness and Mental Illness

Including Facts about Mental and Emotional Health, Depression and Other Mood Disorders, Anxiety Disorders, Behavior Disorders, Self-Injury, Psychosis, Schizophrenia, and More

Edited by Karen Bellenir. 400 pages. 2006. 0-7808-0863-0.

"In both language and approach, this user-friendly entry in the *Teen Health Series* is on target for teens needing information on mental health concerns." —*Booklist, American Library Association, Jan '02*

"Readers will find the material accessible and informative, with the shaded notes, facts, and embedded glos-

sary insets adding appropriately to the already interesting and succinct presentation."
— *School Library Journal, Jan '02*

"This title is highly recommended for any library that serves adolescents and parents/caregivers of adolescents." — *E-Streams, Jan '02*

"Recommended for high school libraries and young adult collections in public libraries. Both health professionals and teenagers will find this book useful." — *American Reference Books Annual, 2002*

"This is a nice book written to enlighten the society, primarily teenagers, about common teen mental health issues. It is highly recommended to teachers and parents as well as adolescents." — *Doody's Review Service, Dec '01*

Sexual Health Information for Teens

Health Tips about Sexual Development, Human Reproduction, and Sexually Transmitted Diseases

Including Facts about Puberty, Reproductive Health, Chlamydia, Human Papillomavirus, Pelvic Inflammatory Disease, Herpes, AIDS, Contraception, Pregnancy, and More

Edited by Deborah A. Stanley. 391 pages. 2003. 0-7808-0445-7.

"This work should be included in all high school libraries and many larger public libraries. . . . highly recommended." — *American Reference Books Annual, 2004*

"Sexual Health approaches its subject with appropriate seriousness and offers easily accessible advice and information." — *School Library Journal, Feb '04*

Skin Health Information for Teens

Health Tips about Dermatological Concerns and Skin Cancer Risks

Including Facts about Acne, Warts, Hives, and Other Conditions and Lifestyle Choices, Such as Tanning, Tattooing, and Piercing, That Affect the Skin, Nails, Scalp, and Hair

Edited by Robert Aquinas McNally. 429 pages. 2003. 0-7808-0446-5.

"This volume, as with others in the series, will be a useful addition to school and public library collections." — *American Reference Books Annual, 2004*

"There is no doubt that this reference tool is valuable." — *VOYA: Voice of Youth Advocates, Feb '04*

"This volume serves as a one-stop source and should be a necessity for any health collection." — *Library Media Connection*

Sports Injuries Information for Teens

Health Tips about Sports Injuries and Injury Protection

Including Facts about Specific Injuries, Emergency Treatment, Rehabilitation, Sports Safety, Competition Stress, Fitness, Sports Nutrition, Steroid Risks, and More

Edited by Joyce Brennfleck Shannon. 405 pages. 2003. 0-7808-0447-3.

"This work will be useful in the young adult collections of public libraries as well as high school libraries." — *American Reference Books Annual, 2004*

Suicide Information for Teens

Health Tips about Suicide Causes and Prevention

Including Facts about Depression, Risk Factors, Getting Help, Survivor Support, and More

Edited by Joyce Brennfleck Shannon. 368 pages. 2005. 0-7808-0737-5.

Health Reference Series

Adolescent Health Sourcebook,
2nd Edition

AIDS Sourcebook, 3rd Edition

Alcoholism Sourcebook, 2nd Edition

Allergies Sourcebook, 2nd Edition

Alzheimer's Disease Sourcebook,
3rd Edition

Arthritis Sourcebook, 2nd Edition

Asthma Sourcebook, 2nd Edition

Attention Deficit Disorder Sourcebook

Back & Neck Sourcebook, 2nd Edition

Blood & Circulatory Disorders
Sourcebook, 2nd Edition

Brain Disorders Sourcebook, 2nd Edition

Breast Cancer Sourcebook, 2nd Edition

Breastfeeding Sourcebook

Burns Sourcebook

Cancer Sourcebook, 4th Edition

Cancer Sourcebook for Women,
3rd Edition

Cardiovascular Diseases & Disorders
Sourcebook, 3rd Edition

Caregiving Sourcebook

Child Abuse Sourcebook

Childhood Diseases & Disorders
Sourcebook

Colds, Flu & Other Common Ailments
Sourcebook

Communication Disorders Sourcebook

Complementary & Alternative Medicine
Sourcebook, 3rd Edition

Congenital Disorders Sourcebook,
2nd Edition

Consumer Issues in Health Care
Sourcebook

Contagious Diseases Sourcebook

Contagious & Non-Contagious Infectious
Diseases Sourcebook

Death & Dying Sourcebook, 2nd Edition

Dental Care & Oral Health Sourcebook,
2nd Edition

Depression Sourcebook

Dermatological Disorders Sourcebook,
2nd Edition

Diabetes Sourcebook, 3rd Edition

Diet & Nutrition Sourcebook,
3rd Edition

Digestive Diseases & Disorder
Sourcebook

Disabilities Sourcebook

Domestic Violence Sourcebook,
2nd Edition

Drug Abuse Sourcebook, 2nd Edition

Ear, Nose & Throat Disorders
Sourcebook, 2nd Edition

Eating Disorders Sourcebook

Emergency Medical Services Sourcebook

Endocrine & Metabolic Disorders
Sourcebook

Environmentally Health Sourcebook,
2nd Edition

Ethnic Diseases Sourcebook

Eye Care Sourcebook, 2nd Edition

Family Planning Sourcebook

Fitness & Exercise Sourcebook,
3rd Edition

Food & Animal Borne Diseases
Sourcebook

Food Safety Sourcebook

Forensic Medicine Sourcebook

Gastrointestinal Diseases & Disorders
Sourcebook, 2nd Edition

Genetic Disorders Sourcebook,
3rd Edition

Head Trauma Sourcebook

Headache Sourcebook

Health Insurance Sourcebook

Healthy Aging Sourcebook

Healthy Children Sourcebook

Healthy Heart Sourcebook for Women

Hepatitis Sourcebook

Household Safety Sourcebook

Hypertension Sourcebook

Immune System Disorders Sourcebook,
2nd Edition